Surgical Management of Cutaneous Ulcers and Pressure Sores

Edited by

Bok Y. Lee, M.D., F.A.C.S.
Professor of Surgery
New York Medical College
Valhalla, NY
Adjunct Professor
Center for Biomedical Engineering
Renssclaer Polytechnic Institute
Troy, NY

Burton L. Herz, M.D., F.A.C.S.
Professor of Clinical Surgery
New York Medical College
Valhalla, NY
Director, Department of Surgery
Sound Shore Medical Center of Westchester
New Rochelle, NY

CHAPMAN & HALL

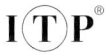 INTERNATIONAL THOMSON PUBLISHING
Thomson Science

New York • Albany • Bonn • Boston • Cincinnati • Detroit • London
Madrid • Melbourne • Mexico City • Pacific Grove • Paris • San Francisco
Singapore • Tokyo • Toronto • Washington

Join Us on the Internet
WWW: http://www.thomson.com
EMAIL: findit@kiosk.thomson.com

thomson.com is the on-line portal for the products, services and resources available from International Thomson Publishing (ITP).
This Internet kiosk gives users immediate access to more than 34 ITP publishers and over 20,000 products. Through *thomson.com* Internet users can search catalogs, examine subject-specific resource centers and subscribe to electronic discussion lists. You can purchase ITP products from your local bookseller, or directly through *thomson.com*.

Visit Chapman & Hall's Internet Resource Center for information on our new publications, links to useful sites on the World Wide Web and an opportunity to join our e-mail mailing list.
Point your browser to: **http://www.chaphall.com**
or **http://www.thomson.com/chaphall/med.html** for Medicine

Cover design: Curtis Tow Graphics

A service of **I T P**®

Chapman & Hall
115 Fifth Avenue
New York, NY 10003

Chapman & Hall
2-6 Boundary Row
London SE1 8HN
England

Thomas Nelson Australia
102 Dodds Street
South Melbourne, 3205
Victoria, Australia

Chapman & Hall GmbH
Postfach 100 263
D-69442 Weinheim
Germany

International Thomson Editores
Campos Eliseos 385, Piso 7
Col. Polanco
11560 Mexico D.F
Mexico

International Thomson Publishing–Japan
Hirakawacho Kyowa Building, 3F
1-2-1 Hirakawacho-cho
Chiyoda-ku, 102 Tokyo
Japan

International Thomson Publishing Asia
221 Henderson Road #05-10
Henderson Building
Singapore 0315

1 2 3 4 5 6 7 8 9 10 XXX 01 00 99 98

Library of Congress Cataloging-in-Publication Data

Surgical management of cutaneous ulcers and pressure sores / edited by Bok Y. Lee, Burton L. Herz.
    p.   cm.
    Includes bibliographical references and index.
    ISBN 0-412-99421-6 (alk. paper)
    1. Bedsores. I. Lee, Bok Y., 1928–   II. Herz, Burton L., 1941–
    [DNLM: 1. Skin Ulcer—prevention & control. 2. Decubitus Ulcer— prevention & control. WR 598 C988 1996]
    RL675.C88   1996
    616.8′45--dc20
    DNLM/DLC
    for Library of Congress   96-8950
                                                            CIP

British Library Cataloguing in Publication Data available

To order this or any other Chapman & Hall book, please contact **International Thomson Publishing, 7625 Empire Drive, Florence, KY 41042.** Phone: (606) 525-6600 or 1-800-842-3636. Fax: (606) 525-7778. e-mail: order@chaphall.com.

For a complete listing of Chapman & Hall titles, send your request to **Chapman & Hall, Dept. BC, 115 Fifth Avenue, New York, NY 10003.**

CONTENTS

PREFACE

With ever increasing health care costs, physicians face the dilemma of providing expensive and prolonged care to those who suffer from the consequences of illness, injury or aging. Pressure ulcers have a tremendous impact on overall well-being and impact on morbidity and mortality. They prolong hospitalization and escalate treatment costs and time. Chronic ulcers of the skin may lead to increased morbidity and mortality in disabled and bedridden patients and are difficult to manage. They have a low frequency of spontaneous healing, and when spontaneous healing does occur, it often produces poor results. The magnitude of the problem of pressure sores increases when one considers the growing population of geriatric patients who will develop skin ulcer secondary to arterial and venous disease. Of the approximately 10,000 new cases of paraplegia and quadriplegia which occur annually in the United States, 50 to 75 percent suffer from pressure sores. Such unfortunate patients, many of who are young adults with spinal cord injuries, require a long-term expenditure of health care resources. The estimated cost of healing a single pressure ulcer range from $2,000 to $40,000. The Agency for Health Care Policy and Research has identified pressure ulcers as one of the seven conditions affecting large number of patients involving relatively expensive treatment and urgently needing strategies for prevention and cost containment. With the increasing age of the population and use of life support technologies *Surgical Management of Cutaneous Ulcers and Pressure Sores* attempts to present state-of-the-art information to the medical community. It is authored by leaders in the development of methods for preventing and managing cutaneous ulcers and pressure ulcers.

Chapter 1 is an overview of society's values and health care costs related to chronic skin ulcers. Chapter 2 offers a detailed history of wound healing through the ages. Chapter 3 presents the anatomy and physiology of the microcirculation and noninvasive methods available for assessment of the cutaneous circulation. Chapter 4 details the basic biology in wound healing. Chapter 5 is an in-depth presentation of the classification of wounds and topical therapies including debridement, cleansing, dressings and adjunctive therapies. Chapter 6 presents the role of nutritional support. Chapter 7 presents skin ulcers caused by arterial and venous disease. Chapter 8 presents recent advances in the diagnosis and management of venous ulcers. Chapter 9 is a complete detailed overview of pressure sores. Chapter 10 is the relationship between mechanical loading. Chapter 11 is a discussion of antimicrobial agents in infected decubitus ulcers. Chapter 12 deals with state-of-the-art surgery for

v

decubitus ulcer. Chapter 13 deals with the special nursing care required for patients with pressure ulcers. Chapter 14 presents a comprehensive approach to treatment of the diabetic foot ulcers. Chapter 15 also reviews diabetic as well as other causes of foot ulcerations. Chapter 16 details the modified plantar medial approach for fasciotomy to treat the diabetic foot with compartment syndrome. Chapter 17 presents techniques in the surgery of pressure sores and Chapter 18 presents the surgical management of difficult pressure ulcers.

Well deserving of appreciation are all the contributors whose efforts have made this book possible. I would also like to thank the many surgical residents who have trained in this program for their special contributions to the *Surgical Management of Cutaneous Ulcers and Pressure Sores.*

A special note of gratitude must be extended to my secretary Teresa Geelan for selfless devotion to this project and to Catherine Felgar and Tracy Tucker at Chapman & Hall for their assistance and cooperation.

CONTRIBUTORS

Nanakram Agarwal, M.D.
Chief, Surgical Intensive Care Unit
Our Lady of Mercy Medical Center
Bronx, NY

David M. Brienza, Ph.D.
University of Pittsburgh
School of Health and Rehabilitation Sciences
Pittsburgh, PA

Marcelo C. DaSilva, M.D.
Department of Surgery, Section of Trauma and
   Critical Care Surgery
The Milton S. Hershey Medical Center
Penn State College of Medicine
Hershey, PA

Thomas M. DeLauro, D.P.M.
Professor, Divisions of Medical and Surgical Sciences
New York College of Pediatric Medicine
New York, NY

Ralph G. DePalma, M.D.
Professor of Surgery/Associate Dean
Department of Surgery
University of Nevada School of Medicine
Reno, NV

James T. Evans, M.D.
Professor of Surgery
Louisiana State University School of Medicine—
   Shreveport
and
Chief, Surgical Service
Overton Brooks VA Medical Center
Shreveport, LA

Randall S. Feingold, M.D.
Assistant Clinical Professor of Plastic and
   Reconstructive Surgery
Albert Einstein College of Medicine
Bronx, NY

V. J. Guerra, M.D.
Former Research Associate
New Rochelle Hospital—Medical Center
New Rochelle, NY

Burton L. Herz, M.D., F.A.C.S.
Professor of Clinical Surgery
New York Medical College
Valhalla, NY
and
Director, Department of Surgery
Sound Shore Medical Center of Westchester
New Rochelle, NY

E. A. Husni, M.D.
Chief, Vascular Surgery
Meridia Hillcrest Hospital
Mayfield Heights, OH

Irfan M. Jameel, M.D.
President, Surgicare Corporation
Gaspe, Quebec, Canada

Milon G. Karmakar, M.D.
New Rochelle Hospital
New Rochelle, NY

Alex J. Keller, M.D.
Assistant Clinical Professor of Plastic Surgery
New York University Medical School
New York, NY

Bok Y. Lee, M.D., F.A.C.S.
Professor of Surgery
New York Medical College
Valhalla, NY
and
Adjunct Professor
Center of Biomedical Engineering
Rensselaer Polytechnic Institute
Troy, NY

**Gordon D. Lutchman, M.D., F.A.C.S. F.R.C.S.
  (Eng.)**
Associate Chairman
Department of Surgery
Coney Island Hospital
Brooklyn, NY

Robert E. Madden, M.D.
Professor of Surgery
New York Medical College
Valhalla, NY

Zahid B. M. Niazi, M.D.
New York Group for Plastic Surgery
Burn Center-Macy Pavilion
Westchester County Medical Center
Valhalla, NY
and
Consultant, Plastic and Reconstructive Surgeon
DeShawar, Pakistan

Lee E. Ostrander, Ph.D.
Associate Professor
Biomedical Engineering Department
Rensselaer Polytechnic Institute
Troy, NY

C. Andrew Salzberg, M.D.
New York Group for Plastic Surgery
Burn Center-Macy Pavilion
Westchester County Medical Center
and
Assistant Professor
New York Medical College
Valhalla, NY

Mary Lou Shannon, Ed.D., R.N.
The University of Texas Medical Branch at Galveston
Galveston, TX

David A. Staffenberg, M.D.
Fellow, Plastic Surgery
Emory University
Atlanta, GA

1

SETTING THE OBJECTIVES: SOCIETAL VALUES

Bok Y. Lee, M.D., and Marcelo C. DaSilva, M.D.

The most important kind of tolerance is tolerance of the individual by society and the state.
————Albert Einstein

Across the United States, there is concern regarding the high and still-increasing costs of health care [1]. Technological advances prolong the lives of older people and save the lives of trauma victims. Health care expenditures were 11.4% to 11.7% of the annual gross domestic product (GDP) in 1987 (approximately $511 billion) [2, 3]. Since 1987, spending has increased further: $666 billion in 1990 (12% GDP), $736 billion in 1991 (13% GDP), approximately $820 billion in 1992 (13.9% GDP) [1, 7]. It is expected to reach $2 trillion by the year 2005 [1,8,9].

There are an estimated 1.5 to 3 million individuals in the United States with pressure ulcers [10]. The incidence of pressure ulcers varies from 2.7% to 29.5% [10, 11]. The incidence of pressure ulcers increases to 60% in quadriplegics and 66% in elderly patients with hip fracture [11]. Other factors that contribute to higher risks for pressure ulcer patients include malnutrition, volume depletion, decreased body weight, anemia, cardiovascular diseases, renal failure, diabetes, major surgery, orthopedic injuries, malignancy, sedation, and fever [6]. The risk of death increases fourfold with the development of a pressure ulcer among geriatric patients [4–6]. Allman et al. reported that there were no differences for age or race. Fecal incontinence, diarrhea, fractures, urinary catheter use, and dementia

were all noted in a significantly greater proportion of patients with pressure ulcers. There was a three-fold increase in pressure ulcers for every gram decrease in serum albumin level [4].

Cost data for pressure ulcers vary widely, but an independent analysis has estimated the cost at $6.4 billion annually [11]. The National Pressure Ulcer Advisory Panel estimates the cost of healing a pressure ulcer at $5,000 to $25,000 [10]. Healing a stage IV pressure ulcer may cost from $25,000 to $75,000 [10]. Approximately 90% of the patients that develop pressure ulcers are age sixty-five or older. Medicare reimbursement pays only for treatment of pressure ulcers accompanied by fever, leukocytosis, infection, and sepsis [10]. Medicare does not pay for prevention. The prevention of pressure ulcers may cost as little as $500 and includes nursing time, special mattresses, skin care, and supplemental nutrition [10]. The cost of preventing pressure ulcers, obviously, is less costly than the treatment.

With health care costs ever increasing, physicians face the dilemma of providing "expensive" and prolonged care to those who suffer from the consequences of illness or aging. On the other hand, physicians must consider society's needs as well as individual patient's requirements in determining appropriate medical care. Defining the care physicians deliver must focus on the physician's sense of obligation to patients. Physicians must not confuse value judgments with medical indications for therapy. Bioethics is concerned with society's view that technologic medical advances are expensive and that elderly or severely debilitated patients have a societal duty to die. When practicing medicine, doctors cannot serve two masters. The master must be the patient [14]. If doctors do not become active in defining what is appropriate medical care, others, including insurance companies, governmental agencies, and the courts, will decide for them [13].

Physicians must be guided by medical ethics based on: *autonomy*, respect for the patient's capacity of self-determination and personal choice; *nonmaleficence*, the obligation not to inflict harm intentionally; *beneficence*, the provision of benefit or promoting well-being; and *distributive justice*, the fair, equitable, and appropriate distribution of medical resources. These principles provide a framework for making medical decisions and interventions [12]. Physicians are empowered to make decisions by society to meet the population's medical needs. Society has questioned the moral obligation to treat all people and the self-regulation of the medical profession. Health care reform measures are designed to provide access, improve quality, and contain costs in providing health benefits. These reform measures include improving quality care by emphasizing prevention and primary care for all American citizens [12]. Cost containment measures include global budgets, managed care and capitation reimbursement methodologies. These plans, with primary care physicians as gatekeepers, restrict extensive testings, therapies, and specialists. These restrictions will be part of the new physician-patient relationship. A health care provider should collaborate with the patient to establish a satisfactory course of therapy. This may include providing, on a limited basis, medical therapies or procedures that, although not of reasonable benefit, are meaningful to the patient and his family. Physicians should remember that the patient is the genitor of society. This empowerment is possible because physicians set high standards and hold all patients' interests in trust. This commitment to patients is not an antiquated concept, but one that should be kept alive to preserve respect and confidence [13].

The physician's duty is to relieve suffering and to prolong life [15, 16].

Medical ethics conflict with the health care cost stability. Managed care may not allow physicians "to do everything they believe may benefit each patient without regard to costs or social considerations" [12, 14]. Physicians may be requested to demonstrate that the things they do produce a benefit "which appreciably improves the patient as a whole," which may not be necessarily reasonable according to society's values [12, 18]. Janson proposes a proportional advocacy. Advocacy argues not for everything possible, but for everything probably beneficial [19]. A patient should never be treated as a means to make others happier or wealthier by his or her demise or just to make medical care more cost effective [16, 17, 20]. If physicians become more interested in societal pressures rather than patients' needs, the reason for treating reversible illnesses, correctly diagnosing, and using new, expensive drugs will diminish. The loss of human dignity, as defined by the patient, will prove more costly to society. Physicians should lead, not follow.

REFERENCES

1. Layon, A. J.; George, B. E.; Hamby, B.; and Gallagher, T. J., Do elderly patients overutilize healthcare resources and benefit less from them than younger patients? A study of patients who underwent craniotomy for treatment of neoplasm, *Crit Care Med* 1995; 23:829–834.

2. Fuchs, V. R., The heath care sector's share of the gross national product, *Science* 1990; 267:534–538.

3. Ginzberg, E., A hard look at cost containment, *N Engl J Med* 1987; 316:1151–1154.

4. Allman, R. M.; Laprade, C. A.; Noel, L. B.; Walker, J. M.; Moorer, C. A.; Dear, M. R.; and Smith, C. R., Pressure sores among hospitalized patients, *Ann Intern Med* 1986; 105:337–342.

5. Norton, D.; McLaren, R.; and Exton-Smith, A. N., *An Investigation of Geriatric Nursing Problems in Hospital*, Edinburgh: Churchill Livingstone, 1975:193–238.

6. Michocki, R. J., and Lamy, P. P., The problem of pressure sores in a nursing home population: Statistical analysis, *J Am Geriatr Soc* 1976; 24;323–6.

7. Burner, S. T.; Waldo, D. R.; and McKusick, D. R., National health care expenditures projections through 2030. *Health Care Finance* 1992; 14:1–29.

8. Aaron, H., and Schwartz, W. B., Rationing health care. The choice before us. *Science* 1990; 247:418–422.

9. Rockefeller, J. D. IV, The Pepper Commission report on comprehensive health care (special report), *N Engl J Med* 1990; 323:1005–1007.

10. Hausman, L. L., Cost containment through reducing pressure ulcers, *Nurs Manage* 1994; 25(7):88R, 88T, 88V.

11. Marwick, C., Recommendations seek to prevent pressure sores, *JAMA* 1992; 268(6):700–1.

12. Luce, J. M., Physicians do not have a responsibility to provide futile or unreasonable care if a patient or family insists, *Crit Care Med* 1995; 23(4):760–6.

13. Sprung, C. L.; Eidelman, L. A.; and Steinberg, A., Is the physician's duty to the individual patient or to society? *Crit Care Med* 1995; 23(4):618–620.

14. Levinsky, N. G., The doctor's master. *N Engl J Med* 1984; 311:1573–1575.

15. Friedlander, W. J., "The Bollinger case": A 79-year-old headline conveys a current medical-ethical dilemma, *Pharos* 1994; 57:34–37.

16. Nilges, R. G., Doctors should lead, not follow, *Bull Am Coll Surg* 1995; 80(6):15–17.

17. Duffy, Y., The indignity of assisted suicide, *Chicago Tribune*, February 13, 1994, Sec. 4, p. 1.

18. Schneiderman, L. J.; Jecker, N. S.; and Jonsen, A. R., Medical futility: Its meaning and ethical implications. *Ann Intern Med* 1990; 112:949–954.

19. Janson, A. R., *The New Medicine and the Old Ethics*, Cambridge: Harvard University Press, 1990.

20. Eisman, B., A new clause in the social contract, *Bull Am Coll Surg* 1994; 79(3):23–25.

2

HISTORICAL ASPECTS OF WOUND HEALING

Bok Y. Lee, M.D., and Marcelo C. DaSilva, M.D.

To primitive and modern alike, ceremonial is a shock-absorber, a mitigating diversion from the change become inevitable.

————Elsie Clews Parsons, 1914.

There have been times when rigorous scholarship and academia in medicine led to great improvement in the quality of healing, and there have been times when medicine disappeared from its own history. Physicians are taught that only what is "relevant" counts and that they should practice medicine in ignorance of their past. But it is through knowledge of the history of our profession that physicians can understand the present and speculate on the future. The history of medicine is not just the history of physicians and their fields of specialization, nor is it just the history of how to treat diseases; it is a history of man's endeavors.

ANCIENT AND PRIMITIVE MEDICINE

Collective investigations of historians, ethnologists, archeologists, and sociologists reveal that phases of social anthropology converge to a single point: instincts of self-preservation and reproduction. Savage man, in his effort to cope with injury and hostile forces, created religious and ethical beliefs based on the necessity to survive. Civilized minds differ from the savage one in regard to evolution. Primitive minds lacked the ability to assign causes for phenomena. The convergence of all medical folklore is animism: the world crawls with invisible spirits that cause disease and death. As savage man advanced, knowledge was gained from experience; there followed herbal medicine, bone setting, and crude surgery as a means of livelihood for some individuals [1]. The history of wound care begins with man's first injury [2], and the art of healing is as old as humanity [3]. Surgery, however, has become a science of recent times.

Primitive surgery was rudimentary. Instruments included such items as leaf-shaped flint or fish teeth. Primitive procedures included "blood letting," abscess emptying, scarifying tissues, trephining skulls, and performing circumcisions. Wounds were dressed with moss[1] or fresh leaves, ashes or natural balsams. The Chinese civilization utilized bread mold, "cupping," and "moxisbution"[2] for the treatment of neurologic and muscle pain [4]. Signs of amputation have been found in prehistoric bones.

[1]Any of various green, usually small, nonvascular plants of the class Musci of the division Bryophyta.

[2]Smoldering, soft wormwood leaves applied at acupuncture site.

During the Bronze and Iron Ages, craftsmanship of metal improved. Surgical saws and files were plentiful from Egypt to Central Europe. Articulated surgical instruments, like scissors, appeared during the Gallo-Roman period.

Development of a rational, scientific concept of disease is essentially modern. Its origin is in the Greek Period as written in the Hippocratic tract on *Ancient Medicine* (circa 430–420 B.C.): "... men came to learn by themselves how their own sufferings came about and cease, ... medicine has long had all its means at hand, and has discovered both a principle and a method, through which the discoveries made during a long period are many and excellent."

History suggests that permanent ignorance and superstition result from oppression of mankind by fanatical "leaders." Essential traits of folk and ancient medicine have been alike; in each case an affair of attraction and spells, plant lore, and psychotherapy exists to reject the effects of supernatural agencies. When this pattern exists, there is no place for development in medicine. The primitive minds had natural standards and were worthy of consideration and scientific respect. "There is nothing men will not do, and there is nothing men have not done to recover their health and save their lives" [5].

PREHISTORIC PHASES

The prehistory of man begins with the origins of highly developed primates in the Oligocene epoch,[3] the transformation of these in the Pliocene epoch,[4] and the extinction of the great mammals and dawn of Old Stone Age culture in the Pleistocene epoch (500,000 B.C.).[5] The question that arises about that period is primarily, What was the relation of prehistoric man to medicine? It began with human and comparative anatomy; innumerable carvings, mural paintings, statuettes, and line engravings of man and animals. Found in caves of the Old Stone Age (Paleolithic[6] period, 150,000 to 35,000 B.C.), these works represented physiological and pathological findings. What were the primary reactions to agonizing wounds, fatal hemorrhage, terrifying diseases, suffocation, and imminent death? From ancient medical German folklore we learn that the reaction was panic. Prehistoric trephining was performed by Neolithic[7] man 10,000 years ago. Cauterization of skull wounds was a common Neolithic practice in northern France and evidence of it was found in a pre-Columbian skull from Peru. North American Indian remains of the pre-Columbian period reveal the results of inflammation of bone. Evidence of lesion of soft tissues in Neolithic man comes from the paleopathology of ancient Egypt.

EGYPTIAN MEDICINE

The oldest records of the history of medicine known are the medical papyri of ancient Egypt. Predating these are well-splinted fractures of the fifth dynasty (2750 to 2625 B.C.). The earliest known physician was Im-hotep of King Zoser's reign (third dynasty, 2980 to 2900 B.C.). A valuable medical papyrus (1600 B.C.) was that found by Edwin Smith [1, 9] at Thebes in 1862, translated by J. H. Breasted. The Smith papyrus contains 48 cases in clinical surgery, examination, semiology, diagnosis, prognosis, and treatment and a glossary of archaic terms. Next, an important medical papyrus was obtained

---

[3]The geologic time and deposits of the epoch in the Tertiary period of the Cenozoic era that extended from the Eocene epoch to the Miocene epoch.

[4]**The five epochs** of the Tertiary period, characterized by the appearance of distinctly modern animals.

[5]The earlier of the two epochs of the Quaternary period, characterized by the alternate appearance and recession of northern glaciation and the appearance of the progenitors of human beings.

[6]Designating the cultural period beginning with the earliest chipped stone tools, about 750,000 years ago, until the beginning of the Mesolithic age, about 15,000 years ago.

[7]The cultural period beginning around 10,000 B.C. in the Middle East and later elsewhere, characterized by the development of agriculture and the making of polished stone implements.

by Georg Ebers [1, 10] at Thebes in 1872 and translated by H. Joachim in 1890, that dates to about 1550 B.C.. The Ebers papyrus documented the first medical vocabulary, surgical methods, drug therapies, and techniques of splitting and bandaging of wounds [3]. The ancient Egyptians understood wound healing. They used honey, or *byt*, frequently, and described it as an aseptic, antiseptic, and antibiotic [3, 8]. The Egyptians believed pus was helpful as along as it was not excessive and they advocated draining suppuration from wounds.

SUMERIAN AND ORIENTAL MEDICINE

Sumerian tablets, which date to 2100 B.C. [6] describe chronic wound care; washing, bandaging, plastering, and otherwise treating wounds. The Sumerians were skilled in mathematics and astronomy and created the decimal system of notation, weights, and measures. Medical practice in Babylon advanced in public esteem and was rewarded with adequate fees, which were carefully regulated by law.

GREEK MEDICINE

The chief of healing in Greek pantheon was Apollo, commonly called Alexikakos (the averter of ills), also known as Pæan, as he treated and cured diseases with the root of the peony. Hence, the epithet "sons of Pæan" was applied to physicians. Legend related that knowledge of medicine was communicated by Apollo and his sister Artemis to the centaur Chiron, son of Saturn. Chiron was entrusted with the rearing and education of the heros Jason, Hercules, Achilles and, in particular, Aesculapius, the son of Apollo by the nymph Coronis [1]. Among the legendary children of Aesculapius by his wife Epione were his daughters Hygieia and Panacea, who assisted in the temple rites and fed the sacred snakes.[8] Aesculapius is commonly represented with the sacred snake entwined around a rod, a miniature Omphalos, and a childish figure called Telesphorus, the god of convalescence.

The classical period (460–136 B.C.) of European medicine begins in the Age of Pericles, and its scientific developments center in the figure of Hippocrates (460–370 B.C.), who gave Greek medicine its scientific principles and its ethical ideals. He was a contemporary of Sophocles, Euripides, Aristophanes, Socrates, Plato, Herodotus, Thucydides, Phidias, and Polygnotus and lived when the Athenian democracy had reached its zenith. Not before or since have so many men of genius appeared within the same limits of space and time. The eminence of Hippocrates is threefold: (1) he dissociated medicine from theology and philosophy, (2) he crystallized the loose knowledge of medicine into a more systematic science, and (3) he gave physicians the highest moral inspiration. Hippocrates revolutionized the fundamentals of wound care by emphasizing the importance of light, stating that examination of a patient should be comfortable for the physician, and emphasizing that the injured area should be compared to the corresponding uninjured area.

The formal writings on *Fractures, Dislocations,* and *Wounds of the Head* may be thought of as modern. Hippocrates argued, in *Wounds of the Head*, for decompressive trephining, even in contusions, and advised simple treatment for an open depressed fracture. In *Wounds*, he infers that wounds should never be irrigated except with clean water or wine. He describes the dry state near the healthy, the wet to the diseased. He prescribes the aseptic advantages of extreme dryness and the avoidance of greasy dressings. This effort would bring the fresh edges of the wound to close apposition. Hippocrates recognized that "rest and immobilization are of capital importance." While describing symptoms of suppuration, he said "In such cases, medicated dressings, if applied at all, should be not upon the wound itself, but around it." If water was used for irrigation, it had to be pure or boiled. The hands and nails of the surgeon were to be clean. Hippocrates gave the first description of healing by first and second intention. He described the operating room environment as well illuminated, and discussed proper patient posture and the presence of capable

---

[8]The ancient Greeks, Egyptians, Cretans, and Hindus venerated the serpent as the companion of many gods.

assistants. About the surgeon's training he said, "War is the only proper school of the surgeon." Behind the phenomena of nature he hypothesized the existence of a tremendous power. Hippocrates founded the bedside method of examining the patient, which is the distinct talent of all clinicians. His method of using the mind and senses as diagnostic instruments, his transparent honesty, his elevated conception of dignity of the physician's duty, and his respect for patients made him the "father of medicine."

After Hippocrates came Aristotle (384–322 B.C.) of Stagira. A pupil of Plato, Aristotle gave medicine the origins of botany, zoology, comparative anatomy, embryology, teratology, and physiology. He named the aorta and regarded the heart as the primary source of heat, sensation, and thought, a view upheld even in Harvey's writings. After the foundation of Alexandria (331 B.C.) Herophilus (335–280 B.C.), grandson of Aristotle, created the great school of anatomy at Alexandria, becoming known as the "father of scientific anatomy." Herophilus made important advances in the study of the nervous system, including sensory and motor nerves. He wrote about wounds of the head, venous drainage of the skull, and the anatomic basis of wounds. Erasistratus (circa 310–250 B.C.) was an experimental physiologist who described the aortic and pulmonary valves, the chordae tendineae of the heart, and the capillary network of arteries and veins. In the third century B.C., Alexandrine medicine was introduced in Mesopotamia, and in this way Syria acquired some of Hippocrates' doctrine via Egypt.

GRECO-ROMAN PERIOD (156 B.C.–A.D. 576)

The northern half of the early Roman Empire was conquered by warriors. The southern half of Italy and Sicily were not occupied by northern invaders, but remained free as Magna Graecia from the sixth century B.C. to the tenth century A.D. Magna Graecia introduced cultural influences that led to the School of Medicine of Salerno. After the destruction of Corinth (146 B.C.), Greek medicine migrated to Rome. The most eminent physicians came from the Schools of Pargamus, Ephesus, Tralles, and Miletus in Asia Minor. Greek medicine was respected in Rome through the personality, tact, and ability of Asclepiades of Bithynia (124 B.C.).

Roman medicine was almost entirely in Greek hands and produced names such as Aurelius Cornelius Celsus (25 B.C.–A.D. 50) who was also known as the "Latin Hippocrates." Celsus was not a physician, but he translated encyclopedia writings on medicine. He was ignored by Roman practitioners, and his work went unrecognized until the Renaissance when *De re medicina* was one of the first medical books printed (1478). *De re medicina* consists of eight books. The first four describe diseases treated by diet and regimen, and the last four describe those amenable to drugs and surgery. The third book contains a definition of insanity (*Insania*) and the first drawing of heart disease. The fourth book contains the four cardinal signs of inflammation: *rubor, tumor, calor*, and *dolor* (redness, swelling, heat, and pain). The fifth book classifies lists of drugs, pharmaceutical methods, and weights and measures. The sixth book describes diseases of the skin and venereal disease. The seventh book is on surgery and describes the use of the ligature for bleeding vessels, management of cancer of the head, neck, and nose, hypertrophic scar, and proper dressing of wounds. Celsus said, "The physician cannot apply the proper therapeutics without a correct diagnosis" [3].

Three Greek surgeons were contemporaries of Celsus: Heliodorus, Archigenes, and Antyllus. Heliodorus described the first ligation and torsion of blood vessels, surgery of hernias, and circular and flap amputations. Archigenes of Apamea used ligatures during surgical procedures. Antyllus treated aneurysms by applying two ligatures and cutting down between them, which became the method of treatment until John Hunter (1728–1793). This ancient period ends with a widely respected Greek physician, Galen of Pergamon (131–201). He founded experimental physiology and was the first experimental neurologist. He was a skilled practitioner, and his theories dominated Western medicine for 1500 years [3]. He was the foremost contributor of experimental physiology prior to William Harvey (1578–1657). He treated wounded gladiators during mortal combats in Pergamon and Rome. During this period he learned about human anatomy, the venous and arterial circulation, and wound healing. Galen wrote that, "The best physician has also to be a philosopher." His theory that suppuration is essential to the healing of wounds led to Arabic notions of healing by second intention. His concept of "*pus bonum et laudibile*" was opposed by Mondeville, Paracelsus, and Paré, and lasted until Lister in 1881 [7].

BYZANTINE PERIOD (A.D. 476–732)

The Western Roman Empire lasted 500 years. The Eastern Empire lasted over 1000 years (395–1453). The downfall of the Western Empire began when the Romans acquired a state where "wealth accumulates and men decay." Degeneration of mind and body, with consequent relaxation of morals, led to mysticism and respect for the supernatural. This paved the way for dogmatism and the mental inertia of the Middle Ages.

The decomposition of the mind, luxury, and sloth in the Eastern Empire became synonymous with the Byzantine Empire. Medical achievement was limited to the preservation of the language, culture, and literary texts of the Greeks. The habit of compilation established by Greek and Roman writers was expressed in four industrious compilers. Oribasius (325–403) wrote a treatise on medicine, *Euporista*, that was the most popular during the Dark Ages. Aetius of Amida, in the sixth century, described for the first time the ligation of the brachial artery above the sac for aneurysm, which evolved into the Hunterian method (1786).

MOHAMMEDAN AND JEWISH PERIODS (732–1096)

The Middle Ages were first influenced by Arabic authors, such as Rhazes (860–932), who described smallpox and measles. Haly ben Abbas, a Persian, was the author of the *Almaleki*, containing an anatomical section that was the only source of knowledge at Salerno from 1070–1170. Ibn Sina or Avicenna (980–1037), "the Prince of Physicians,"

recommended wine as a wound dressing and was the first to describe the preparation and properties of sulfuric acid and alcohol.

During the second period of the Middle Ages, medicine greatly prospered during the Spanish dynasty (655–1236). Abulkasim, called Albucasis (1013–1106), was the author of a medico-surgical treatise called *Altasrif* (Collection), which contained three books. The first discussed the use of cautery; the second contained detailed descriptions of lithotripsy, amputations for gangrene, the treatment of wounds, and management of phlegmon and carbuncle; and the third book dealt with fractures and dislocations.

Closely associated with Mohammedan medicine is the Jewish influence upon European medicine. During the Middle Ages and long after, the destiny of the Jewish physicians in Europe was protected by monarchy and clergy. They were utilized as teachers in the Schools of Salerno and Montpellier because of their scientific knowledge. The prohibition of Jewish physicians by Popes Paul IV (1555–1559) and Pius V (1566–1572) was lifted by Pope Gregory XIII in 1584. It was not, however, until the beginning of the modern industrial movement that Jewish physicians had access to the universities.

MEDIEVAL PERIOD (1096–1438)

The Middle Ages are described as a period of conflict between feudalism and ecclesiasticism, or Church and State. The School of Salerno was the first independent medical school. It aroused the healing art from 500 years of stagnation. Salerno was known by Romans as the ideal health resort. Its medical teachings produced surgeons like Roger (Ruggiero Frugardi) of Palermo and Roland (Rolando Capelluti) of Parma. Roger studied many important areas in medicine, one being the healing of wounds by second intention. The medical school of Salerno was abolished by Napoleon in November 1881.

The authority on surgery in the fourteenth and fifteenth centuries was Guy de Chauliac (1300–1368). He introduced medical education at Toulouse, Montpellier, and Paris, and taught a special course in anatomy at Bologna, becoming the most erudite surgeon of his time. He believed in resecting cancer at an early stage with a knife. Guy de Chauliac wrote *Wounds and Fractures* in 1363 and included instructions on bandaging, suturing, compresses, drains, and the treatment of keloids [3]. Despite his knowledge and clinical experience, he is known as a reactionary in wound healing. He stated that, "The healing of a wound must be accomplished by the surgeon's interference: salves, plasters and other interventions."

Another pupil of the School of Montpellier was Arnold de Villanova (1235–1311) of Spain, who described suture materials and their differences. He wrote, in relation to wound healing, "In large wounds one should use sutures, and silk thread should be tied at short distances . . . a collection of pus is best dissolved by incision and cleaning out the purulent material, to put off the opening of an abscess brings many dangers with it . . . where veins and arteries are notably large, incision and deep cautery should be avoided."

During the Middle Ages, the Crusades aroused nationhood, an idea of citizens against barons. In the struggle between collectivism and individualism, intellectual independence was ostracized if it did not agree with Church or State. Popes and kings supported advances in medicine by building universities and hospitals, and by encouraging individuals. This, however, was done by suppression of experimental science. Until the Renaissance, there was neither induction nor experimentation.

THE RENAISSANCE (1453–1600)

Humanistic revival of classical art, architecture, literature, and science originated in Italy in the Fourteenth through the Sixteenth centuries and later was spread throughout Europe. Known as the Renaissance, it marked the transition from medieval to modern times. Many factors led to the defeat of individualism by authority inflicted upon mankind, gunpowder being the most important. The use of gunpowder and bullets during the Renaissance eventually led to the end of feudalism. It changed the role of surgeons into an active and aggressive one. Resurgence of Greek culture was brought by the Byzantine scholars into Italy after the fall of Constantinople (Istanbul) in 1453. This Renaissance revival reached its peak with the medical leaders of the Sixteenth century. These leaders were Parcelsus, Vesalius, and Paré.

Philippus Aureolus Theophrastus Bombastus von Hohenheim, or simply Parcelsus (1493–1541), was the forerunner of chemical pharmacology and therapeutics. His coarseness of fiber often hindered his ability to think "straight and see clear." The son of a physician, he had a peculiar "disaffection" for those who disagreed with his views and writings. He was one of the few who advanced medicine by debating about it. He traveled all over Europe, collecting information from regional folklore. Practically the only asepsist between Mondeville and Lister, he taught that nature heals wounds. As a theorist, Paracelsus believed in the descent of living organisms from primordial ooze, anticipating Darwin's observation that "the strong war down and prey upon the weak." Andreas Vesalius (1514–1564), was a commanding figure in European medicine after Galen and before Harvey. He introduced anatomy as a living science. He taught students to dissect and inspect the partis in situ, and wrote *De Fabrica Humani Corporis* in 1543. He was the first to diagnose and describe aneurysm of the abdominal and thoracic aorta (1551). Disregarded by his old teacher, Sylvius, and persecuted by his contemporary colleagues, Vesalius burned his manuscripts and left Padua to work as a court physician to Emperor Charles V [1].

Ambroise Paré (1510–1590), a barber's apprentice, worked as a dresser at Hotel Dieu in Paris. He became an army surgeon in 1537. He was the only "Protestant" to be spared (by royal mandate) at St. Bartholomew. Paré's contribution to medicine related to treatment of gunshot wounds: "diseases not curable by iron are curable by fire." During the Battle of Villaine, Paré's supply of boiling oil was depleted and he applied milder treatments to amputation wounds. He practiced with meticulous cleanliness and epitomized these words: "I make the wound, God heals it," ending dogma of laudable pus.

SEVENTEENTH CENTURY: THE AGE OF INDIVIDUAL SCIENTIFIC ENDEAVOR

In the Seventeenth century, medicine produced physicians such as William Harvey (1578–1657), who graduated from Padua. Not since Vesalius had a body of works by one writer so influenced modern medicine. Harvey reviewed theories of blood in motion, showed their inadequacy, and proceeded to prove that the heart acts as a muscular force-pump in propelling blood continuously and in a cycle. For Harvey, the primary necessity underlying all his actions was personal observation. He wrote to Riolan: ". . . by my observations and experiments, and not to demonstrate by causes and probable principles, but to confirm it by sense and experience, as by a powerful authority, according to the rule of the anatomists [11]." He published *De Motu Cordis* in 1628.

The introduction of the microscope was made in the last half of the seventeenth century by Anton van Leeuwenhoek (1632–1723), a Dutch naturalist, who devoted his private life to studying natural history. He had 247 microscopes, and observed small particles in ordinary pond water, calling them "animalcules." Leeuwenhoek was the first to describe spermatozoa, red blood cells, sarcolemma, and microorganisms in the teeth, and he accurately described the morphology of bacterial chains and clumps. He demonstrated capillary anastomosis between the arteries and veins, which Malpighi observed in 1660, completing Harvey's demonstration. The greatest microscopist was Marcello Malpighi (1628–1694), the founder of histology and professor of anatomy at Bologna and Pisa. He discovered the rete mucosum, or Malpighian layer of skin, and he demonstrated pulmonary capillary anastomosis between arteries and veins and capillaries (1660). Prior to Harvey, respiration was regarded as a means of refrigeration and not combustion. Malpighi demonstrated that blood changes from venous to arterial in the lungs, but did not correlate how or why humans breathe. Robert Boyle (1627–1691) demonstrated the necessity of air for life and combustion through experiments involving flames and animals. In 1665, Robert Hooke (1635–1703), in his treatise *Micrographia*, described microscopic units that made up cork, naming these units "cells." In 1667 he proved that by attaching a bellow to the trachea of a dog with an open thorax, life could be maintained by artificial means. Antoine-Laurent Lavoisier (1743–1794) discovered oxygen as the true element in the interchange of gases in the lungs. Lavoisier demonstrated that respiration is the analog of combustion, the chemical products of carbon dioxide and water.

EIGHTEENTH CENTURY: THE AGE OF THEORIES AND SYSTEMS

John Hunter (1728–1793), a Scottish surgeon, came to London in 1748 and was taken in by his brother, William Hunter (1718–1783), who was also a surgeon. During the expedition of Belleisle (1761) John Hunter acquired a unique knowledge of gunshot wounds. He was the first to classify healing by *primary and secondary intention* and to describe granulation tissue in healing wounds. As a surgical pathologist, he described shock, phlebitis, pyemia, and intussusception and studied inflammation, gunshot wounds, and surgical treatment related to the vascular system. In 1790, he first introduced artificial feeding via a flexible tube passed into the stomach. He described inflammation as not a disease, but a nonspecific response that has a "salutary" effect on its host. John Hunter recognized the possibility of tissue acceptance for transplants [3]. He referred to a female calf, the nonidentical twin of a male, which matured into a sterile cow lacking immunogenicity. This antedated the works of Carrel, Guthrie, and Sir Peter Brian Medawar on tissue transplantation and acquired immunologic tolerance, respectively. Hunter's position in science is based upon the fact that he was the founder of experimental and surgical pathology as well as comparative physiology and anatomy.

NINETEENTH CENTURY: THE BEGINNING OF SCIENCE

Great industrial and social-democratic movements of man followed the political revolutions in America and France and intensified feelings for intellectual and moral liberty. The publication of works such as Helmholtz's *Conservation of Energy* (1847) and Darwin's *Origin of Species* (1859) led to true advancements in medicine. Physics, chemistry, and biology were finally studied as objective laboratory sciences. Prior to 1850 and afterwards, advancements in medicine primarily came from France, as Germany as recovering from the Thirty Years War. Virchow published *Cellular Pathology*, which described new forms of disease.

Theodor Schwann (1810–1882), born near Dusseldorf, described the constitution of tissues: "The elementary parts of all tissues are formed of cells in an analogous, though very diversified, manner. . ." His cell theory was published in 1839. He discovered the sheath of neurons that bear his name. Schwann proved necessity of air for development in the embryo, and also addressed spontaneous generation. In 1836, he proved that putrefaction was produced by living organisms. Following research by Schleiden and Schwann, cells became the primary subject of investigation. Virchow (1858) published works on the continuity of cellular development and its importance in pathology. The cell became known as the structural and physiological unit in all living organisms. Anatomic studies became more progressive and more histologic. The "seats and causes" of disease were regarded as cellular elements of the body. Jacob Henle (1809–1885), a German pathologist, is recognized as the identifier of epithelial tissues of the body (1836–1837). He maintained that a physician's duty was to prevent and cure disease, and he believed disease to be a deviation from normal physiologic processes. He published *Allgemeine Anatomie* in 1841, a book on microscopic histology.

The rise of modern medicine includes a German pathologist, Rodolf Virchow (1821–1902), the founder of cellular pathology. Virchow graduated in Berlin in 1843. He was the first to observe leukocytosis. Virchow described the "body as a cell-state in which every cell is a citizen," and in 1856 created the doctrine of embolism. He articulated the cell theory in 1858: "Every animal appears as a sum of vital units, each of which bears in itself the complete characteristics of life." A pupil of Virchow, Julius Cohnheim (1839–1884) made microscopic observations of initial vasodilatation and changes in blood flow and subsequent edema caused by increased vascular permeability. He demonstrated, in opposition to Virchow, that an essential feature of inflammation included passage of white blood cells through walls of capillaries and that pus and pus cells are formed away from blood. Diapedesis was described by Addison; however, Cohnheim's investigations traced the migration of stained leukocytes.

Advances in scientific medicine during the second half of the nineteenth century were characterized by the introduction of the biological or theory of evolution by Charles Robert Darwin (1809–1882). Darwin graduated from Cambridge and worked for twenty years prior to publishing *On the Origin of Species by Means of Natural Selection* (1859). Darwin's work in biology introduced cellular pathology, bacteriology, and parasitology, which had been previously referred to as the germ theory. Louis Pasteur (1822–1895) graduated in chemistry in 1847 from the École normale in Paris. His work included writings on molecular asymmetry (1848), fermentation (1857), spontaneous generation (1862), preventive vaccinations (1880), and discovery of the anaerobic and aerobic characteristics of bacteria. In November 1877, Robert Koch (1843–1910), after working with bacillus anthrax, published methods of fixing and drying bacterial films. He used cover-slips for staining and photographing as well as identification and comparison. Joseph Lister (1827–1912), an English surgeon, graduated from the University of London in 1852, becoming house surgeon and a professor at the University of Glasgow. Lister, interested in the high mortality from surgical infections, which included his own 45% mortality rate for amputations, was attracted by Pasteur's work and experimented with zinc chloride and sulfites. He stumbled by "chance" upon carbolic acid, which was used to disinfect sewage in Carlisle. In 1867 he published the results of two years' work *On the Antiseptic Principle in the Practice of Surgery*. In 1874, Lister sent Pasteur a letter acknowledging his work in relation to antiseptic surgery.

Claude Bernard (1813–1878), born in Saint Julien (Rhone), a physiologist from France, is regarded as a founder of experimental medicine, that is, the artificial production of disease by chemical and physical manipulation. His achievements include the discovery of effects of vasodilator and vasoconstrictor nerves on circulation.

The theory of evolution, combined with the cell theory, provided the intellectual framework that developed biology into an experimental science. It branched into biochemistry and genetics. In 1865, Austrian monk Gregor Mendel described the basic rules of heredity, but it was not until 1900 that his theory was widely accepted. Friedrich Miescher, in 1871, isolated what may have been DNA from the nuclei of dead white blood cells. Elie Metchnikoff (1845–1916), a Russian biologist, demonstrated how amoeboid cells in connective tissues and blood engulf solid particles and bacteria, destroying them by phagocytosis. He called them "phagocytes" and related their function as scavengers. He described inflammation as the effect of phagocytosis to the site of injury by chemotaxis. He upheld the theory of immunity as phagocytosis.

MODERN PERIOD

Ancient surgeons were able to care for wounds and hemorrhage by cleansing and bandaging. Paul Ehrlich's (1854–1915) lock-and-key theory of antigen-antibody recognition was instrumental in understanding immunochemical principles of wound healing. He developed the humoral theory of wound healing. Sir Thomas Lewis established that chemical substances, locally induced by injury, mediated the vascular changes in inflammation. In 1897, Eduard Buchner demonstrated that chemical transformation could be performed by cell extracts.

By 1900, 16 of the 20 standard amino acids that form proteins had been identified. That same year, Emil Fischer proposed the correct mechanism for formation of chemical links in protein: peptide bonds between adjacent amino acids. In 1935, threonine was the last amino acid discovered.

In 1928, while studying staphylococcus variants, Sir Alexander Fleming (1881–1955) observed that a mold contained in one of his cultures caused the bacteria in its vicinity to undergo lysis. The mold belonged to the genus *Penicillium notatum* and was named penicillin. Fleming's career was devoted to investigating human defenses that control bacterial infection [12]. Alexis Carrel's (1873–1944) and C.

C. Guthrie's work on the effects of exudation on fibroblast proliferation found in an inflammatory site suggested that humoral substances present within the inflammatory environment stimulated tissue repair. Their studies led to research in growth factors, cytokines, substrates, hormones, cell-to-cell communication, and the effects of inflammation on cell function and replication.

Sir Peter Medawar, in 1944, devised three characteristics of immune system responsiveness: recognition of non-self, memory, and specificity. He examined the histology of rejection and suggested that the mononuclear cell (lymphocyte) had an important role in allograft destruction [13]. Studies by Paul Ehrlich led to immunoassays. Names in molecular biology include Michael Tswett and his analytical methods and Martin Synge's partition chromatography. In 1953, Frederick Sanger reported the complete amino acid sequence of human insulin [14, 15]. Myles Partridge separated pure amino acids using column chromatography, and others contributed to the identification, isolation, and sequencing of proteins. In 1951, Linus Pauling suggested the helical arrangement for certain parts of protein chains.

The modern era of molecular cell biology, concerned with how genes govern cell activity, began in 1953 when James D. Watson and Francis H. C. Crick postulated the double-helical structure of DNA [16]. In 1961, François Jacob and Jacques Monod suggested that protein products of certain genes regulate activity of other genes. Soon after, proof that mesenger RNA (mRNA) carries information from DNA to protein-synthesizing machinery, discovery of the genetic code, and discovery that proteins are translated by transfer RNA (tRNA) and ribosomes were reported [17]. Technical advances in molecular biology in the 1970s were greatest in analysis and manipulation of DNA. Enzymes that are able to cut DNA were discovered. These enzymatic scalpels are called restriction endonucleases, and their discovery accounts for DNA cloning and sequencing. Throughout the years, the cell has become an organism in which the controlled and integrated actions of genes produce specific sets of proteins that build characteristic structures and carry out specialized enzymatic activities, preserving the species and perpetuating the process of life.

Man's concept of the cell has come a long way from its original characterization as a simple unit of living matter.

REFERENCES

1. Garrison, F. H., *An Introduction to the History of Medicine*, 4th ed., Philadelphia: W. B. Saunders, 1929.

2. Wideman, D. M.; Rovee, D. T.; and Alvarez, O. M., Wound dressings: Design and use, In I. K. Cohen, R. F. Diegelmann, W. J. Lindblad, eds., *Wound Healing; Biochemical and Clinical Aspects*, Philadelphia: W. B. Saunders, 1992:562–580.

3. Brown, H., Wound healing research through the ages, In I. K. Cohen, R. F. Diegelmann, W. J. Lindblad, eds., *Wound Healing; Biochemical and Clinical Aspects*, Philadelphia: W. B. Saunders, 1992:5–18.

4. Weingarten, M. S., Obstacles to wound healing, *Wounds* 1993; 5(5):238–244.

5. Holmes, O. W., *Medical Essays*, Boston, MA, 1883.

6. Caldwell, M. D., Topical wound therapy—An historical perspective, *J Trauma* 1990; 30(S12)S116–S122.

7. Lister, J., An address on the treatment of wounds, *Lancet* 1881; 863:901.

8. Majno, G., *The Healing Hand: Man and Wound in the Ancient World*, Cambridge, MA:Harvard University Press, 1975.

9. Breasted, J. H., *The Edwin Smith Surgical Papyrus*, Chicago: University of Chicago Press, 1930.

10. Ebbell, B., *The Papyrus Ebers. The Greatest Egyptian Medical Document*, London: Oxford University Press, 1937.

11. Whitteridge, G., *William Harvey and the Circulation of the Blood*, New York: Neale Watson Academic Publications, 1971.

12. Gilman, A. G., Rall, T. W.; Nies, A. S.; and Taylor, P., *Goodman and Gilman's The Pharmacological Basis of Therapeutics*, 8th ed., New York and Oxford:Pergamon Press, 1990:1065.

13. Amos, D. B., and Sanfilippo, F., The immunology of transplants antigens, In David C. Sabiston, Jr., ed., *The Biological Basis of Modern Surgical Practice*, 14th ed., Philadelphia: W. B. Saunders, 1991:346.

14. Brown, H.; Sanger, F.; and Kitai, R., The structure of pig and sheep insulins, *Biochem J* 1955; 60:556–565.

15. Sanger, F., Sequences, sequences, and sequences, *Ann Rev Biochem* 1988; 57:1–28.

16. Watson, J. D., and Crick, F. H. C., Molecular structure of nucleic acids. A structure for deoxyribose nucleic acid, *Nature* 1953; 171:737–738.

17. Darnell, J.; Lodish, H, and Baltimore, D., *Molecular Cell Biology*, 2nd ed. New York: Scientific American Books, 1990:1–15.

3

NONINVASIVE EVALUATION OF THE CUTANEOUS CIRCULATION

Bok Y. Lee, M.D., and Lee E. Ostrander, Ph.D.

INTRODUCTION

The body's microcirculation, or system of capillaries, is responsible for the delivery of nourishment and the removal of waste products. The assessment of the cutaneous circulation can provide insight to the cause and management of many pathological conditions, particularly diseases affecting the peripheral vascular system. In this chapter we present a brief review of the anatomy and physiology of the microcirculation and a review of methods available for the noninvasive assessment of the cutaneous circulation.

ANATOMY OF THE MICROCIRCULATION

In human skin, there is a dense system of capillary loops in the papillae of the corium that empties into a subcapillary venous plexus that contains a major fraction of the cutaneous blood volume. The microvascular bed is a subunit of the circulatory system and is composed of vessels less than 100 µm in diameter. The microvascular bed (Figure 3-1) begins with the terminal arteriole, with vessel walls

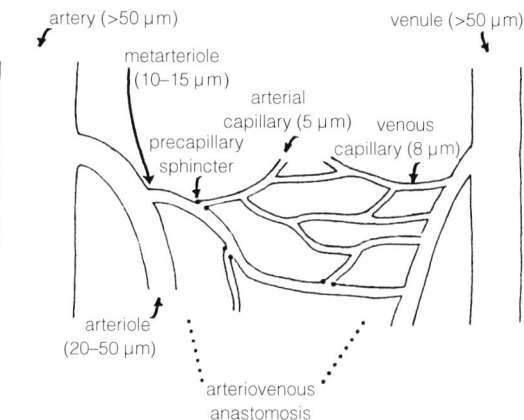

Figure 3-1. Diagrammatic representation of a microcirculatory unit.

composed of an inner layer of epithelium, an internal elastic lamina, and a surrounding sheath of at least two continuous layers of vascular smooth muscle cells. Arterioles, which arise from the terminal arteries, have a single continuous layer of vascular smooth muscle. Next are the metarterioles, with a single discontinuous layer of vascular smooth muscle cells. The metarterioles often have a band of vascular smooth muscle cells at the origin, the precapillary sphincter. The capillaries arise from the metarterioles and consist of a single layer of endothelial cells and a basement membrane surrounded by a fine, reinforcing network of reticular collagen fibers. The capillaries are classified as being either arterial or venous, depending on whether they are closer to the metarterioles (arterial capillaries) or the draining collecting venules (venous capillaries).

The walls of the capillaries function as a selectively permeable membrane. Endothelial cells that form a single layer range from 0.1 to 3 μm in thickness (Figure 3-2). Between the cells is an intercellular space of about 100 Å in width. Almost all spaces have a constricted area about 40 Å wide. Within the cells are many small vesicles that continually join with the inner and outer cell membranes, contributing to the transport of materials across the capillary walls.

In the microcirculation, sympathetic vasoconstrictor innervation usually extends only as far as the arterioles but in some instances may be found in the metarterioles. Metarterioles in general, as well as precapillary sphincters, are under local control, being influenced by tissue waste products, oxygen deprivation, or other factors. These vessels usually show a rhythmic vasomotion of alternating vasodilation and vasoconstriction. Arteriole changes in vessel caliber are more irregular. Venules, in general, receive few sympathetic vasoconstrictor nerves.

In terms of function, the microvascular bed can be divided into (1) resistance vessels—arterioles, metarterioles, and precapillary sphincters—which together control organ blood flow; (2) exchange vessels—the capillaries; and (3) reservoir vessels—venules and veins.

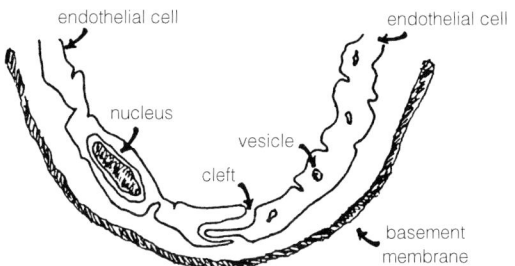

Figure 3-2. Diagrammatic representation with electron microscopy of a cross section through a capillary.

PHYSIOLOGY OF CAPILLARY PERFUSION

Perfusion and function of the capillaries are regulated and affected by a number of factors. Vasoconstriction or vasodilation alters the diameter of the arterioles and therefore influences the amount of blood flow that enters the capillaries. Vasoconstriction and vasodilation are regulated by both sympathetic and parasympathetic fibers and catecholamines such as epinephrine and norepinephrine. Additionally, pharmacologic agents (e.g., alpha stimulators, beta blockers) will affect arteriolar diameter. In many tissues, arteriovenous shunts may open to cause a complete bypass of the capillary bed. Increases in cardiac output elevate arterial blood pressure and increase capillary blood flow. Elevation in arterial blood pressure caused by arteriolar constriction, however, decreases capillary blood flow. The presence of precapillary sphincters also influences the amount of blood reaching the capillaries, and it is possible that capillaries may open and close because of the intrinsic contractibility of capillary endothelial cells. Such capillary constriction and dilation are independent of action by the arterioles. Essential components appear to be anoxia and histamine production. A capillary is closed from 60 to 95% of the time; therefore, as few as 5% of all capillaries are open at any one time, although the open 5% are constantly being changed. Thus, all capillaries are perfused in turn.

Blood viscosity is an important factor in capillary blood flow. Viscosity is influenced by plasma protein concentration and hematocrit, among other factors such as capillary size. Capillaries vary in size from 4 to 10 μm in diameter and are thus frequently much smaller than red blood cells, which average 7 μm in diameter. Red blood cells are required to deform themselves to pass through a capillary and are therefore a factor in blood viscosity. Blood viscosity decreases as capillary size diminishes, promoting capillary blood flow. However, this is a limited phenomenon, because at a critical diameter, capillary blood flow dramatically decreases as blood viscosity sharply increases, possibly because of the sticking of red blood cells in the capillaries. The deformability of red blood cells can be adversely affected by bacterial endotoxins, swelling of the cells by fluid absorption, and low pH.

An important factor in the noninvasive evaluation of the cutaneous circulation is tissue pressure. Severe increases in tissue pressure can virtually shut off capillary flow. Total tissue pressure is typically close to atmospheric. External pressure increases interstitial fluid pressure, which, at about 12 mm Hg, increases capillary arteriolar pressure, leading to filtration of fluid from the capillaries, edema, and autolysis. Unrelieved pressure is a primary cause of pressure sore formation.

The permeability of the capillary membrane can be expressed as the amount of water per minute that is forced through the membrane at a given pressure. Most exchange between blood and extracellular fluid takes place through the clefts between the cells of the capillary wall because of the presence of a hydrophobic layer of lipoprotein in the cell wall.

The plasma volume and the volume of the interstitial space are controlled by factors at the capillary level: plasma oncotic pressure, hydrostatic pressure, oncotic pressure of the interstitial fluid, and hydrostatic pressure of the interstitial space. Plasma oncotic pressure develops because of the restricted passage of large molecules such as proteins. Albumin makes up 51% of the plasma proteins. Because of its high concentration and relatively low molecular weight, it is primarily responsible for determining the oncotic pressure. Other plasma proteins include globulin (17%), fibrinogen (4%), and other miscellaneous proteins (28%). The plasma oncotic pressure is approximately 25 mm Hg. The capillary hydrostatic pressure ranges from 32 mm Hg at the arterial capillaries to about 15 mm Hg at the venous capillaries. The midcapillary hydrostatic pressure is about 25 mm Hg. The interstitial fluid oncotic pressure is assumed to be very small. The tissue hydrostatic pressure is similarly difficult to measure, but is about 1.8 mm Hg.

NEURAL CONTROL OF CUTANEOUS BLOOD FLOW

Determinants of cutaneous blood flow include the direct, local, and reflex effects of central and peripheral heating. Cutaneous resistance vessels have a significant regulation by the sympathetic nervous system, and one factor regulating the cutaneous vascular resistance is the frequency of the impulses over the sympathetic nerve fibers that are tonically vasoconstrictive. At normal room temperature, the cutaneous resistance vessels demonstrate basal tone (vascular resistance independent of innervation). In contrast, cutaneous arteriovenous anastomoses possess little basal tone and are regulated by a tonic neural discharge. The elimination of this tonic neural discharge produces a maximum passive dilation. In the thigh and calf of a cool subject, a weak vasoconstrictor tone is maintained; active vasodilation, however, takes over when the subject is heated.

The heating or cooling of cutaneous areas induces vasomotor changes in the skin that are partly due to the return of heated or cooled blood to central areas (e.g., the hypothalamus) that may mediate vasomotor responses. In humans, central thermoreceptors are quite sensitive; for example, a 0.15°C increase in oral temperature reflexly dilates the hand.

Baroreceptors also exert an influence over the cutaneous resistance vessels. Carotid sinus hypertension causes a reflex vasodilation. Baroreceptors also play a role in the intense cutaneous vasoconstriction that accompanies severe hemorrhage.

At the beginning of exercise, veins and the cutaneous resistance vessels constrict, but then relax as the central body temperature rises. The extent of the increase in skin blood flow during exercise is a result of the competing drives for vasoconstriction caused by the exercise and vasodilation caused by the generation of heat by the exercising muscles.

The primary response of the cutaneous circulation to an elevation in skin temperature is a four- to fivefold increase in flow. This response is under direct control, as this increase in flow occurs even with denervation. If one cools the whole body, cutaneous vasoconstrictor tone increases, depressing the local effects of heating. Thus, for example, local heating of the hand with lowered body temperature produces a lesser increase in skin blood flow than the same heat intensity applied at a normal body temperature. The vasodilation of heated skin paradoxically adds heat to the body as heat is gained when the surface to deep body temperature gradient is reversed. The high skin flow, however, does remove heat from the underlying skin, preventing burning. As mentioned, cold constricts cutaneous blood vessels, and the response to local cold is greater in a cold person than in a warm one. At about 15°C in a cold subject, hand blood flow is minimized. If, however, the local temperature is brought to below 10°C, the intense vasoconstriction of the fingers or toes is interrupted by the "hunting reaction" (periods of vasodilation). Induced vasodilation is free of sympathetic control but does seem to rely on a somatic nerve supply, probably through an axon reflex, where nerve impulses from a sensory ending pass to an effector organ along the divisions of a nerve fiber without passing through a nerve cell.

Cutaneous vasomotor tone can also be affected by a single stroking of the skin with a finger or other blunt object. A "white reaction" appears caused by blood being mechanically forced from the venous plexi. A more forceful mechanical stimulation causes "triple response." A red line appears initially, due to dilation, followed by a flare, probably due to an axon reflex. With strong enough stimulation, a wheal develops secondary to increased permeability of the capillaries, leading to the loss of fluid and protein.

The veins of the skin have a rich sympathetic innervation and are more responsive to sympathetic stimulation than resistance vessels, although this difference is associated with a difference in structure. Veins, however, are similar to the resistance vessels in that they are under vasoconstrictor control. Local skin cooling decreases venous compliance, and healing has minimal direct effect on compliance. With a cool body temperature, the cutaneous veins constrict proportionately to the severity of the exercise.

NONINVASIVE ASSESSMENT OF CUTANEOUS CIRCULATION

Skin survival can be adversely affected by a variety of pathological conditions that diminish cutaneous circulation and interfere with tissue maintenance and healing [1–3]. The skin is one of the few directly visible organs of the body. The first line of circulatory assessment is therefore to observe the appearance of the skin, the temperature of the skin, and the presence of blanching and of intraoperative wound bleeding. These can be combined with hands-on examination including palpation and pulse findings [4, 5]. The data may differentiate the circulatory status of skin in full health and skin that is dead. However, there is a middle range of uncertain tissue status, particularly in patients with difficult healing. Examples of these problem cases are seen with diabetes and peripheral vascular disease. The cutaneous tissues also can offer an element of undesired suprise. The failure of the circulation in cutaneous tissue can be silent; the loss or impending loss may not be visibly apparent until hours or even days after the damage has occurred. For these reasons, more sophisticated and quantitative methods deserve consideration in order to monitor and assess the circulation in the cutaneous tissue where risk of tissue loss exists. The methodologies employ a variety of physical principles for their success, including the use of optical methods [6], radioisotope indicators, and electrochemical sensing.

CUTANEOUS PERFUSION

Circulatory assessment may occur by noninvasive measurement of blood perfusion within the skin. Several methods are described here.

XENON 133 WASHOUT

The use of xenon 133 by Moore and others [7–9] has provided excellent results, but has not received widespread clinical acceptance. The technique of xenon 133 washout requires the injection of a radioactive substance into the body. As described by Malone et al. in the selection of amputation level [9], patients are placed supine and allowed to equilibrate for 15 minutes at a room temperature of 22 to 27°C. The xenon 133, dissolved in saline (0.05 ml; 100 to 500 μc), is injected intradermally in two parallel injections, 2 cm apart medial and lateral to a point indicated by the surgeon. The needle is kept in place for about 10 seconds, and a slight pressure is applied over the injection site for about 5 seconds.

The activity of the xenon 133 is monitored for 10 minutes. A computer generates time-activity curves for the xenon's disappearance. The cutaneous blood flow is calculated using the Kety-Schmidt treatment of the Fick flow equation:

$$\frac{\text{skin blood flow in milliliters}}{\text{100 grams of tissue per minute}} = \frac{10\alpha K}{P}$$

where K is the slope constant of xenon 133, α is the blood-skin coefficient for xenon 133, and P is the specific gravity of skin. Using this technique, local skin blood flow in the range of 0.6 to 2.2 ml per 100 grams of tissue per minute has been found to be indicative of good healing.

LASER DOPPLER

Another method for perfusion measurement employs Doppler frequency shifts of laser light. The laser Doppler method continues to be a subject of further research study, and the instrumentation is commercially available. An advantage of this technique is that readings are obtained rapidly. Laser Doppler is sensitive to blood flow velocity in capillaries, but may not always be as specific as fluorometry to blood flow changes [10]. Laser Doppler can produce artifacts, in which zero blood flow may result in a nonzero reading because of random movement of blood cells.

In a variant of the laser Doppler method, heat is applied to the skin in the area of the laser Doppler sensing element. With this version of the Doppler system, the accuracy in predicting the healing outcome for ischemic wounds has been reported as similar to that for transcutaneous oxygen measurement (described later in this chapter) [11]. Another study reported that laser Doppler velocimetry in combination with measurement of platelet-derived growth factor served as a prognostic indicator for the healing of ulcers and ischemic lesions of the lower limb [12].

FLUOROMETRY

Fluorometry is a method that contributes to the direct observation of blood circulation in the tissues. Measurement requires the introduction of fluorescein dye into the vasculature, where it becomes distributed by the circulation of the blood. An ultraviolet light source illuminates the skin and excites the dye in the vessels lying beneath the surface of the skin. The dye fluoresces, thereupon emitting light of a yellow-green appearance that can be observed visually. The assessment of circulation is limited by several factors, such as skin coloration, the timing of dye injection and of observation, and the limitations of the eye in observing gradations of light intensity. Therefore, instrumented and quantitative versions of the fluorometric method have been investigated.

Quantitative measurement of the fluorescence has been reported by Silverman and colleagues for assessing skin flap survival, skin viability prior to amputation, and intestinal viability [13–18]. The perfusion fluorometer quantifies the tissue fluorescence. A light source in the blue wavelengths of 450 to 500 nm is transmitted via a fiber optic cable to illuminate a selected tissue site. The transmitted light excites the fluorescein within the tissue in an area of approximately 2.5 cm^2 beneath the tip of the probe. The fluorescein emits light in the range of 520 to 660 nm, a portion of which is directed via fiber optics back to the fluorometer. The returning light travels to a photomultiplier tube and electronics, which produces a direct and quantitative readout of dye fluorescence. Fluorometry is not a continuous reading. In most subjects, the dye is tolerated well, but a few subjects will show a reaction to it. Bolus fluorescein injection has a reported 0.6% incidence of anaphylactoid reactions [19, 20].

PERFUSION PRESSURE

Another set of techniques for assessing cutaneous circulation makes use of the pressure with which the blood enters the tissues. The basic measurement concept is an application of pressure to the skin surface to balance the driving pressure of the blood. Instrumentation is then applied to identify the minimum pressure at which perfusion of the tissue ceases or the maximum pressure at which perfusion is reestablished. The perfusion may be monitored in this test by any of several methods, including radioisotope clearance, laser Doppler, and photoplethysmography. Of these various methods, one study reported that the most accurate measurement used radioisotope clearance, and that laser Doppler was the simplest to use. Low agreement with the other methods was observed for the photoplethysmographic method [21]. As with any test method, however, the quality of results will depend upon the technique used and the quality of the particular instrumentation employed.

HOLSTEIN'S ISOTOPE TECHNIQUES

Holstein used the degree of external pressure required to halt isotope washout [22–25]. As with the xenon 133 washout method previously described, this technique is somewhat time consuming and requires injection of a radioactive substance. Holstein et al. dissolved [^{133}I] antipyrine (4-[^{133}I]-iodoantipyrine) in sterile water and histamine diphosphate and injected the combination intradermally (0.1 ml). The gamma emission was measured for about 3 to 5 minutes, when external pressure was increased to give a stepwise decrease in the washout rate. Pressure increments of 20 to 40 mm Hg were observed for about 3 minutes, and then 5-mm Hg increases were observed for about 5 minutes at each level. The "flow cessation external pressure" is estimated as a pressure 3 mm Hg above the last pressure that allowed detection of a minimal washout. Using this technique, Holstein et al. [23] found the skin perfusion pressure in normal subjects to be about 10 mm Hg lower than systemic mean arterial blood pressure. In the assessment of wound healing in blow-knee amputations, Holstein et al. [25] have reported a skin perfusion pressure > 30 mm Hg to yield the highest postoperative success, and a perfusion pressure < 20 mm Hg to yield poor results.

SKIN PERFUSION PRESSURE USING LASER DOPPLER

Another recent variant on measurement of skin perfusion pressure replaces the radioactive indicator of perfusion with measurements of perfusion using the laser Doppler flowmeter [26]. The laser Doppler system measures perfusion more shallowly than does the isotope, but the laser Doppler system is much simpler to apply—no radioactive materials are used, and measurement can be done more rap-

idly. Studies with this system suggest that prediction of wound healing following amputation is practicable. The measurement method was applied to assess the outcome for 53 amputations ranging from major amputations to toe amputations. A pressure of 30 mm Hg or better showed a prediction of healing of 90%; a value of less than 30 mm Hg had a healing failure of 75%.

CUTANEOUS PRESSURE PHOTOPLETHYSMOGRAPHY

Cutaneous pressure photoplethysmography has also been reported as advantageous in measuring cutaneous perfusion pressure for determining amputation level and predicting the results of revascularization [27–29]. Cutaneous pressure photoplethysmography does not directly rely on the shape of the arterial pulse of the main trunk arteries because the critical pressure readings occur where waveforms begin or cease, independent of wave shape.

One study evaluated 25 patients and 9 normal subjects with this technique. Of the 25 patients, 10 were postoperative amputees (follow-up of 3±3 years), studied to determine the cutaneous perfusion pressure required to maintain a healed stump. Five of the patients were candidates for bypass surgery (disabling claudication), and the remaining 10 patients were prospective amputees (gangrene). Bypass patients were followed up for 3±1 month, and postoperative amputees for 4±3 months.

The cutaneous pressure photoplethysmograph senses blood flow in the skin at various skin-bearing pressures with the use of a hand-held probe. The photoplethysmograph probe contains a small light source and a photosensitive cell that responds to light reflected from the cutaneous vascular bed. A recorder prints out a permanent waveform (Figure 3-3). A pressure sensor within the probe is calibrated using a known loading force on the surface of the probe, and the skin-bearing pressure is directly shown on a digital display in millimeters of mercury. In use, the probe is placed at the site desired, and a waveform is obtained. The waveform is obliterated with the manual application of gradually increasing pressure (Figure 3-4). When the pressure is gradually released, the pressure reading at the

Anterior   Posterior

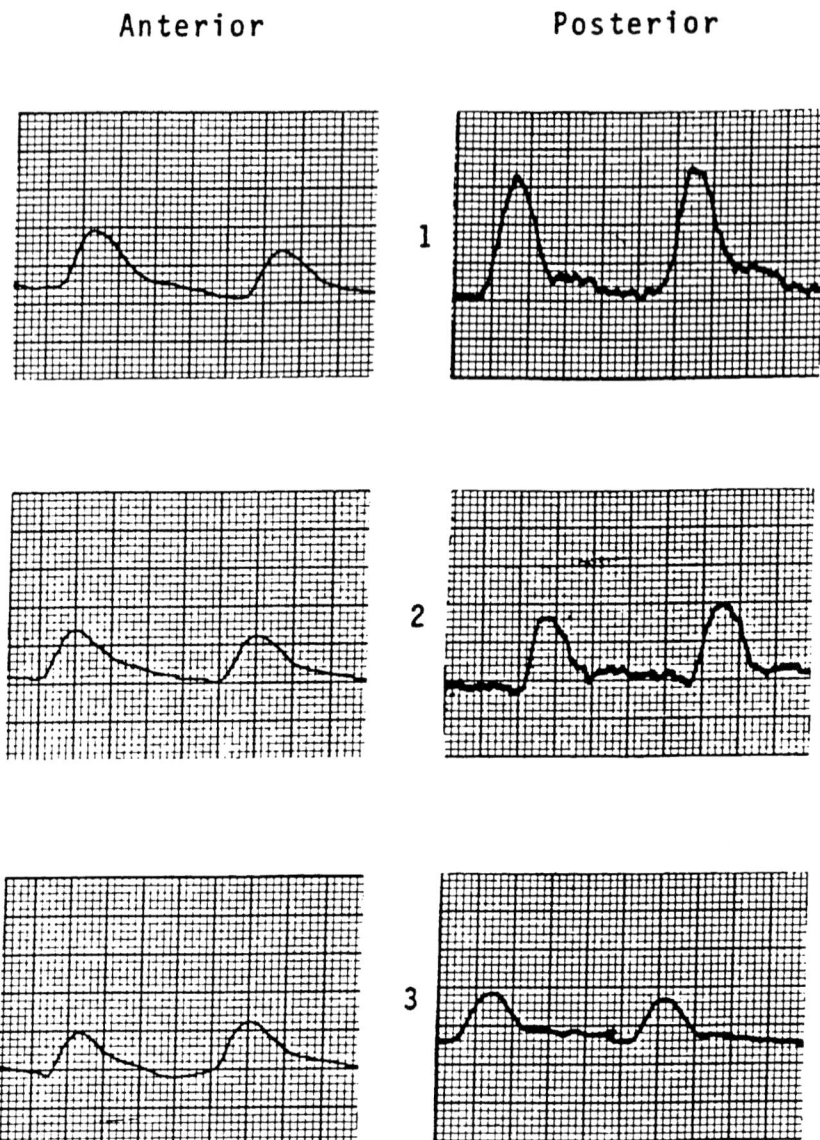

Figure 3-3.   The photoplethysmographic waveform is printed and becomes a permanent part of the patient's record.

point when the photoplethysmographic waveform returns is recorded as the cutaneous pressure.

In the retrospective study of amputees, cutaneous pressure photoplethysmographic measurements were made above the knee and at the stump. For the prospective patients (amputees and bypass patients) and the normal subjects, measurements were made at four locations: the chest, 10 cm proximal to

the knee joint, at midcalf, and over the dorsum of the foot.

The cutaneous pressures obtained are shown in Table 3-1. In normal subjects, a dorsum of foot: chest index greater than 1.0 was obtained. In the five patients with disabling claudication, an index of > 0.50 was obtained preoperatively. Postoperatively, an increase in the index to > 0.80 was

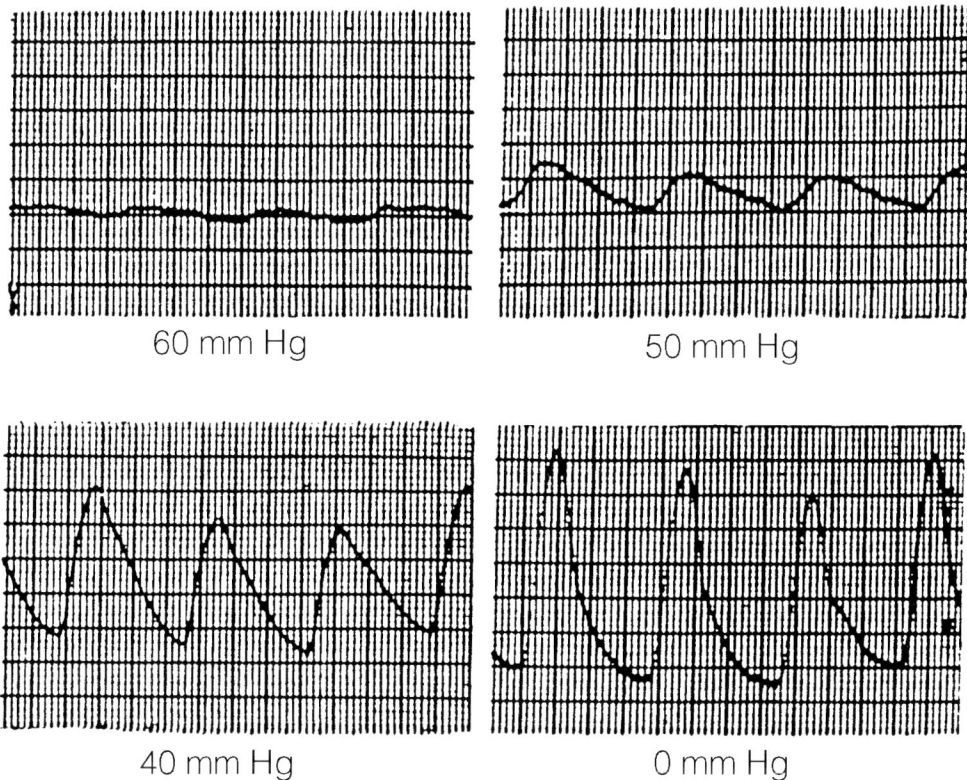

Figure 3-4. With the application of pressure the cutaneous pressure photoplethysmograph waveform is obliterated; the pressure at which the waveform returns with gradual release of pressure is the cutaneous pressure.

Table 3-1. Cutaneous Pressure Photoplethysmographic Measurements in Predicting Outcome of Amputation or Revascularization

Subjects	Chest	Cutaneous perfusion pressure (mm Hg) Above knee	Midcalf	Dorsum of foot
Normal (*N*=9)	144.8±35.0	146.0±35.4	149.9±38.6	150.9±41.0
Claudication (*N=5*)				
Preop	140.2±30.4	130.3±51.0	110.3±48.1	73.4±26.2
Postop	121.3±64.0	111.0±30.9	116.0±39.1	98.0±56.1
Prospective amputees[a] (healed, preop) (*N*=7)	119.6±19.4	108.9±21.8	89.7±32.8	41.1±19.9
Prospective amputees[b] (nonhealed) (*N*=3)	—	—	40.7±8.1 (postop)	27.3±17.5 (preop)
Retrospective amputees (*N=10*)	—	122.0±46.3	91.2±30.1	—

Source: Katsamouris et al. [32].

[a]One patient had above-knee amputation.

[b]Midcalf pressure at level of amputation.

accompanied by excellent clinical improvement. Nine of the prospective amputees had below-knee or more distal amputations: six had primary healing and three required revision. One patient with an above-knee amputation healed primarily. In the seven healed patients, the preoperative indices were > 0.90 above knee, > 0.70 at midcalf, and < 0.35 at the dorsum of the foot. In the four patients with below-knee amputation, the dorsum of the foot index was < 0.25 and was > 0.60 at the level of amputation. At the level of amputation the cutaneous pressure was 78.0±30.1 mm Hg in healed patients preoperatively and increased to 90.0±4.0 mm Hg postoperatively. In contrast, three patients without primary healing had a cutaneous pressure of 40.7±8.1 mm Hg at the level of amputation and 27.3±17.5 mm Hg over the dorsum of the foot preoperatively. Postoperatively, no improvement was seen (mean change: −1.0±1.4 mm Hg). In two patients with healed distal amputation (one Syme's and one digital amputation), preoperative dorsum of the foot cutaneous pressure was 57.0±7.1 mm Hg, which increased to 65.0±29.6 mm Hg postoperatively. In the ten retrospective amputees (all below-knee), above knee cutaneous pressure was 122+46.3 mm Hg and midcalf pressure was 91.2+30.1 mm Hg (very similar to the cutaneous pressure at the stump of the prospective amputees).

medicine and more recently has been applied to evaluating the cutaneous circulation of adults [30–33]. Transcutaneous oxygen measurements ($TcPO_2$) reflect changes in tissue perfusion and metabolic status. The technique is relatively simple and noninvasive, involving the application of a small sensing unit to the surface of the skin. The electrode within the sensor contains a heating unit that elevates the skin temperature, causing localized hyperemia. Oxygen within the blood diffuses through the skin and is sensed by an oxygen-sensing electrode. In 49 patients, Katsamouris et al. [32] demonstrated that in successful revascularization procedures $TcPO_2$ increases significantly, whereas it remains unchanged or decreases in the presence of poor results (Table 3-2). In a further study of 10 patients monitored intraoperatively, $TcPO_2$ increases of 4 to 50 mm Hg immediately following reestablishment of flood flow were associated with good results. Cina et al. [31] have also found $TcPO_2$ to successfully identify the presence of vascular disease and distinguish among different levels of severity (Table 3-3). Using $TcPO_2$ measurements, Rhodes and Cogan [33] have found, following otherwise successful revascularization, that nonhealing foot ulcers that remain so are "islands of ischemia" caused by microangiopathy, scarring, or a discontinuity of pedal artery flow. Franzeck et al.

OXIMETRY

Another way to assess cutaneous circulation is to measure the oxygen present within the cutaneous layers. If circulation is poor in the presence of normal tissue metabolic loading, or if the delivered oxygen levels are low, the oxygen levels of the blood within the tissue will be low.

TRANSCUTANEOUS OXYGEN TENSION

The measurement of transcutaneous oxygen tension has long been an integral part of neonatal

Table 3-2. Transcutaneous Oxygen Tension Measurements Over the Dorsum of the Foot Pre- and Postoperatively (7 days postoperatively)

| Diagnosis | Transcutaneous oxygen tension | | | | | |
| | Good results | | | Poor results | | |
	Preop	Postop	N	Preop	Postop	N
Claudication	46±8	60±10[a]	14	41±5	41±2[c]	3
Rest pain	15±10	53±13[a]	15	25±7	22±8[c]	4
Impending gangrene	5±3	45±11[b]	3	6±1	8±7[c]	2
Ischemic ulcer	21±19	52±13[a]	6	43±24	24±3[c]	2

Note: All values in millimeters of mercury.

Source: Katsamouris et al. [32].

[a] $p<.001$.

[b] $p>.05$.

[c] $p<.03$.

Table 3-3. Transcutaneous Oxygen Tension Measurements in Distinguishing Severity of Peripheral Vascular Disease

Subjects	Transcutaneous oxygen tension (mm Hg)		
	Chest	Calf	Foot
Normal[a] (N =10)	65±6	64±8[c]	64±8[d]
Claudication (N=26)	64±15	52±10	46±10[d]
Rest pain (N=19)	65±8	40±10[b]	17±9[d]
Impending gangrene (N=10)	60±9	26±17	5±2

Source: Cina et al. [31].

[a]Normal subjects > 45 years of age; TcPO$_2$ inversely correlated (P<.005). The difference between younger and older than 45 years was significant (P<.01).

[b]P <.015 (P value between adjacent values vertically).

[c]P <.003 (P value between adjacent values vertically).

[d] P <.001 (P value between adjacent values vertically).

[30] have additionally reported TcPO$_2$ measurements of 36.5±17.5 mm Hg to be predictive of primary healing of an amputation, whereas failed amputations had TcPO$_2$ measurements in the range of 0 to 3 mm Hg.

The transcutaneous measurement is predominantly a measurement of arterialized blood reaching the skin, and does not necessarily reflect venous status. Roszinski and Schmeller found that in chronic venous insufficiency, the TcPO$_2$ measurements did not correlate with tissue intracutaneous measurements determined with needle probes, and concluded that skin damage in patients with chronic venous insufficiency is not necessarily associated with hypoxia [34].

SUBCUTANEOUS OXYGEN TENSION

Rather than measuring oxygen through the skin, a catheter containing an oxygen sensor can be inserted into the skin layers. The sensor can be an oxygen-sensing polarographic electrode or one of the more recent devices, such as an oxygen-sensing fluorescence-quenching optode [35]. Because this method is invasive, its primary use has been as a research tool. In clinical studies of this method, it has been described as a reliable indicator of blood loss and peripheral perfusion [36].

NEAR INFRARED REFLECTANCE OXIMETRY

The illumination of tissues for medical purposes goes back as far as 1912, with a light torch applied to illuminate soft tissue (diaphanography) and visualize lesions within the breast [37]. Today's successful use of pulse oximetry followed from these early origins. However, pulse oximetry has been used primarily for transmission of light through tissue thickness, where pulsatile changes of blood within the tissue can be monitored.

In the early use of reflectance spectrography, the surface of the skin was flooded with light, and instrumentation was used to quantitatively measure the returning light [38,39]. However, reflectance methods using light flooding do not measure as deeply as methods using point light sources. The results of experimental studies and modeling have shown that the depth to which photons travel can be related to parameters of surface reflectance, and to the optical properties of the biological medium. Measurements of oxygen in deeper layers of cutaneous tissue now appear possible using methods known, respectively, as time-resolved and space-resolved reflectance spectroscopy.

The time-resolved method is also described as photon time of flight measurement [40]. This method selectively examines the distribution of photon travel times between a point of photon incidence on the skin surface and another point at which is placed a photon-capturing detector. Space-resolved methods look instead at the averaged intensity of returned light generally distributed over multiple distances from light source to detector.

Because oxygenation of the blood is wavelength dependent, the application of two or more light wavelengths (usually red and infrared) in combination with reflectance of up to a few centimeters can be used to measure oxygenation via light reflectance at depth within the biological tissue. The method remains sensitive to other chromophores such as carboxyhemoglobin and methemoglobin. However, additional light wavelengths may assist in reducing the effect of these artifacts on oxygen measurement [41].

OTHER METHODS

Nuclear magnetic resonance principles, upon which magnetic resonance imaging is based, also provide a means for tracking perfusion [42]. Because capillary perfusion follows a tortuous path and the linear velocity is low, phasing techniques suitable for large vessels are not applicable. However, tracking of a bolus of injected contrast material is possible.

Included in the category of other methods is the evaluation of wound healing through wound histology. If the circulation is impaired, one would expect that the cutaneous wound healing would be impaired. The test consists of applying a Simplate II bleeding-time device to create standardized wounds within the skin. The authors [43] have concluded that the method allows evaluation of tissue repair performance with relative safety even for patients with peripheral vascular disease and diabetes mellitus.

REFERENCES

1. Silver, I. A., Cellular microenvironment in healing and nonhealing wounds, Chapter 4 in *Soft and Hard Tissue Repair*, Hunt, Heppenstall, Pines, Rovee, eds., New York:Praeger, 1984.

2. Knighton, D. R.; Oredsson, S.; Banda, M.; and Hunt, T. K., Regulation of repair: Hypoxic control of macrophage mediated angiogenesis, Chapter 3 in *Soft and Hard Tissue Repair*, Hunt, Heppenstall, Pines, Rovee, eds., New York:Praeger, 1984.

3. Kerrigan, C. L., and Daniel, R. K., Skin flap failure: Pathophysiology, *Plast Reconstr Surg* 1983; 72:76.

4. Romano, R. L., and Burgess, E. M., Level selection in lower extremity amputations, *Clin Orthop* 1971; 74:177.

5. Lee, B. Y.; Trainor, F. S.; Kavner, D.; Crisologo, J. A.; Shaw, W.; and Madden, J. L., Assessment of the healing potentials of ulcers of the skin by photoplethysmography, *Surg Gynecol Obstet* 1972; 148:232.

6. Lubbers, D. W., Optical sensors for clinical monitoring, *Acta Anaesthesiol Scand Suppl* 1995; 104:37–54.

7. Moore, W. R., Determination of amputation level: Measurement of skin blood flow with xenon 133, *Arch Surg* 1973; 107:798.

8. Moore, W. S.; Henry, R. E.; Malone, J. M.; Daly, M. J.; Patton, D.; and Childers, S. J., Prospective use of xenon Xe133 clearance for amputation level selection, *Arch Surg* 1981; 116:86.

9. Malone, J.; Leal, J. M.; Moore, W. S.; et al., The "gold standard" for amputation level selection. Xenon 133 clearance, *J Surg Res* 1981; 30:449.

10. Liu, A. J.; Cummings, C. W.; and Trachy, R. E., Venous outflow obstruction in myocutaneous flaps: Changes in microcirculation detected by the perfusion fluorometer and laser Doppler, *Otolaryngology—Head and Neck Surgery* 1986; 94:165.

11. Padberg, F. T., Jr.; Back, T. L.; Hart, L. C.; and Franco, C. D., Comparison of heated-probe laser Doppler and transcutaneous oxygen measurements for predicting outcome of ischemic wounds, *J Cardiovasc Surg* 1992; 33:715–722.

12. Martins, R., and Rao, S., Laser Doppler velocimetry and platelet-derived growth factor as prognostic indicators for the healing of ulcers and ischaemic lesions of the lower limb, *Cardiovasc Surg* 1995; 3:285–90.

13. Ostrander, L. E.; Lee, B. Y.; Silverman, D. A.; and Groskopf, R. A., Constant infusion fluorometry to predict flap survival, *Decubitus* 1988; 2:40.

14. Sloan, G. M., and Sasaki, G. H., Noninvasive monitoring of tissue viability, *Clin Plast Surg* 1985; 12:185.

15. Silverman, D. G.; Rubin, S. M.; Reilly, C. A.; Brousseau, D. A.; Norton, D. J.; and Wolf, G. L., Fluorometric prediction of successful amputation level in the ischemic limb, *J Rehabil Res Dev* 1985.

16. Silverman, D. G.; Rubin, S. M.; Reilly, C. A.; Brousseau, D. A.; Norton, K. J.; Bartley, E.; and Neufeld G. R., Fluorometric quantification of low dose fluorescein delivery to predict amputation site healing, *Surgery* 1987; 101:335.

17. Silverman, D. G.; Cedrone, F. A.; Hurford, W. E.; Bering, T. G.; and LaRossa, D. D., Monitoring tissue elimination of fluorescein with the perfusion

fluorometer: A new method to assess capillary blood flow, *Surgery* 1981; 90:409.

18. Weisman, R. A.; Pransky, S. M.; Silverman, D. A.; Lyons, K. M.; Denneny, J. C. III; Vidas, M. D.; and Kimmelman, C. P., Clinical assessment of flap perfusion by fiberoptic fluorometry, *Ann Otol Rhinol Laryngol* 1985; 94:226.

19. LaPiana, F. G., and Penner, R., Anaphylactoid reaction to intravenously administered fluorescein, *Arch Opthal* 1968; 79:161.

20. Stein, M. R., and Parker, C. W., Reactions following intravenous fluorescein, *Am J Opthal* 1971; 72:861.

21. Malvezzi, L.; Castronuovo, J. J., Jr.; Swayne, L. C.; Cone, D.; and Trivino, J. Z., The correlation between three methods of skin perfusion pressure measurement: Radionuclide washout, laser Doppler flow, and photoplethysmography, *J Vasc Surg* 1992; 15:823.

22. Holstein, P., and Lassen, N. A., Radio-isotope-clearance technique for measurement of distal blood pressure in skin and muscles, *Scand J Clin Lab Invest Suppl* 1973; 128:143.

23. Holstein, P.; Lund, P.; Larsen, B.; and Shoemacker, T., Skin perfusion pressure measured as the external pressure required to stop isotope washout: Methodological considerations and normal values on the legs, *Scand J Clin Lab Invest* 1977; 37:649.

24. Holstein, P.; Doney, H.; and Lassen, N. A., Wound healing in above-knee amputations in relation to skin perfusion pressure, *Acta Orthop Scand* 1979; 50:59.

25. Holstein, P.; Sager, P.; and Lassen, N. A., Wound healing in below-knee amputations in relation to skin perfusion pressure, *Acta Orthop Scand* 1979; 50:49.

26. Adera, H. M.; James, K.; Castronuovo, J. J., Jr.; Byrne, M.; Deshmukh, R.; and Lohr, J., Prediction of amputation wound healing with skin perfusion pressure, *J Vasc Surg* 1995; 21:823–9.

27. Lee, B. Y.; McCann, W. J. Jr.; Trainor, F. S.; Thoden, W. R.; and Kavner, D., Noninvasive assessment of wound healing potentials and determination of amputation level, *Contemp Surg* 1980; 17:20.

28. Lee, B. Y.; Thoden, W. R.; Madden, J. L.; and McCann, W. J. Jr., Cutaneous pressure photoplethysmography: A new technique for noninvasive evaluation of peripheral arterial occlusive disease, *Contemp Surg* 1984; 25:39–43.

29. Lee, B. Y.; Ostrander, L. E.; Thoden, W. R.; and

Madden, J. L., Use of cutaneous pressure photoplethysmography in managing peripheral vascular disease, *Contemp Surg* 1987; 30:58.

30. Franzeck, U. K.; Talke, P.; Bernstein, E. F.; Fronek, A.; and Goldbranson, F. L., Transcutaneous PO_2 measurements in peripheral arterial occlusive disease, In *Microcirculation and Ischemic Vascular Diseases: Advances in Diagnosis and Therapy*, K. Messmer, ed., Chicago:Abbott Laboratories, 1981:160.

31. Cina, C.; Katsamouris, A.; Megerman, J.; Brewster, D. C.; Straghorn, E. C.; Robinson, J. G., and Abbott, W. J. M., Utility of transcutaneous oxygen tension measurements in peripheral vascular disease, *Int Cardiovasc Soc* 1983 (abstract).

32. Katsamouris, A. N.; Cina, C.; Robinson, J.; Megerman, J.; Straghorn, E.; Brewster, D. C.; and Abbott, W. M., Intra- and postoperative assessment of revascularization procedures utilizing a transcutaneous PO_2 electrode, *Surgical Forum* 1983; 34:461.

33. Rhodes, G. R., and Cogan, F., "Island of ischemia": Transcutaneous PO_2 (PO_2tc) documentation of pedal malperfusion following lower limb revascularization, *Seventh Annual Surgical Symposium 81* 1983 (abstract).

34. Roszinski, S., and Schmeller, W., Differences between intracutaneous and transcutaneous skin oxygen tension in chronic venous insufficiency, *J Cardiovasc Surg* 1995; 36:407–13.

35. Hopf, H. W., and Hunt, T. K., Comparison of Clark Electrode and optode for measurement of tissue oxygen tension, *Oxygen Transport to Tissue* 1994; 345:841–7.

36. Powell, C. C.; Schultz, S. C.; Burris, D. G.; Drucker, W. R.; and Malcolm, D. S., Subcutaneous oxygen tension: A useful adjunct in assessment of perfusion status, *Crit Care Med* 1995; 23:867–73.

37. Cutler, M., Transillumination as an aid to diagnosis of breast lesions, *Surg Gynecol Obstet* 1929; 48:721.

38. Afromowitz, M. A.; Callis, J. B.; Heimbach, D. M.; DeSoto, L. A.; and Norton, M. K., Multispectral imaging of burn wounds: A new clinical instrument for evaluating burn depth, *IEEE Trans Biomed Eng* 1988; 35:842.

39. Jones, B. M.; Sandes, R.; and Greenlagh, R. M., Monitoring skin flaps by colour measurement, *Brit J Plast Surg* 1983; 36:88.

40. Chance, B.; Nioka, S.; Kent, J.; McCully, K.; Fountain, M.; Greenfeld, R.; and Holtom, G., Time re-

solved spectroscopy of hemoglobin and myoglobin in resting and ischemic muscle, *Analyt Biochem* 1988; 174:69.

41. Findlay, G. H., Carbon monoxide poisoning: Optics and histology of skin and blood, *Brit J Derm* 1988; 119:45.

42. Altobelli, S. A.; Caporihan, A.; Fukushima, E., and Majors, P. D., Liquid flow velocity determination by NMR imaging, IEEE Engineering in Medicine and Biology Society 11th Annual Conference 1989, p. 50.

43. Olerud, J. E.; Odland, G. F.; Burgess, E. M.; Wyss, C. R.; Fisher, L. D.; and Matsen, F. A., A model for the study of wounds in normal elderly adults and patients with peripheral vascular disease or diabetes mellitus, *J Surg Res* 1995; 59:349–360.

4

THE BIOLOGICAL BASIS OF WOUND HEALING

Marcelo C. DaSilva, M.D. and Bok Y. Lee, M.D.

Man can learn nothing unless he proceeds from the known to the unknown.

———Claude Bernard

MOLECULAR BIOLOGY OF COLLAGEN SYNTHESIS AND DEGRADATION

COLLAGEN STRUCTURE AND SYNTHESIS

Collagen is the major class of insoluble fibrous protein in the extracellular matrix and in connective tissue. Fibroblasts are spindle-shaped cells with an oval nucleus, and are rich in mitochondria and rough endoplasmic reticulum (RER). Fibroblasts originate from undifferentiated stem cells located along blood vessels in tissues. They are stimulated by cytokines secreted by macrophages in the wound. There is evidence of at least 13 distinct types of collagen (Table 4-1). Fibroblasts, osteoblasts, and chondroblasts are able to synthesize collagen. In spite of diversity, essentially all collagen molecules possess a common structural central core, characterized by a high proportion of triple helices. These are flanked at both ends by non-triple helical or globular domains.

Chromosomal localization of genes coding for 13 of the chains are distributed among 7 chromosomes in the human genome. Transcription of protein-coding genes (DNA) into heterogeneous nuclear RNA (hnRNA) are catalyzed by RNA polymerase II (Figure 4-1, A). RNA polymerase II

Table 4-1. Collagen Types

Type	Chains	Localization
I	$[\alpha1(I)]2 [\alpha2(I)]$	Skin, tendon, bone, etc.
II	$[\alpha1(II)]3$	Cartilage, vitreous humor
III	$[\alpha1(III)]3$	Skin, muscle, etc., frequently together with type I
IV	$[\alpha1(IV)2 [\alpha2(IV)]$	All basal laminas
V	$[\alpha1(V)] [\alpha2(V)] [\alpha3(V)]$	Most interstitial tissues; associated with type I
VI	$[\alpha1(VI)] [\alpha2(VI)] [\alpha3(VI)]$	Most interstitial tissues; associated with type I
VII	$[\alpha1(VII)]3$	Epithelia
VIII	$[\alpha1(VIII)]3$	Some endothelial cells
IX	$[\alpha1(IX)] [\alpha2(IX)] [\alpha3(IX)]$	Cartilage associated with type I
X	$[\alpha1(X)]3$	Hypertophic and mineralizing Cartilage
XI	$[\alpha1(XI)] [\alpha2(XI)] [\alpha3(XI)]$	Cartilage
XII	$[\alpha1(XII)]$	In vicinity of collagens I and III
XIII	$[\alpha1(XIII)]$	Synthesized by certain tumor cell lines

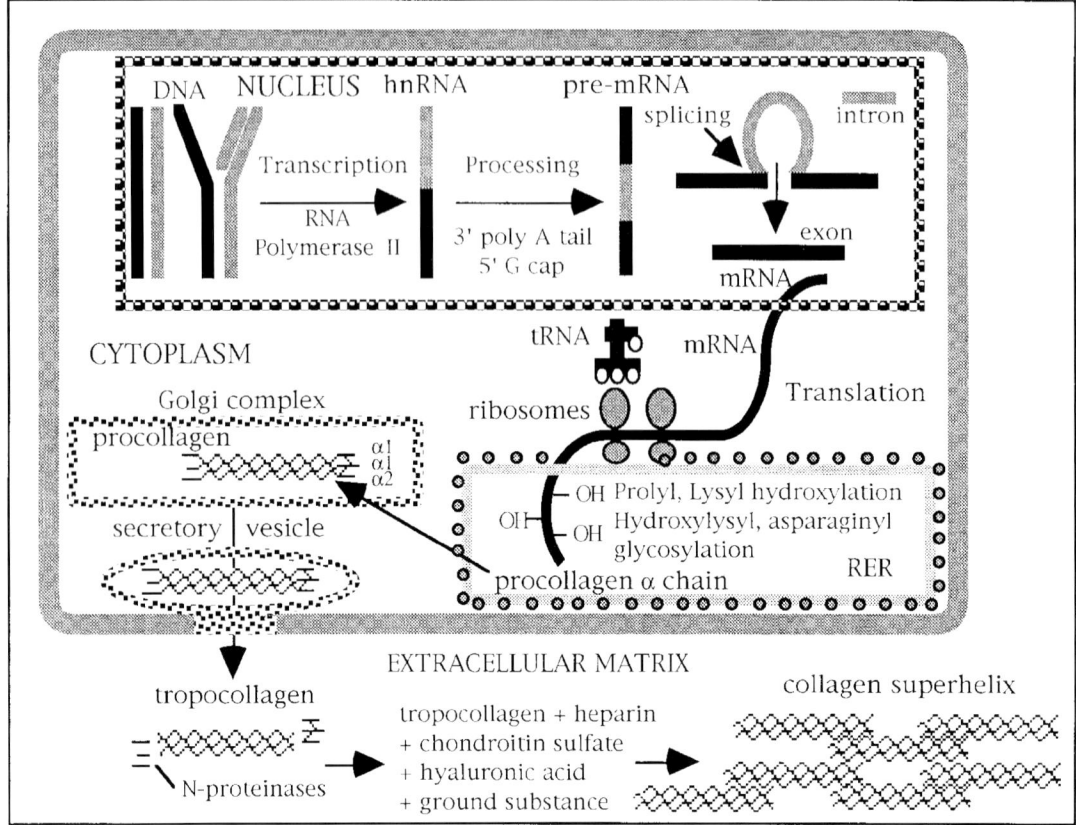

Figure 4-1.   Collagen synthesis.

recognizes a start sequence, called the TATA *box,* located in a fixed position approximately 25–35 bases upstream from the RNA start site. The protein factor that helps RNA polymerase II to recognize the TATA *box* and assist the enzyme to begin transcription is $TF_{11}D$, which binds to the TATA *box* region. Two other gene sequences aid in the transcription of hnRNA; (1) the promoter-proximal sequences, CCAAT and GGGCG present in 10 to 15% percent of genes and located upstream from the start site, and (2) gene activators, called enhancers, that boost transcription when placed either close to, or at great distances from, the start site. There also are stimulatory proteins (SP1) that bind to the GGGCG box (promoter sequences) and aid in transcription.

Studies show that hnRNA and mRNA share distinctive features, suggesting that hnRNA is a pre-

cursor to mRNA, forming a complex methylated structure, 7-methylguanylate (m^7G), at the 5′ prime end of the mRNA molecule called *cap*. This aids in translation of mRNA and insertion of approximately 200–250 nucleotides to the 3′-hydroxyl end of the mRNA molecule, called the *poly A* tail. The *poly A* tail is a posttranscriptional addition to hnRNA that accumulates in polyribosomal mRNA[1]. The presence of the *poly A* tail is not a requirement for mRNA to enter the cytoplasm and direct protein synthesis; however, no eukaryotic mRNAs lacking the *poly A* tail have been found entering the cytoplasm[1] (Figure 4-1, B).

Not all primary hnRNA transcripts are cleaved and spliced in the nucleus to yield mature mRNAs. Splicing, the final step in mRNA processing, involves removing intervening and noncoding sequences called introns by small nuclear ribonucleoproteins, spliceosomes. Introns refer to the primary transcript (DNA) not included in finished mRNA. An exon, a primary transcript[1], exits the nucleus and reaches the cytoplasm as part of an mRNA molecule (Figure 4-1, C). Mechanisms of RNA transport to cytoplasm are unknown at present. It is likely that the nuclear pore acts as a passageway for molecules between the nucleus and cytoplasm.

The first cytoplasmic event in the initiation stage of collagen synthesis is attachment of a free molecule of methionine to the end of a tRNA by specific methionyl-tRNA synthetase. There are two types of $tRNA^{met}$, but only the $tRNA_i^{met}$ initiates protein synthesis (translation). In cytoplasm, a eukaryotic cell's $tRNA_i^{met}$, along with a molecule of GTP and a small ribosomal subunit, bind to mRNA at a specific site often located near the AUG initiation codon. Recognition of the 5′ end of the mRNA occurs first. More than 90% of the AUG initiation signals are from the first (the 5′-most) AUG in the mRNA molecule[1]. Initiation of collagen translation in eukaryotic mRNAs involves: 1) recognition of the 5′ prime end cap, and (2) location of a consensus sequence surrounding the AUG initiation codon. With help from proteins called *initiation factors* (IF), a complex of $mRNA-Met-tRNA_i^{met}-GTP$-small ribosomal subunits form. In eukaryotic cells, a large initiation factor (eIF-4) helps small subunits to bind to the end of mRNA and begin searching for the AUG initiation codon. After AUG is located and bound, large subunits join the complex $mRNA-Met-tRNA_i^{met}-GTP$-small ribosomal subunit, initiating translation (Figure 4-1, D).

For the newly synthesized peptide chain to grow requires an *elongation factor* (EF) properly positioned on a second amino-acyl-tRNA on the ribosome molecule. Two ribosomal sites need to be occupied: (1) site A, which binds incoming amino-acyl-tRNA, allowing the new amino acid to grow, and (2) site P, which contains the peptidyl-tRNA complex. The *first* amino acid to the chain, Met-$tRNA_i^{met}$, enters the P site. The *second* amino acid in the chain, glycine-$tRNA^{gly}$, binds to the A site, forming a peptide bond between the carboxyl group of glycine-$tRNA^{gly}$, thus forming dipeptide methionyl-glycine-$tRNA^{gly}$. Energy for the translocation of peptidyl-tRNA comes from the hydrolysis of GTP. The role of the ribosome is collagen molecule

translation is to provide binding sites to aminoacyl-tRNA to correct codon-anticodon matching before an activated amino acid is brought close to peptidyl-tRNA. Selection of the correct aminoacyl-tRNA for elongation of the chain is a time-consuming part of protein synthesis. As amino acid sequences are attached, a polypeptide chain is formed.

In mRNA molecules there are three bases, UAG, that signal termination of translation. This codon, as well as codons UAA and UGA, signal release of peptidyl-tRNA complex on recognition by protein *termination factors* (TF). When peptidyl-tRNA is released, ribosomes disengage from mRNA and divide into two subunits. The whole cycle begins again, resulting in synthesis of procollagen molecules (Figure 4-1, E).

Each procollagen chain has coiled subunits: two alpha one I chains and one alpha two I chain. Disulfide bonds as well as triple helices form in RER. Several intrachain and five interchain disulfide bonds connect C-terminals of three procollagen chains. There are also short segments on either side of procollagen chains that do not assume triple-helical conformation. These segments cross-link two lysine or hydrolysine residues at the C-terminal of one chain and with two at the N-terminal of an adjacent chain, stabilizing the side-by-side arrangement.

At the molecular level, collagen is defined as a protein containing lengthy domain(s) of triple-helical conformation. This spatial configuration is possible because there is repetitive Gly-X-Y in participating chains, and every third amino acid is glycine, whose side chains contain H^+. Positions X and Y can be occupied by any amino acid, however, the stabilization of the chain is provided by the presence of prolyl and hydroxyprolyl residues. These specific proline residues are hydroxylated by *prolyl 4-hydroxylase* and *prolyl 3-hydroxylase* in the RER. Lysine residues are hydroxylated by *lysyl hydroxylase*. Vitamin C, molecular oxygen, ferrous iron, and alpha-ketoglutarate are a requirement for successful hydroxylation of proline by *prolyl hydroxylase*. Protein glycosylation also occurs in RER as *galactosyl-glucose* is linked to hydroxylysine residues, allowing transport of synthesized procollagen across the plasma membrane. Following pro-alpha-collagen chains synthesis and modification

Table 4-2.   Enzymes Involved in Collagen Synthesis and Degradation

Enzyme	Function	Cofactors
Prolyl hydroxylase	Hydroxylates proline	Ascorbic acid, and O_2
Lysyl hydroxylase	Hydroxylates lysine	α-Ketoglutarate, Fe^{2+}, O_2, Cu^{2+}
Procollagen peptidase	Cleaves nonhelical peptides	
Tissue collagenase	Cleaves collagen	

in the RER, chains are assembled into trimers and translocated to the Golgi complex (Figure 4-1, F). In the Golgi apparatus, procollagen is packaged into secretory vesicles that fuse to the cell membrane, releasing procollagen into the extracellular space (Figure 4-1, G). The enzymes involved in collagen synthesis and degradation are listed in Table 4-2.

The second feature of collagen, as a protein, is its capacity for self-assembly into aggregates supporting elements in the extracellular matrix. Collagen is secreted, as procollagen, with linear alpha-chain residues at the C-terminal into the extracellular space. These nonhelical extensions interfere with subsequent aggregation of collagen fibrils cleaved by collagen type-specific N-proteinases. The molecule produced is tropocollagen (Figure 4-1, H). Tropocollagen aggregates with mucopolysaccharides; heparin, chondroitin sulfate, hyaluronic acid, and ground substance in the extracellular space. Collagen monomers spontaneously assemble into fibrils, forming quaternary structures of collagen. Collagen monomers associate by lateral interactions when a telopeptide region of one fibril interacts with the triple-helical region of adjacent molecules (Figure 4-1, I). Collagen fibers are stabilized by intermolecular cross-links that provide tensile strength and insolubility. Gram for gram, type I collagen is stronger than steel[1]. Collagen fibril is an extraordinarily effective structural element for maintaining integrity of connective tissue[2].

COLLAGEN DEGRADATION

Connective tissue is dynamic. Fibrillar collagen is essentially insoluble in physiologic circumstances. Nature has provided an extremely effective, organized, enzymatic degradation of collagen in wound healing. Degradation of interstitial and basement membrane collagen is the process controlling growth, development, morphogenesis, remodeling, and tissue repair.

Collagen degradation occurs in extracellular and in intracellular spaces. Ten percent or more of newly synthesized collagen degrades intercellularly under normal conditions. Extracellular fibrillar collagen is cleaved by collagenases that act almost exclusively with collagen. Products of this cleavage are soluble in solvents and are thermally unstable. The consequence is rapid solubilization and denaturation of collagen. Collagenases are responsible for the committed step in degradation. Regardless of other enzymes present in the extracellular milieu, degradation cannot occur until collagenase is activated, to begin its catalytic action. Human skin collagenase is synthesized and secreted by cells as zymogen or proenzyme. Procollagenase is incapable of catalytic activity until activated by a variety of reagents. The exact physiological mechanisms of conversion of procollagenase into collagenase zymogen is unknown.

Enzymes are tightly bound to collagen fibrils, making them difficult to remove from collagen molecules. Two systems have been associated with collagenase activation: (1) limited trypsin activation, and (2) organomercurial compounds promoting conformational change in collagenase. Studies show that collagenase inhibitors are produced by the same cells that synthesize collagenase. These inhibitors have been identified and named *Tissue Inhibitor of Metallo Proteinases* (TIMPs). The best-characterized inhibitor of collagenase is a glycoprotein that is approximately 20,000 daltons in mass and found in human skin fibroblast. Unlike the enzyme collagenase, TIMPs are secreted from cells as fully functional molecules that do not require cofactors or cleavage[3].

Glucocorticoids are the most predictable regulators of collagenase production. Steroids may inhibit collagenase synthesis at the level of mRNA transcription. *Vitamin A,* a retinoid, appears to inhibit collagenase production by amplifying collagenase inhibitor (TIMP) production in human fibroblasts. *Phenytoin,* an antiepileptic drug, decreases collagen degradation instead of increasing collagen deposition, causing gingival hyperplasia in 20 percent of patients. The mechanism of phenytoin on the regulation of collagenase remains unknown. *Platelet-derived growth factor* (PDGF) stimulates the new synthesis of collagenase. Epidermal growth factor (EGF) induces collagenase production. *Transforming growth factor-β* (TGF-β) blocks EGF, inhibiting synthesis of procollagenase. It also induces TIMP synthesis and blocks activation of procollagenase by serine proteases, which enhances collagen deposition. *Interleukin-1* (IL-1) stimulates collagenase production. These regulatory factors of collagen synthesis, degradation, and remodeling seem to balance. The exact mechanisms of collagen metabolisms remain unknown[3].

EPIMORPHIC REGENERATION VERSUS TISSUE REPAIR

An important function of a living organism is its capacity of self-repair. All tissues are able to repair injuries, except teeth. Organisms have to differentiate between self and non-self to accomplish repair. The ability to recognize self from foreign substances, to recognize physiological and morphological deviations, is a fundamental function of the immune system. Chemical reactions correct imbalances at the molecular level. Tissue proliferation and atrophy provide stability at the cellular and tissue levels. These biological processes function to maintain constancy of the *milieu intérieur* and they provide the primary condition for freedom and independence of existence[4].

Repair and regeneration functions are inseparable from the morphological functions. In *embryogenesis,* structural development (tissue morphology) precedes physiological competence. In *regeneration,* there is morphological outgrowth and functional restoration. Structures will regenerate unless nonfunctional. In regeneration, the distinction between morphology and physiology is not so defined. Tissue *repair* is a stopgap reaction designed to reestablish continuity of interrupted tissues. Repair begins when severed or injured parts form scar tissue. Repair is accomplished by (1) *proliferation,* (2) *migration,* and (3) *differentiation* of injured cells. Epithelial tissue heals primarily

by cellular migration, whereas mesodermal tissue repair forms in cellular aggregates that migrate into the lesion and redifferentiate.

In *epimorphic regeneration,* there is direct replacement of an amputated appendage by a direct outgrowth from the injured tissue, reconstituting morphology and function. Processes of tissue repair and epimorphic regeneration do have similarities: (1) both are initiated by trauma, (2) both require normal tissue in order for renewal to proceed, and (3) both are accomplished by a combination of cell migration, proliferation and redifferentiation. However, the similarities are outnumbered by differences that distinguish restorative reactions toward healing[5].

Repair of internal tissue occurs in the absence of epidermal participation. Epimorphic regeneration requires epidermal wound healing. In tissue repair, loss of cellular specialization does not prevent cells from redifferentiating into a different tissue, such as scar tissue. In epimorphic regeneration, the degree of dedifferentiation is remarkable, and development is not limited to extensions in the stump. A new structure is formed with its own location and function. Epimorphic regeneration always occurs in a proximodistal direction, requiring functional nerves to ensure competence of the new structure. In tissue repair, differentiation proceeds at the same time in all locations, distally and proximally. Denervated limbs can heal injuries, reunite severed tendons, and heal integumental lesions.

Tissue repair is a universal phenomenon. Most organs and tissues in the human body carry this basic biological process, which is designed to restore morphological integrity and continuity of interrupted parts. Epimorphic regeneration is, rather, a selective phenomenon reflecting an evolutionary adaptation or an exaggerated version of tissue repair.

There are two evolutionary landmarks in the history of vertebrate evolution: (1) successful transition from aquatic to terrestrial habitats, and (2) elevation of metabolic rates to establish a homeothermic condition. Almost all adaptation processes have been associated with a decline in regenerative capacity, which has been replaced by tissue repair. Terrestrial vertebrates who walk on land cause their ambulating members to be more susceptible to repeated injury. The only mammalian appendages capable of regeneration are those not bearing weight or under constant mechanical pressure.

Another factor involved with the "loss" of the regenerative process during adaptation is the elevated metabolic rate of mammals that feed frequently. Mammals starve to death if they cannot find nourishment, particularly water. A mammal without a leg is at great risk, and regeneration would take months. The animal would either starve or be killed by predators. Tissue repair, therefore, is advantageous for survival and is accomplished by epidermal migration, epithelization, wound contraction, and scar formation, which provides tensile strength and tissue continuity. There is no advantage to regenerate a structure if survival is undetermined[6]. Animals can live without epimorphic regeneration but cannot live without tissue repair. Therefore, it seems our ancestors may have sacrificed their regenerative abilities in exchange for more primitive processes of tissue repair in order to survive.

NORMAL MECHANISMS OF WOUND HEALING

Despite basic research and a sound biological knowledge of the principles of wound healing, empirical knowledge seems to predominate. Many physicians feel a sense of helplessness when applying scientific knowledge to wound healing. Physicians have a responsibility to understand a great deal about the biochemistry, molecular biology, and cell physiology of the individual events that lead to wound healing (Figure 4-2).

THE INFLAMMATORY OR SUBSTRATE PHASE (0–4 DAYS)

Physiological and biochemical responses to injury begin with inflammation. Inflammation is the reaction of vascularized living tissue to local injury[7]. Inflammatory response is closely intertwined with the process of repair. It includes phagocytosis of the damaging agents and neutralization of noxious stimuli by specialized cells. This remains true whether the injury is an aseptic surgical incision

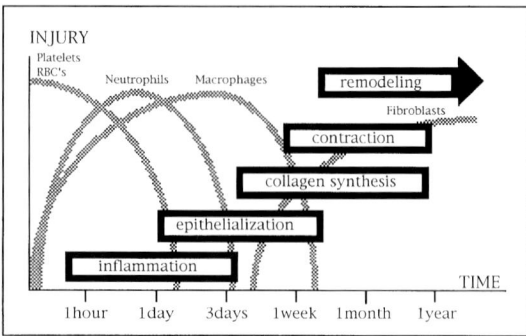

Figure 4-2. Phases of wound healing.

or a traumatic contaminated injury. Only the reaction of blood vessels characterizes inflammation in higher forms of life. Inflammation and repair contain injuries and promote repair, without which infection would be relentless, wounds would not heal, and tissue would remain as festering sores. However, repair may be harmful and disfiguring.

After injury, organisms react with intense, acute, and localized response to minimize trauma. Initially, transient vasoconstriction of arterioles and capillaries occurs and then disappears within 3 to 5 seconds. This response lasts longer in more severe injury and burns. Plugging of capillaries with erythrocytes and platelets that adhere to damaged endothelium and exposed collagen rapidly decreases hemorrhage. Leukocyte margination to the injured endothelium soon follows. Tissue mast cells release histamine and serotonin, reversing vasoconstriction and increasing blood flow and intravascular hydrostatic pressure, usually within 15 minutes (Figure 4-3). Slowing of the blood flow is brought about by increased permeability of the microvasculature. There is transudation of protein-poor fluid and leukocytes in the extracellular space, causing an increase in interstitial oncotic pressure. The result of these vascular changes is called *edema*. Together the injured cell membranes activate phospholipase, releasing arachidonic acid, and forming prostaglandins E_1 and E_2 (PGE_1 and PGE_2) and kinins released by kallikrein (Figure 4-4).

Three types of vascular responses are demonstrated during the ebb phase of inflammation. The *immediate-transient* response is evoked by histamine and other mediators in small and medium

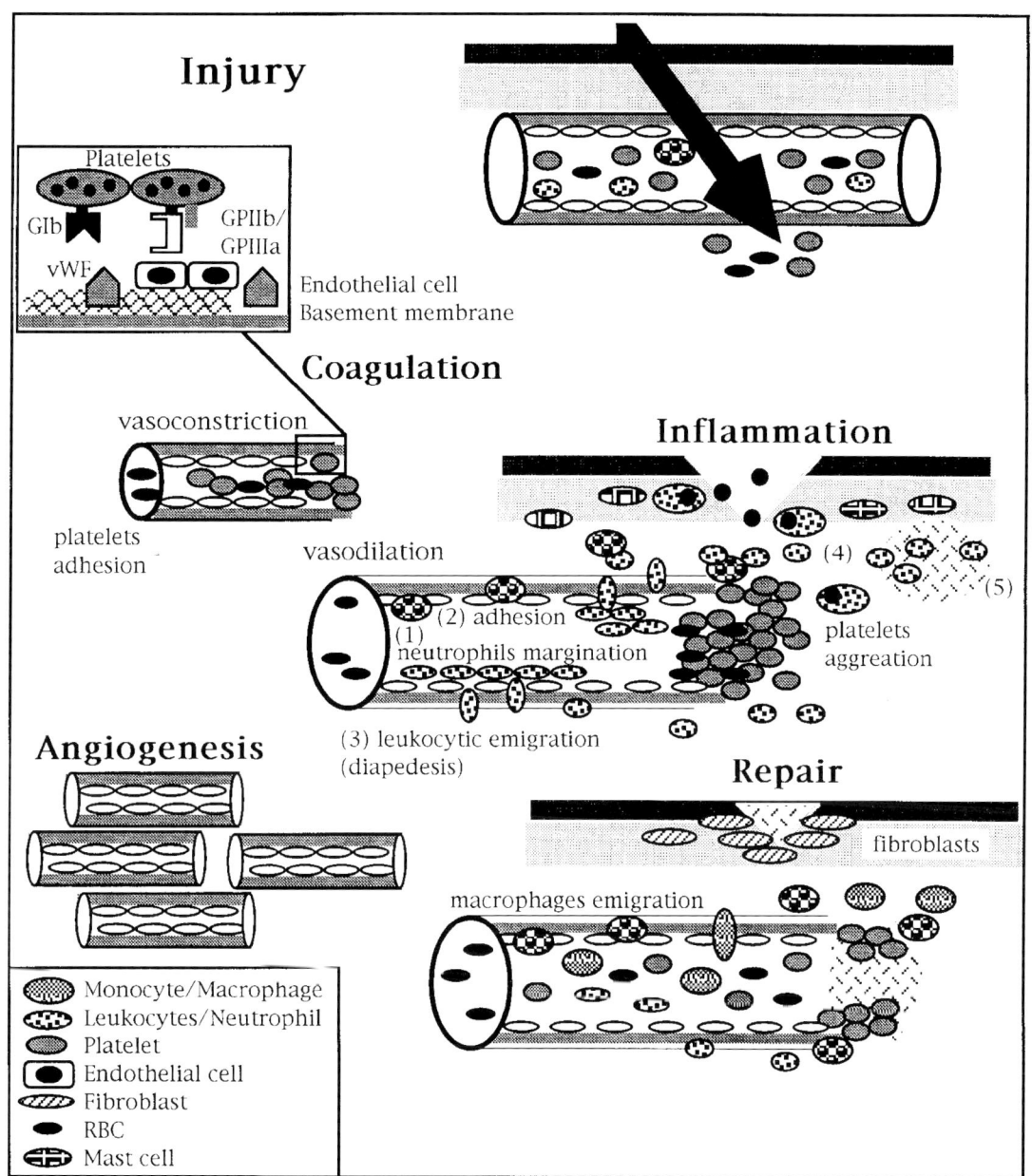

Figure 4-3. Cellular phases of inflammation.

venules and lasts up to 30 minutes. The *immediate-sustained* reaction is found in severe injuries and is associated with endothelial cell necrosis at all levels of microcirculation, including venules, capillaries, and arterioles. This reaction, which may last for days, repairs the damaged vessels. The third reaction is a *delayed-prolonged response,* which last for several hours or days and involves venules and capillaries. It is caused by mild-to-moderate thermal injury, x-ray or UV light irradiation, certain bacterial toxins, and delayed (type IV) hypersensitivity reactions. Macroscopically, these events rep-

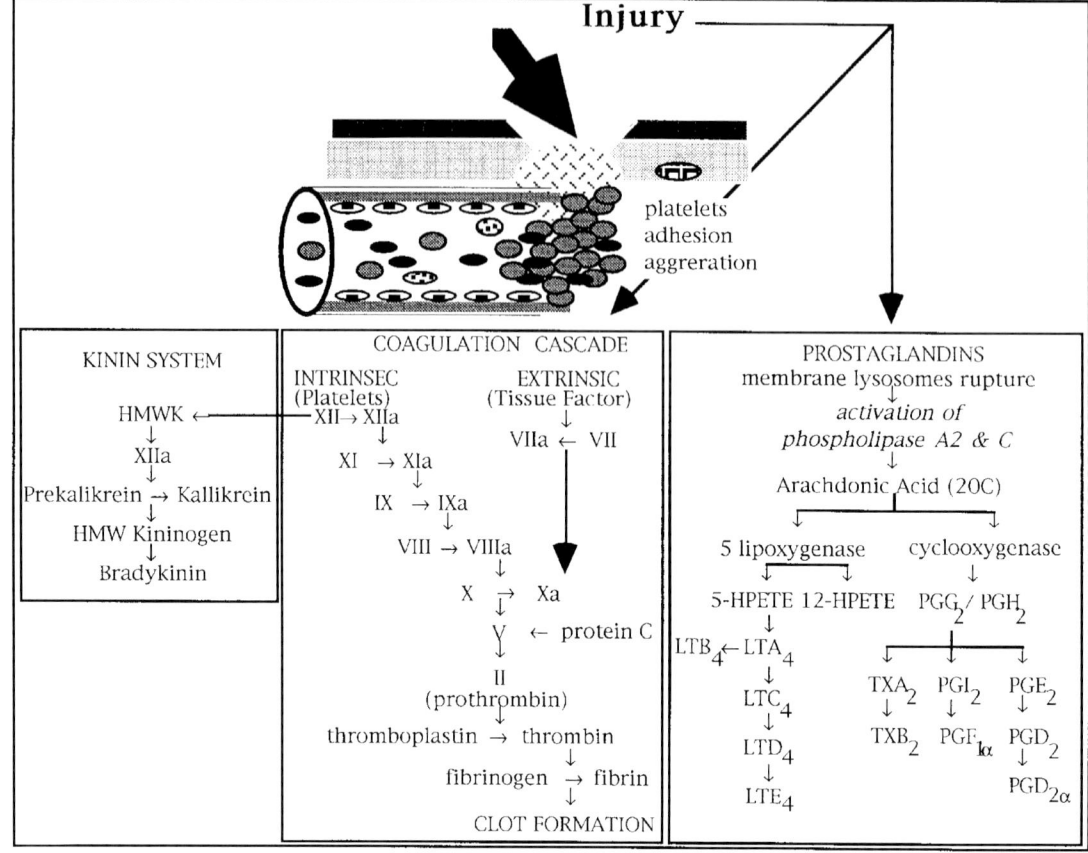

Figure 4-4. Metabolic pathways of wound healing.

resent classic signs of inflammation: redness, swelling, warmth, and pain as described by Celsus 2000 years ago.

The cellular phase of inflammation is characterized by invasion of vascularized connective tissue by circulating cells. Vascularized connective tissue consists of basement membranes, various types of collagen, elastin, proteoglycans, and glycoproteins (fibronectin and laminin). Circulating cells involved in inflammation include neutrophils, monocytes, eosinophils, lymphocytes, basophils, and platelets. Connective tissue cells are mast cells, tissue fibroblasts, and macrophages. Accumulation of leukocytes, neutrophils, and macrophages is most important in the inflammatory reaction. The sequence of these leukocytic events are (1) margination, (2) adhesion, (3) emigration toward a chemotactic agent, (4) phagocytosis and intracellular deg-

radation, and (5) extracellular release of leukocyte products (Figure 4-3).

Neutrophils are the first cells to cross the endothelial membrane. They predominate in the first 6 to 24 hours, engulf foreign material, and neutrophils digest debris. Although neutrophil function is important in defense mechanisms, they are not essential in wound healing. **Monocytes** replace neutrophils in 24 to 48 hours in the wound environment and function as immunoreactants. Activated **macrophages** are most important in the healing process. Macrophages are scavenger cells that release monokines, biological mediators. These mediators regulate the action of other inflammatory cells and stimulate fibroblasts to initiate collagen synthesis. **Fibroblasts** are specialized cells that differentiate from resting mesenchymal cells in connective tissue. During the first three to five days after the injury, their primary function is to synthesize collagen. Scar tissue that is reopened and closed shows immediate onset of collagen synthesis. The result of the inflammatory phase is hemostasis at the injury site. Hemostasis sets the stage for the next phase of the wound healing process.

THE PROLIFERATIVE PHASE (2–22 DAYS)

The proliferative phase begins within two days of injury and can last up to three weeks, in wounds closed by *primary intention*. The main activities during the proliferative phase are (1) epithelization, (2) neoangiogenesis, (3) collagen synthesis, and (4) fibroplasia.

Epithelization

Renewal of the epithelial layer is called epithelization. Events of epithelization are (1) detachment, (2) migration, (3) proliferation and (4) differentiation[8]. The layer above the dermis is the basal layer, followed by the granular layer and then the stratum corneum. Within 24 hours of injury, the basal cell layer thickens, the basal cells detach, and these cells migrate into the wound. Forty-eight hours after closure there is complete migration of basal cells across the wound line. Division begins, causing upward migration and reconstitution of the epidermis.

In open wounds and burns, basal cells migrate along and underneath the wound. This migratory phase is characterized by loss of contact inhibition between adjacent cells and dedifferentiation. Dedifferentiation is the phenomenon through which mature basal cells return to their embryological stage. They are still able to reestablish contact inhibition, upward migration, and secretion of keratin.

Neoangiogenesis

As blood coagulates, it releases chemotactic factors that attract neutrophils (0–24 hours) and macrophages (24–48 hours) to the wound environment. Macrophages release chemotactic factors that enhance the migration of myofibroblasts. Chemotaxis is the unidirectional migration of cells toward an attractant. Chemotactic factors include both exogenous and endogenous substances (Table 4-3). The

Table 4-3. Chemical Mediators of Inflammation

	Cells	Plasma proteases
Preformed	*Newly synthesized*	
Histamine	Prostaglandins	Complement system: C3a, C5a, C5b–C9
Serotonin	Leukotrienes	Kinin system
Lysosomal enzyme	PAF Cytokines	Clotting/fibrinolytic system

most important chemotactic agents for neutrophils are bacterial byproducts, C5a, and leukotriene B_4 (LTB_4), a product of the arachidonic acid pathway via 5-lipoxygenase (Figure 4-4 and 4-5). Activated platelets release chemotactic factors TGF-β and PDGF for macrophages.

Myofibroblast migration and the subsequent release of growth factors into the wound promote capillary sprouts just behind the wound edges. This leads to the appearance of newly functioning capillary loops, fibroblasts, and collagen in the extracellular matrix. As the wound heals, granulation tissue appears on the third day. Newly formed capillaries differentiate into venules and arterioles; and fibrillar collagen is remodeled, and the matrix becomes less acellular.

Physiologically, capillaries only proliferate during embryological development, ovulation, menstruation, inflammation, and tissue repair. Endothelial cells in mature blood vessels do not divide or migrate. Neoangiogenesis usually begins as outgrowths from preexisting venules, endothelial cell migrations, and proliferation. Newly formed capil-

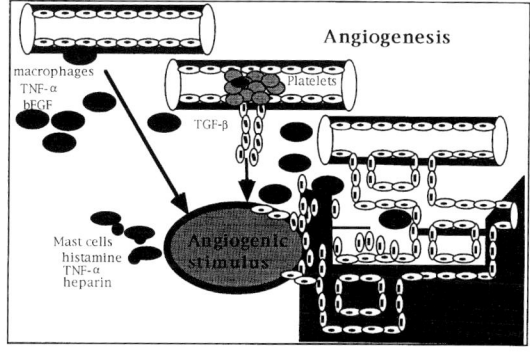

Figure 4-5. Neoangiogenesis.

laries lack the well-formed basement membranes, and within hours of exposure endothelial cells in preexisting vessels begin to produce enzymes degrading the vascular basement membrane at the side facing the stimulus. Endothelial cells begin migration within 24 hours of angiogenic stimulus across the degraded basement membrane (Figure 4-5), dividing and differentiating. These cells come together and form a tubular lumen, which then connects with an adjacent neovessel. This gives rise to a branching vascular network. As vessels mature, extracellular matrix components are deposited to form a new basement membrane. In skin flaps, neocapillaries cross the wound edges, connecting with each other and reestablishing blood flow across the wound within three days of initial insult[9–12]. Vascularization in vivo can be divided into two classes based on the morphology of new vessels: (1) in tumors, arteriovenous malformations, and hemangiomas, the vasculature has tortuous thin-walled vessels, dilated endothelial-lined lacunae, and copious arteriovenous connections; and (2) in development and wound healing, there is an active remodeling of new vessels that eventually differentiate into arteries and capillaries. Some vessels in the network regress. The cause of this regression is not known. Likewise, the morphological differences between neovascularization, tumor growth, and arteriovenous malformation remain unexplained[13].

In summary, the angiogenesis cascade in wound healing is similar in development to that of tumor neovascularization. There is a balance, however, between cellular components, biomolecular modulators of repair, chemotactic factors, growth factors, and angiogenesis factors during neoangiogenesis in wound healing. Cells that produce angiogenic modulators during inflammatory response are platelets, macrophages, and mast cells. Activated *platelets* release TGF-beta (a chemoattractant for macrophages), PDGF (a chemoattractant for macrophages and a stimulator of vascular smooth muscle cells), and angiogenic factors stored in the basement membrane (Figure 4-5). *Macrophages* produce direct-acting angiogenesis (first-class) factors: TNF-alpha (tumor necrosis factor) and basic FGF (fibroblast growth factor). *Mast cells* are not essential for angiogenesis but release histamine, TNF-alpha, and

heparin, which stimulate the synthesis and secretion of other angiogenic factors (Figure 4-5).

Inflammatory responses following injury lead to degradation of basement membrane followed by endothelial cell migration, angiogenic factor(s), proliferation, and lumen formation. Angiogenic factors are classified as either first or second-class angiogenic-factors. *First-class factors,* which have a direct effect on endothelial cell migration include FGF, TGF-alpha, macrophage-derived growth factor (MDGF), TNF-alpha (cachectin), and wound angiogenic factor (WAF). *Second-class factors,* or indirect angiogenic factors, include angiogenin and TGF-beta (Table 4-4). Studies show that heparin interacts with angiogenic factors; these are called heparin-binding angiogenic factors. They include tumor angiogenesis factor (TAF), endothelial cell growth factor (ECGF), retinal- and eye-derived growth factor (RDGF), and cartilage-derived growth factor (CDGF). Some growth factors interact and bind to heparin, regulating angiogenesis in vivo, and some involve the selective release of growth factors from extracellular matrix deposits.

The extracellular matrix is the arena of inflammatory response and neoangiogenesis. The first substance found in the matrix is fibrin. Dvorak and others [14–16] have shown that *fibrin* causes endothelial cells to retract and migrate, promoting tumor angiogenesis and wound neovascularization. *Hyaluronic acid* and *fibronectin* also enhance neoangiogenesis in the wound environment. *Hyaluronic acid* predominates during the early granulation phase and is replaced between the fifth and tenth day by chondroitin sulfate and dermatan sulfate[17]. *Fibronectin* is deposited from plasma with fibrin and is produced by endothelial cells and macrophages. It is the initial structural fibril secreted by fibroblasts and acts as the template for collagen deposition. Fibronectin contains binding receptors

Table 4-4. Angiogenic Factors

First Class	Second Class
βFGF	Angiogenin
TGF-α	TGF-β
TNF-α (cachectin)	
WAF (wound angiogenic factor)	

for heparin; this binding dramatically increases angiogenesis. The growth factors that are currently available have been used clinically to accelerate healing in chronic, nonhealing wounds.

Collagen Synthesis

After the inflammatory reaction has subsided, fibroblasts, spindle-shaped cells with oval nuclei, become increasingly abundant in the wound environment. These cells synthesize and secrete collagen molecules. Convincing evidence of fibroblasts as collagen secreting cells comes from Ross's experiments with parabiotic rats[18,19]. Neovascularization causes endothelial cells to migrate toward the wound site. These cells contain a potent plasminogen activator. As fibroblasts advance into the injured area, intense fibrinolysis occurs, destroying the fibrin network and allowing collagen deposition.

Collagen types I and III are involved in dermis regeneration, and type II collagen is found in cartilage for the remodeling of basement membrane in epidermal lesions. Type III collagen and procollagen are found in the early phases of normal wound repair, usually within the first 24 to 48 hours. After 72 hours, there is a substantial increase in type I collagen along with mature fibroblasts at the injury site. The early appearance of type III collagen has been associated with the deposition of fibronectin[20].

Another study has suggested that an increase of type IV collagen forms the scaffold of epidermal basement membranes and reconstitutes the collagenous network that is the hallmark of normal epidermal wound healing. Type V collagen has been associated with the migration and movement of capillary endothelial cells during angiogenesis[20,21]. Ultimately, the acellular, fiber-rich scar tissue contains fibrils derived from type I collagen molecules[20].

Fibroplasia

Fibroplasia is the production of fibrous protein in the wound. More than 50% of the protein found in scar tissue is collagen, with the remainder distributed as elastin and reticulin. During the first three to four weeks of wound healing, epithelial cells and fibroblasts produce collagenase, which controls the amount of scar tissue. By the fourth or fifth week, the absolute number of wound fibroblasts has decreased, and the rich capillary network generated by neoangiogenesis has shrunk to a few capillaries. The ratio of collagen synthesis to degradation reaches a balance, and the wound enters a phase of collagen maturation. This phase continues for months. Glycoprotein and mucopolysaccharide levels decrease, and new capillaries eventually disappear. In some wounds, scars enlarge, producing massive keloids or hypertrophic scars. In others, the color fades, bulk decreases, and normal pigmentation returns, the scar almost disappears. The gross appearance of remodeling scars suggests that collagen fibers are altered into different patterns over time.

MATURATION AND REMODELING PHASE (21 DAYS TO 2 YEARS)

The conversion of fragile collagen fibrils converted into insoluble, strong collagen fibers is called maturation or remodeling. Maturation of collagen produces the physical characteristics of scar tissue[8]. Collagen cross-linking is the covalent bonding between collagen peptide chains, it is an important step in collagen maturation. Collagen cross-linking increases strength in two ways: (1) *intramolecular* cross-linking formed by covalent bonding between peptide chains produced by *lysyl oxidase,* and (2) cross-linking formed as an *intermolecular* bond by a Schiff base reaction. Wounds become stronger with time. The rate of wound strength determines what suture material should be used, when sutures should be removed, and how quickly the patient's activity level should be resumed. The two most common parameters for measuring wound strength are *tensile* and *burst* strength. Collagen maturation dramatically increases the *burst strength* of the scar three to nine weeks after injury. It measures the load required to break the wound regardless of dimension. The *tensile strength* measures the load per cross-sectioned area of rupture. By the twenty-first day *burst strength* has reached over 1 kg per linear cm[18].

Maturation of collagen occurs by an increasing density and cross-linking of the collagen fibers, and occurs for up to one year. Wound repair, although strong, converts an elastic, pliable tissue to an inelastic and brittle one. During maturation there is a constant turnover of collagen molecules brought about by collagenase. Collagenase is secreted by fibroblasts, neutrophils, and macrophages. Collagenase is responsible for collagenolysis, a process of hydrolysis. Wound *remodeling,* as seen by the surgeon, is a change in texture, thickness, and color of a healing wound. The burst strength of the scar is more important than the cosmetic appearance. Collagen appears in the wound environment three to seven days after injury. The scar strength increases on day 3 as the content of collagen in the wounded tissue continues to increase. At nine weeks after injury, a scar has 70% the burst strength of normal skin; this increases to 90% at six months. Wounds continue to gain strength at a relatively constant rate for over one year. However, despite prolonged strength gain, wound tissue rarely regains the strength of normal tissue.

CHRONIC INFLAMMATION

Acute inflammation may result in repair; i.e. complete morphologic and functional restoration, or it may lead to healing by scarring, which occurs after substantial tissue destruction. Abscess formation, particularly in infections with pyogenic organisms, is another outcome of wound healing. Finally, the initial inflammatory reaction may progress to chronic inflammation.

Chronic inflammation follows an acute inflammatory response by persistence of the inciting stimulus or by defective wound healing. It may also result from repeated insult or insidiously as a low-grade smoldering inflammatory response such as rheumatoid arthritis or chronic pulmonary disease. The end result of chronic inflammation is infiltration of the wound environment by macrophages, fibroblast proliferation, angiogenesis, fibrosis, tissue destruction associated with loss of function, and in some instances granuloma formation. Chronic inflammation may present in a number of ways: (1) with diverse morphologic variations, (2) as a serous inflammation such as a pleural effusion, and (3) as a fibrinous inflammation with large amounts of plasma proteins. These may appear as, for example, fibrinogen, such as from a fibrinous pericarditis,

or a purulent inflammation, an abscess, or an ulcer. An ulcer is a local defect or excavation of the surface of an organ or tissue produced by sloughing of inflammatory necrotic tissue. It may result from poor circulation, chronic inflammation of the lower extremities of older patients, or pressure sores in bedridden spinal cord injury patients. Chronic ulceration is characterized by fibroblastic proliferation, scarring, and accumulation of lymphocytes, macrophages, and plasma cells at the ulcer margin.

GROWTH FACTORS AND CYTOKINES

Recombinant DNA technology has made possible the production of these peptides in pure form and in pharmacological quantities[22]. Growth factors and cytokines act as messengers in wound healing. Experimental data continue to accumulate demonstrating ability of these substances to influence migration populations of macrophages and PMNs (polymorphonuclear leukocytes) to the wound. Growth factors can function in an endocrine, a paracrine, or an autocrine fashion. Endocrine factors affect a target cell at a distance and are carried via the bloodstream. Paracrine factors are released by one cell and affect a different cell in the vicinity. Autocrine factors are released by a cell and affect the function of that same cell. However, the ability of a cell to respond to a growth factor depends on whether or not the target cell has receptors for that specific growth factor. Conservation of growth factor peptide sequences between species suggests evolutionary preservation for fundamental physiological reasons and supports an essential role for these substances as biological regulators of cell division and differentiation.

Tissue repair is initiated by the release of growth factor peptides such as TGF-β, TGA-α, PDGF, βFGF, and TNF (see table 4-5). Wound healing aims to produce granulation tissue and replace it with mature scar tissue. Studies suggest that peptide growth factors act as a cascade leading to wound healing[23]. Angiogenesis is a critical event in forming granulation tissue. TGF-β, βFGF, and TNF are potentially angiogenic. Only FGF is chemotactic or mitogenic for endothelial cells in vitro, suggesting an indirect action by other peptides. Clinical research on the application of growth factors to

Table 4-5. Growth Factors and Cytokines[1]

Factor	Source	Target	Action
TGF-β	Platelet	Fibroblast	Mitosis, chemotaxis, collagen synthesis
	Macrophage Lymphocyte Bone Kidney	Macrophage	FGF, PDGF, TNF, IL-1 synthesis
TGF-α	Platelet	Epithelial cell Mesenchymal cell	Fibroblast proliferation
	Keratinocyte	Fibroblast	
	Macrophage	Endothelial cell	
PDGF	Platelets	Fibroblast	Mitosis, chemotaxis, collagen synthesis
	Macrophage Endothelial cell	Smooth muscle cell Glial cell	Mitosis, chemotaxis
aFGF, bFGF/	Macrophage	Endothelial cell	Angiogenesis
HBGF	Cartilage	Fibroblast	Collagen synthesis
		Chondrocyte	Collagen synthesis
	Brain	Glial cell	
EGF	Saliva	Epithelial cell	Mitosis, chemotaxis
		Endothelial cell	Mitosis
		Fibroblast	Mitosis, chemotaxis
		Smooth muscle cell	
AGF	Macrophage	Endothelial cell	
EDF	Epithelial cell Fibroblast	Epithelial cell	
MAF	T lymphocyte	Macrophage	
MDGF	Macrophage	Fibroblast Smooth muscle cell	
FGF	Macrophage	Fibroblast	
IGF-I/Sm-C	Hepatocyte	Fetal tissue	
	Fibroblast	Fibroblast	Fibroplasia
TNF	Macrophage	Fibroblast	Mitosis, PGE$_2$ release, collagen synthesis
		Macrophage	Pyrogen
IL-1	Macrophage	Fibroblast	Proliferation Arachidonic acid Collagen synthesis Increase collagenase/ hyaluronidase activity
		Epithelial cell	Chemotaxis
		Neutrophil	Chemotaxis
		Monocyte	Chemotaxis
		Synovial cell	Chemotaxis
IL-2	T lymphocyte	?	
MIF	T lymphocyte	Macrophage	

Source: Adapted from McGrath., M.H., Peptide growth factors and wound healing, Clin Plast Surg 1990; 17: 421–432.

[1]TGFα/β: transforming growth factor alpha/beta; PDGF: platelet-derived growth factor; a/bFGF: acid/basic fibroblast growth factor; HBGF: heparin-binding growth factor; EGF: epidermoid growth factor: MAF: macrophage growth factor; MDGF: manocyte/macrophage-derived growth factor; IGF-I: insulin-like growth factor; Sm-C: Somatomedin-C; TNF: tumor necrosis factor; IL-1/2: interleukin one/two; MIF: macrophage inhibitor factor;

stimulate wound healing is of paramount importance, especially where the morbidity and mortality are significant, as in diabetic patients, those using glucocorticoids, radiation, or chemotherapy, or in the management of chronic wounds.

TYPES OF WOUND HEALING

Wound healing represents a highly dynamic, integrated series of cellular, physiological, and biochemical events. Although all wounds heal by the same processes, clinical wounds are of two distinct types: simple closed wounds, and open wounds with or without tissue loss. Wounds are classified into four general categories according to the healing process: (1) primary healing, (2) delayed primary healing, (3) secondary healing, and (4) healing partial-thickness skin wounds[24].

Closed wounds heal by inflammation, epithelization, neoangiogenesis and collagen maturation and remodeling. Open wounds with or without tissue loss and acute or chronic wounds are a clinical challenge because they differ from incised and sutured wounds. The phases of healing for closed wounds also take place for healing of open wounds. In open wounds, contraction and epithelization assume a more important role than in closed wounds. *Wound contraction* is an energy-dependent process that decreases the size of a wound by active movement of the tissue. *Contracture,* on the other hand, refers to a permanent state resulting from the process of tissue contraction. For example, small wounds on the hand and on the heel of the foot heal by contraction. Likewise, large open wounds heal by contraction, not by epithelization. In extensive cutaneous burns or in large tissue loss, contraction may lead to irreversible loss of morphology and function and may result in death.

Gabbiani[25] was the first to describe cells within the wound environment with structural properties of both fibroblasts and smooth muscle cells. He named these myofibroblasts. Myofibroblasts contain a well-developed actin microfilament system containing densely packed areas of RER. The origin of these cells is unclear, but data suggest that they are fibroblast derived[25]. They appear in the wound on the third day after injury, reach a maximum level by the twenty-first day, and disappear when contraction is completed. Collagen has no role in wound contraction. Studies show that in animals with scurvy, as well as in open wounds treated with collagen cross-link inhibitors, the wounds contracted.

PRIMARY HEALING

Primary healing occurs when a wound is closed within hours by sutures, staples, or adhesive strips. Integrity and long-term strength are provided by collagen, and epithelization plays a minor role. Epithelial cells cover the wound surface, protecting it against bacterial invasion.

DELAYED PRIMARY HEALING

Delayed primary healing wounds are closed after some period of time, either because the wound edges are poorly delineated, or contamination precludes safe primary closure, or for both reasons. First, wounds should be classified according to level of contamination (Table 4-6). Infected wounds should not be closed primarily; they should be cleansed and healed by secondary healing. Wounds with intermediate degrees of contamination can be cleaned through judicious wound debridement and irrigation and then closed by delayed primary heal-

Table 4-6. Classification of Wound Contamination

Classification	Rate of infection	Type of wound
Clean	1.5–5.1%	Atraumatic, uninfected; no entry of GU, GL, or respiratory tract
Clean-contaminated	7.7–10.8%	Entry of GU, GI or respiratory tract; minor break in technique
Contaminated	15.2–16.3%	Traumatic wounds, gross spillage from GI, entry into infected urine, and bile;
Dirty	28.0%–40.0%	Drainage of abscess; debridement of soft tissue

ing. The first three or four days after injury or surgery, open wounds should be managed with moist sterile gauze dressings, after which the wound edges are approximated with sutures or adhesive strips. This technique is extremely important in managing crush injury wounds, gunshot wounds, or bowel contamination of the soft tissue.

SECONDARY HEALING

When a full-thickness wound is not closed mechanically, it heals by the secondary healing process: that is, by the natural biologic forces of wound contraction. Contraction may help or hinder the functional healing process. Skim wounds contract by stretching the surrounding skin to close the defect, not by producing new skin. After about three days, the dermal edges begin moving toward each other. In a rectangular or square defect, midpoints on the sides move more rapidly than the corners, forming a stellate scar (Figure 4-6).

HEALING OF PARTIAL-THICKNESS SKIN WOUNDS

Partial-thickness wounds include damage to the epithelium and a superficial portion of the dermis. Epithelization, the major mechanism of wound repair in partial-thickness skin loss, occurs at the margins and over the entire surface of the wound from epithelial cells in hair follicles and sebaceous glands. Epithelial cells must have a true dermal or pseudodermal bed to survive. Epithelial cells migrate from skin appendages. The basilar layer elongates and migrates across the denuded surface within 24 hours of injury. These cells must bind to the substrate, must respond to chemotactic factors, and must have cytoskeletal machinery making movement possible. Epithelial binding is provided by fibronectin, vitronectin, epibolin, and collagen

types I, III, and IV. Migration of marginal cells into the wound clears a path for epithelial cells to migrate. Epithelial cell mitosis begins within 72 hours after injury. Simultaneously, basal epithelial cells divide and join the migrating sheet. When migrating epithelial cells contact other epithelial cells, mitosis stops. This is called contact inhibition. Cell maturation begins with differentiation and keratin synthesis, and in many circumstances the rete pegs regenerate. Growth factors such as EGF, β-FGF, and IL-1 also stimulate epithelial proliferation. No contraction and little collagen deposition occur in these wounds.

WOUND MANAGEMENT

PRIMARY CLOSED WOUNDS

Primary wound closure should be limited to clean wounds. Wounds with counts of more than 1 times 10^5 bacteria per gram of tissue should not be primarily closed. Wounds should not be closed under excessive tension, and skin edges should be slightly everted so that the final mature scar is flat. Sutures should be placed in tissues that have significant tensile strength such as fascia and dermis. The choice of sutures is not as important as the general principles of closure. A dressing should protect the wound and absorb drainage during the first 48 hours. After an epithelial seal is present, the dressing can be removed to allow for inspection of the incision.

PRIMARY OPEN WOUNDS

Acute wounds too large to close primarily should be closed with a split-thickness skin graft. In selected cases, such as areas with exposed bone or tendons, a flap may be used.

CHRONIC OPEN WOUNDS

The most important aspect of management of chronic wounds is to correct the underlying disease. Direct wound care is the next step. If the wound contains an eschar, debridement is paramount. If bacterial counts are greater than 1 times 10^5 bacteria per gram of tissue, topical antibiotics may promote

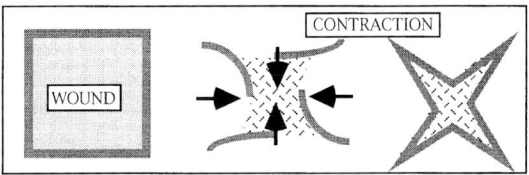

Figure 4-6. Wound contraction.

healthy granulation tissue. Wounds with areas of healthy granulation tissue may heal by contraction and epithelization. Those wounds with a large open area may be closed with a split-thickness skin graft.

WOUND DRESSINGS

OCCLUSIVE DRESSING AND OXYGEN

The primary objective of wound care is to promote healing with the best results combining function and cosmetics. The principal function of a dressing is to provide an optimal healing environment. Wound healing is a dynamic physiologic process involving different phases that overlap and share defined temporal cellular characteristics. To optimize healing, familiarity with the changes occurring in phases of tissue repair is important. During the inflammatory phase, wounds must be protected from further damage, the infection must be controlled and the debris cleared. In the second, or proliferative phase, formation of fibrovascular granulation and epithelization occur. The last phase involves remodeling and maturation of scar tissue.

Hemostasis limits blood loss, decreases dissemination of microbes and toxins, and releases chemotactic and growth factors into the wound environment. A simple compression dressing promotes hemostasis, limits edema, reduces pain, and improves gas and solute exchange between blood and tissue. Infection is contamination of tissues by pathogens that cannot be controlled by body defenses. A dressing, therefore, can not sterilize a wound but can decrease infection by preventing overgrowth and colonization. Wound debris may be removed by debridement, irrigation, and absorption of exudate into a dressing.

Dressings designed for the *proliferative* and *remodeling* phases of wound healing are based on hydration and oxygen tension. An occlusive dressing is defined as one that has the ability to transmit gas and water vapor from the wound surface to the atmosphere. An occlusive dressing affects the epidermis and dermis and limits tissue desiccation and secondary mechanical damage. By maintaining a moist environment, the epidermal barrier function

is rapidly restored. A scab forms when exudate dries, incorporating inflammatory cells, wound debris, and a layer of desiccated normal tissue. In open wounds, epithelization is delayed because epithelial cells are forced to migrate underneath the eschar, as opposed to a moist occluded wound bed. Occlusion can be detrimental and must be closely monitored. It is contraindicated in infected and highly exudative wounds and should be used judiciously in immunocompromised patients.

Perfusion and oxygenation are vital to repair. Oxygen inhibits anaerobic growth, promotes production of free radicals by scavenger cells, and inhibits macrophage angiogenic function. Increasing tissue PO_2 enhances microbial clearance and promotes fibroblast metabolism. Rates of epithelization underneath dressings correlate with their moisture vapor transmission rates, not with their oxygen permeability[26]. Occlusive dressings should be applied on clean wounds, carefully monitored, and used on patients whose underlying pathology has been addressed.

TYPES OF WOUND DRESSINGS

Wound dressings are classified as *primary* and *secondary*. A *primary* wound dressing is in direct contact with the wound, absorbs, and prevents infection, adhesion, and dryness. A *secondary* dressing is placed over a primary dressing to further protect, absorb, compress, and occlude the wound. An example is the placement of sterile gauze over a sheet of xeroform gauze on a split-thickness skin graft donor site. Dressings can be absorbent, nonadherent, occlusive/semiocclusive, hydrophilic/hydrophobic, hydrocolloid, and hydrogel types. Dressings should absorb ooze. They should be used during the acute phase of inflammatory reaction during the first 72 hours. Substances used for dressings include cotton, wool, sponge, chitin and chitosan (exoskeletons of crustaceans), laginates, pectin, gels of polymers of polyoxypropylene and polyethylene oxide, gelatin, carboxymethylcellulose, karaya gum, and starch. Nonadherent dressings are designed not to stick. Examples of these dressings are gauze impregnated with paraffin and petroleum jelly. A secondary dressing may be needed, as the impregnant agent wears off, to seal the wound edge and prevent desiccation. Occlusive/semiocclusive dressings provide an excellent environment for a clean, minimally exudative wound. Film dressings are waterproof, permeable to water vapor, and resistant to microbes. Adhesive films are also used to protect areas vulnerable to pressure, friction, or shear ulceration.

Hydrophilic/hydrophobic dressings are composite. A primary hydrophilic layer absorbs exudate. A second hydrophobic layer, which is waterproof, prevents leakage. Hydrocolloid/hydrogel dressings combine the benefits of occlusion and absorbency. Hydrocolloids consist of gumlike material such as guar or karaya, sodium carboxymethylcellulose, and pectin. They form complex structures with water, they cause fluid absorption by particle swelling, and they have a wet tack (adhesion to wet surface) and a dry tack (adhesion to dry surface) that seal the wound. Hydrogels are complex lattices (framework made of polymers overlapped in a regular, crisscross pattern) that trap water like a molecular sponge. Hydrogels allow a high rate of evaporation without compromising wound hydration and are useful in treating burn patients. Absorbable materials are degraded in vivo and comprise collagen, gelatin, and oxidized cellulose. They are particularly useful internally as hemostats. Collagen and gelatin have been used as wound dressings. The most commonly applied medications are antimicrobials. Neosporin ointment contains polymyxin B, bacitracin-zinc, and neomycin. Zinc oxide ointments enhance epithelization up to 20%. Table 4-7 provides a brief summary of wound dressings.

Wound dressing and management is complicated by the different types of dressings for different types of wounds. It is important that physicians, surgeons, nurses, and other health professionals to develop a clear understanding of the type of dressings used on wounds and provide proper care to patients (Table 4-7).

LOCAL AND SYSTEMIC FACTORS AFFECTING WOUND HEALING

The aging process affects normal wound healing[27]. Fibroblast synthetic activity, collagen synthesis, and cross-linking are slowed. Decreased cellular activity also delays epithelization. Both underlying pulmonary and circulatory problems affect wound perfusion, oxygenation, and healing in the elderly. Anemia, blood loss, and oxygen tension affect wound healing in different ways. Prolonged low oxygen tension in tissue impairs healing. Adequate tissue perfusion is more important than the oxygen-carrying capacity of blood for normal wound healing.

Hypovolemia, vasoconstriction, and elevated blood viscosity may have profound detrimental effects on local oxygen tension, whereas acute hemorrhage or anemia may not alter tissue oxygen tension. Local hyperthermia increases partial pressure of subcutaneous oxygen causing a threefold increase in perfusion. Hypoxia and hyperoxia promote neovascularization. Wound oxygen tension depends primarily on blood flow and secondarily on concentration of inspired oxygen[13]. Soon after injury, there is local vasoconstriction, causing hypoxia, which stimulates angiogenesis. The bursting of capillaries in connective tissue causes hyperoxia especially at the wound edges. Normal wound healing requires adequate oxygen delivery to tissues. Enhancing the oxygen supply causes more rapid accumulations of collagen, increases angiogenesis, and generally accelerates normal wound healing.

Atherosclerosis is a common cause of inadequate wound perfusion. In the diabetic patient, chronic ischemic limb in association with neuropathy is the main determinant of limb loss. The end results of poor wound perfusion are impairment of neutrophil function and decreases in collagen synthesis and cross-linking. Chronic nonhealing wounds exhibit low oxygen tension, decreased tensile strength, and increased susceptibility to infection.

Repeated trauma will interfere with healing. This is particularly true in patients with neurologic impairments, such as spinal cord injury patients or diabetics with neuropathy. Tissue pressure exceeding 32mmHg to the skin causes collapse of the capillaries and decreases blood flow[27]. The presence of foreign bodies, whether exogenous or pieces of devascularized tissue, also interferes with wound healing.

Bacterial invasion interferes with the inflammatory and proliferative phases of wound healing.

Table 4-7.   Wound Dressings

Classification	Composition	Indications	Functions	Brand names
Films	Semiocclusive (polyurethane or copolyester)	Acute partial- or full-thickness wounds Nondraining primarily closed wounds	Water vapor permeable Water and bacteria impermeable Provides moisture	Op-site Biocclusive Tegaderm Blisterfilm Visulin
Hydrocolloids	Hydrophilic colloidal matter (guar, karaya, gelatic, cellulose)	Acute, chronic partial- or full-thickness wounds Stage I and IV decubitus ulcers	Absorbs fluid Debrides soft necrotic tissue by autolysis Promotes granulation and epithelization	Cutinova hydro, J&J Ulcer dressing, Ultec, Restore, Intrasite, Duoderm
Hydrogels	80%–99% water Cross-linked polymer	Acute, chronic partial-thickness wound with minimal exudate	Moist environment Decreases pain Does not adhere to the wound	Vigilon Geliperm Elastogel Intrasite Gel
Foams	Hydrophylic or hydrophobic Nonocclusive Polyurethane or gel film-coated	Acute, chronic partial-thickness wounds that have high secretion, requiring debridement	Debrides High affinity absorbancy Water vapor permeable	Cutinova Plus Lyofoam Allevyn
Impregnates	Fine mesh gauze moistured, antibacterial, Nonadherent	Acute, chronic partial-thickness wounds with minimal/moderate exudate	Non adherent promotes epithelization; antibacterial requires secondary dressing	Aquaphor-Gauze Adaptive Biobrane Scarlet red
Absortive powders, pastes	Starch, colloidal copolymers particles	Chronic full-thickness wounds with large exudative secretion	High absorbancy Debrides necrotic and fibrous tissue from the wound	Spand-Gel Geliperm Envisan paste Bard Absorption Dressing Duoderm granules Hydrogran Hollister Exudate Absorber

Source: Adapted from [26].

Contamination is the presence of bacteria from skin or other sources within a wound. Infection causes macrophages and neutrophils to release inflammatory mediators and free radicals, leading to intense tissue destruction. The healing process is severely impaired in wounds containing more than 1 times 10^5 bacteria per gram of tissue[27].

Poor wound healing can be caused by nutritional deficiencies through hypoproteinemia and deficiencies of critical amino acids, particularly cystine, which is essential for collagen synthesis. Wound slowly gained strength in animals fed a protein-free diet for a prolonged time period. The protein depletion effect on wound healing in humans remains unknown[18,28,29]. Protein deficiencies, leading to decreases in fibroblast proliferation, collagen synthesis, and angiogenesis, are common in the nursing home population suffering from chronic wounds and decubitus ulcer. The association of vitamin deficiencies and scurvy were first documented in the sixteenth century. In 1932, vitamin C (ascorbic acid) deficiency was identified as the cause of scurvy. Vitamin C is an essential cofactor in collagen cross-linking. Vitamin A deficiency decreases the host immunity and increases susceptibility to infection. A vitamin B complex deficiencies also cause immune deficits. Zinc, iron, and copper deficiencies may result in impairment of wound healing[27], because they are required as coenzymes for metabolic pathways during collagen synthesis.

DISEASES THAT PREDISPOSE TO CHRONIC WOUNDS

DIABETES MELLITUS

Diabetic patients are susceptible to injury due to neuropathy and prolonged healing or nonhealing wounds. Wounds related to diabetic microangiopathy cause decreased tissue perfusion and lower oxygen tension. Atherosclerosis is more common in diabetics and involves the tibial vessels in the lower extremities. Atherosclerosis is the most common complication of diabetes, developing in 84% of patients diagnosed with diabetes who survive more than 20 years. Neuropathy, prevalent in 50% of diabetics after 25 years, leaves these patients more prone to injury and gait disturbances[27]. These diabetic sensory neuropathies can be devastating.

Approximately 6 million people in the United States have diabetes. Diabetes is responsible for 38,000 deaths each year. This number reaches 300,000 deaths annually when vascular complications are added. Diabetic patients are 20 times more likely to develop gangrene than nondiabetics[30–32]. Approximately 20% of all diabetics are admitted to hospitals for foot problems[33], and up to 10% of diabetics have a major amputation during their lifetime. Eighty percent of the amputations performed in the United States occur in diabetics[32,33]. The average length of stay for treatment of diabetic foot lesions, gangrene, and amputation varies from three to six weeks. The annual economic impact estimated at more than 14 billion dollars in 1989 includes medical expenses and lost time from work[30].

Immune defense mechanisms, as well as metabolic pathways involved in wound healing, are impaired in diabetics. The best treatment for diabetic patients with chronic nonhealing ulcers is prophylaxis through adequate control of their underlying disease.

CHRONIC VENOUS STASIS ULCERATION

The occurrence of chronic ulcers secondary to chronic venous disease is common. It affects 1.5% of the United States population[27]. More than 500,000 people in this country suffer from chronic venous ulcers[34]. Venous stasis ulcers are caused by chronic venous insufficiency, recanalization of deep veins with persistent deformity, and incompetence of the valves. Valvular insufficiency can be primary, secondary, or both.

The exact mechanisms that elevate venous pressure and to venous ulceration are unknown. The arteriovenous shunting theory postulates that arteriovenous fistulas in the dermis shunt blood away from areas of high venous pressure[35]. The fibrin cuff theory suggests that fibrinogen leaks out of capillaries, polymerizes around the capillaries, and acts as a barrier of oxygen diffusion[36]. Another theory suggests that white blood cells trapped in capillaries activate and release inflammatory mediators. This results in fluid and protein loss in interstitial spaces, thickening and liposclerosis of subcutaneous tissues, and tissue destruction. Whatever the mechanism, there is an increase in interstitial hydrostatic pressure along with capillary leakage of red blood cells and inflammatory white cells which produces the characteristic "brawny", nonpitting edema. When distal perforating veins become incompetent, additional pressure with progressive skin atrophy causes chronic stasis ulceration of the lower extremity.

ISCHEMIC ULCERS

Ischemic ulcers of the lower extremities are usually healed by correction of the underlying arterial occlusive disease. The most common indication for amputation in the United States is chronic arterial occlusive disease. Ischemic (dry) and infectious (wet) gangrene remain common indications for amputation especially in patients with chronic nonhealing ulcers. If restoration of arterial inflow is not possible, management is often difficult.

SMOKING

Smoking interferes with wound healing by decreasing tissue perfusion. It promotes vasoconstriction of capillary beds, binds to hemoglobin molecules and delivers CO_2 (carbon dioxide) to the wound environment instead of oxygen.

CANCER

Patients with cancer have impaired wound healing for a number of reasons. Cancer alters host metabolism in several ways: (1) glucose turnover may increase, (2) protein catabolism may accelerate, and (3) protein breakdown in muscle and hepatic utilization of amino acids increases. Vitamin C, utilized by some tumors, interferes with hydroxylation of proline and lysine residues in collagen synthesis. Patients with cancer present with cachexia, which results in either decreased caloric intake, increased energy expenditure, or both. This protein malnutrition status renders cancer patients anergic and lacking immunologic reactivity. Macrophages do not migrate or function normally. The abnormal inflammatory response and immunologic reactivity may be susceptible to severe systemic and local infection.

STEROIDS AND IMMUNOSUPPRESSION

Adrenocortical steroids hinder wound contraction and epithelization, inhibit macrophage migration and fibroblast proliferation, and decrease collagen synthesis and angiogenesis. Inflammatory cells, particularly macrophages, are affected by steroids. All aspects of steroid-induced healing impairment, except for wound contraction, can be reversed by dosages of 25,000 IU vitamin A per day[8].

RADIATION

Radiation damages the DNA of cells in exposed areas. Initially, radiation produces inflammation and desquamation of the skin in a dose-dependent fashion. Healing responses are abnormal. Fibroblasts migrate but have abnormal multiple vacuoles, irregular RERs, and degenerating mitochondria and cytoplasmic crystalline inclusion bodies. Collagen synthesis is also abnormal, and tissues become fibrotic. The media of dermal blood vessels thickens and becomes occluded. After acute inflammation subsides, the skin becomes grossly firm and is covered by a thin, fragile epidermis. Radiation tissue is also susceptible to infection. The effects of radiation seem more intense in wound-related complication rates. Vitamin A is used to reverse the side effects of irradiation on tissue. In many cases, a skin or myocutaneous flap is required in irradiated areas with wound defects to provide adequate blood supply for the wound healing process.

CONTROLLING THE HEALING AND SCARRING PROCESS

Tissue repair heals wounds and reestablishes tissue integrity quickly and effectively. On occasion, controlled healing prevents dehiscence and evisceration of an abdominal incision. Control of the rate of epithelization of open wounds can, for example, reduce mortality in burn patients and prevent fibrous stricture of the esophagus following lye burns.

Alexis Carrel noted that extracts of embryonic tissues increased the mitotic activity of cultured fibroblasts. Researchers later discovered that dried cartilage powder affects healing by producing significant increases in the breaking strength of animal and human wounds[18]. In bone remodeling, local electrical field changes appear to influence bone matrix architecture[18]. Electrical fields can direct molecular orientation in vitro; however, their influence on collagen fibers and scars remains unknown. Tension and stress also produce significant changes in scars.

Metabolic inhibitors of protein synthesis, such as puromycin and actinomycin D, decrease collagen synthesis. Providing supernormal amounts of ascorbic acid or methionine fails to accelerate gain in strength. Increase in oxygen tension stimulates healing. Hydroxylation of proline by peptidyl proline hydroxylase requires molecular oxygen, α-ketoglutarate, ascorbic acid, and ferrous iron. Ferrous iron chelators selectively inhibit the synthesis of collagen in tissue culture preparations, but no clinical data currently exist. Cells grown in a nitrogen atmosphere fail to hydroxylate procollagen, and the secretion of collagen stops.

Lathyrogens, such as β-aminopropionitrile (BAPN), inhibit intermolecular covalent cross-linking in newly synthesized collagen molecules. β-aminopropionitrile prevents the formation of lysine-derived aldehydes by inhibiting the enzyme lysyl amine oxidase. Collagen molecules are synthesized and excreted at normal rates, but the aggregated fibers fail to form cross-links. Penicillamine is a powerful copper chelator that chelates aldehydes preventing aldol condensation reactions or Schiff formation. In animals, systemic administration of BAPN and penicillamine inhibits the gain in strength in incised wounds.

Growth factors, the biological regulators of cell division and differentiation, are synthesized in pure form and in pharmacological quantities through recombinant DNA technology. In experiments on animals, growth factors are capable of reversing deficient wound healing caused by diabetes, glucocorticoids, irradiation, and chemotherapy[22]. Studies have shown that TGF-β and PDGF act as chemotactics for monocytes and fibroblasts, and FGF is a chemotactic for fibroblasts. TGF-β stimulates transcription of mRNA for procollagen and matrix proteins. Basic FGF and PDGF increase collagenase production essential for collagen remodeling. FGF is also mitogenic and chemotactic for endothelial cells in vitro, suggesting a role in neoangiogenesis. Researchers have applied EGF to open wounds in single doses without any effect in wound strength. In humans, the first clinical trials using daily applications of 5 mg EGF to the anterior abdominal wall did not improve healing.

The application of growth factors at the wound site should develop a conceptual cascade, explaining the interaction between cellular elements and messenger peptides within the healing milieu. Effective control of the healing process in humans has not been achieved. In time, manipulation of impaired healing will control scar formation and wound contraction by applying local growth factors.

The first report of successful serial subcultivation of human keratinocytes appeared in 1975[37,38]. Initial clinical use of a cultured epithelial autograft (CEAU) was reported in 1977 on burn patients[39]. Autologous epithelial cells from split-thickness skin were fractionated and cultured on an irradiated porcine dermis substrate, generating a piece of confluent epithelium that was then transplanted on the burn. This technology lacked the ability to expeditiously generate large amounts of epithelium. By 1980, human keratinocyte sheets were successfully transplanted into immunodeficient mice. This was accomplished by the addition of EGF to the culture medium. Next, the epithelial sheet (1 to 2 cell layers thick at its periphery) was separated without damage from the culture dish by using the enzyme dispase, which completely separates the graft while leaving the structure and growth potential intact. The first clinical application of cultured epithelial autograft was reported in 1981 on two severely burned patients[39,40]. In 1988, a CEAU prepared by Rheinwald and Green became commercially available (BioSurface Technology, Inc, Cambridge MA), expanding the scope and application of this therapy nationwide. Clinical studies revealed that it was possible to accelerate endogenous epidermization of partial-thickness wounds, such as leg ulcers, using topical applications of cultured allogeneic grafts (CEALs). Although CEAL are known to be immunologically rejected within a short period of time after graft placement, their brief contact is enough to stimulate re-epithelization from keratinocyte sources in the wound base and/or at the periphery of the wound. Whether applied as permanent grafts (CEAU) or as wound healing promoters (CEAL), cultured keratynocytes have been reported as treating rheumatoid ulcers. Buerger's disease, pyoderma grangrenosum, decubitus ulcers, amputation, stump ulcers, surgical degloving, and split-thickness skin graft donor sites. The CEAU can be matched by selection of donor skin with similar properties for the target recipient site, such as specialized epithelium for weight-bearing for the buttocks of bedridden patients. Long-term results indicate that a CEAU regenerates a stable normal epidermis. It also modulates healing in subadjacent connective tissues of the wound bed, which induces dermal regeneration[41].

WOUND HEALING AND THE IMMUNE SYSTEM

Wound healing is a complex cascade of biochemical and cellular events designed to restore tissue integrity and continuity following injury[42]. It is evident that cellular compartments of the immune system play a major role in regulation of phases of wound healing. The spatial and temporal interweavings of events and the way in which one biological step affects others remain unknown.

The immune system allows hosts to recognize foreign (non-self) materials including bacteria and viruses, soluble proteins, and neoplastically altered autologous cells. It consists of a cellular compartment (neutrophils, monocytes/macrophages, and lymphocytes) and a humoral component (immunoglobulins). The thymus regulates the development of T lymphocytes located in the cortex of the thymus. Migration progresses from the cortex to the medulla, and the lymphocytes differentiate into mature, immunocompetent cells. The medulla contains small mature thymocytes in the process of leaving the gland. There is evidence that suggests B lymphocyte maturation occurs within the fetal liver and bone marrow. A mature B lymphocyte does not secrete antibodies until stimulated by antigens.

T cells are classified as inducer cells, helper cells, cytotoxic cells, and suppressor cells, among others. Macrophages, fibroblasts, dendritic cells, or endothelial cells present antigen to T helper lymphocytes in association with class II MHC (major histocompatibility) antigens, causing activation and clonal expansion of the T-helper subset. These reactions are dependent upon endogenous synthesis and release of effector molecules and proteins (lymphokines and monokines).

Macrophages are the most important cells in wound healing; and thus they play a major role in the immunological events that lead to tissue repair. They become activated in the wound environment. Rappolee[43], using polymerase chain reaction and amplification, has shown that wound macrophages express mRNA for TGF-α, TGF-β and IL-1α. Leibovich and Ross[44] showed that guinea pigs treated with antimacrophage serum plus steroids had impaired wound debridement and fibroplasia. The major monokines released by activated macrophages are IL-1 and TNF-α. Macrophage secretions have also influenced in vitro fibroblast chemotaxis, proliferation, and collagen synthesis. The proliferative effects of IL-1 on fibroblasts show secondary induction of PDGF synthesis and release from fibroblasts.

In another in vivo study IL-1 enhanced collagen deposition[45].

Currently, there is little information regarding T cell activation during normal repair. Two lymphokines with significant effects on endothelial cell behavior are INF-γ and TGF-β. INF-γ has an immune modulatory effect on endothelial cells, affecting class I and II MHC antigen expression. INF-γ also acts as an inhibitor of fibroblast proliferation and collagen synthesis. TGF-β is a potent fibroblast chemotactic molecule inducing monocyte chemotaxis and secretion of fibroblast growth factors including IL-1. It is also present in large quantities in the wound environment, modulating fibroblast activity directly on monocyte function and growth factor secretion. Subcutaneous injection of TGF-β in newborn mice increased formation of granulation tissue. In vivo administration of human recombinant IL-2 in rats augmented wound breaking strengths with parallel increase in collagen deposition. Fibroblast-activating factor (FAF) has been described in humans as a product of activated T lymphocytes. Lymphokines can exert both stimulatory and inhibitory signals on all aspects of fibroblast activity.

Because monokines and lymphokines can both stimulate and inhibit fibroblast function, a fine balance must exist between them. An imbalance in the production of these factors can lead to wound healing failure. A thorough understanding of the cascade and its interrelations will provide a biochemical tool for correcting disorders of wound healing.

REFERENCES

1. Darnell, J., Lodish, H., Baltimore, D., eds.; *Molecular Cell Biology,* 2nd ed., New York: Scientific American Books, 1990:283.

2. Phillips, C., and Wenstrup, R. J., Biosynthesis and genetic disorders of collagen. In I. K. Cohen, R. F. Diegelmann, W. J. Lindblad, eds.; *Wound healing: Biochemical and Clinical Aspects.* Philadelphia: W. B. Saunders, 1992:152–176.

3. Jeffrey, J. J., Collagen degradation. In I. K. Cohen, R. F. Diegelmann, W. J. Lindblad, eds.; *Wound*

healing: Biochemical and Clinical Aspects. Philadelphia: W. B. Saunders, 1992:177–193.

4. Pick, J., *The Autonomic Nervous System,* Philadelphia: Lippincott, 1970:3–21.

5. Goss, R. J., Regeneration versus repair, In I. K. Cohen, R. F. Diegelmann, W. J. Lindblad, eds.; *Wound healing: Biochemical and Clinical Aspects,* Philadelphia: W. B. Saunders, 1992:20–39.

6. Goss, R. J., Why mammals don't regenerate or do they? *News Physiol Sci* 1987; 2:112–115.

7. Robbins, S. L., Cotran, R. S., Kumar, V., eds., *Inflammation and Repair. Pathologic Basis of Disease,* 3rd ed., Philadelphia: W. B. Saunders, 1989:39–71.

8. Peacock, J. L.; Lawrence; and Peacock, E. E., Jr., Wound healing. In J. P. O'Leary, L. R. Capote, *The Physiologic Basis of Surgery,* Baltimore, MD: Williams and Wilkins, 1993: 95–111.

9. Ausprunk, D. H.; Folkman, J., Migration and proliferation of endothelial cells in preformed and newly formed blood vessels during tumor angiogenesis; *Microvasc Res* 1977; 14:53–65.

10. Ausprunk, D. H.; Boudreau, C. L.; and Nelson, D. A., Proteoglycans in the microvasculature, II. Histochemical localization in proliferation capillaries of the rabbit cornea, *Am J Pathol* 1981; 103:367–375.

11. Nakajima, T., How soon do venous drainage channels develop at the periphery of a free flap? A study on rats. *Brit J Plast Surg* 1978; 31:300–308.

12. Tsur, H.; Danniler, A.; Strauch, B., Neovascularization of skin flaps: Route and timing. *Plast Reconst Surg* 1980; 66:85–93.

13. Whalen, G. F., Zetter, B. R., Angiogenesis, In I. K. Cohen, R. F. Diegelmann, W. J. Lindblad, eds; *Wound healing; Biochemical and Clinical Aspects.* Philadelphia: W. B. Saunders, 1992: 77–95.

14. Dvorak, H. F.; Harvey, V. S.; and Estrella, P., Fibrin containing gels induce angiogenesis. Implications for tumor stroma generation and wound healing. *Lab Invest 1987*; 57:673–686.

15. Dvorak, H. F.; Van DeWater, L.; and Bitzer, A. M., Procoagulant activity associated with plasma membrane vesicles shed by cultured tumor cells, *Cancer Res* 1983; 43:4434–4442.

16. Dvorak, H. F.; Senger, S. R.; and Dvorak, A. M., Fibrin as a component of the tumor stroma: Origins and biological significance, *Cancer Metast Rev* 1983;2:41–73.

17. Bentley, J. P., Rate of chondroitin sulfate formation in wound healing, *Ann Surg* 1967; 165:186–190.

18. Madden, J. W.; Arem, A. J., Wound healing: Biologic and clinical features, In David C. Sabiston, Jr., ed, *The Biological Basis of Modern Surgical Practice,* 14th ed., Philadelphia: W. B. Saunders, 1991: 164–177.

19. Ross, R.; Everett, N. B.; and Tyler, R., Wound healing and collagen formation, VI. The origin of wound fibroblast studied in parabiosis, *J Cell Biol* 1970; 44:645.

20. Miller, E. J. and Gay Steffen, Collagen structure and function. In I. K. Cohen, R. F. Diegelmann, W. J. Lindblad, eds; *Wound Healing: Biochemical and Clinical Aspects,* Philadelphia: W. B. Saunders, 1992: 130–151.

21. Hering, T. M.; Marchant, R. E.; Anderson, J. M., Type V collagen during granulation tissue development, *Exp Mol Pathol* 1983;39:219.

22. Kingsnorth, A. N.; Slavin, J., Peptide growth factors and wound healing, *Brit J Surg* 1991; 78:1286–1290.

23. Hunt, T. K., Prospective; a retrospective perspective on the nature of wounds. *Prog Clin Biol Res* 1988; 266:13–20.

24. Cohen, I. K.; Diegelmann, R. F., Wound healing, In L. J. Greenfield, M. W. Mulholland, K. T., Oldham, G. B., Zelenock, *Surgery: Scientific Principles and Practice,* Philadelphia: J. B. Lippincott, 1993; 86–102.

25. Gabbiani, G., The role of contractile proteins in wound healing and fibrocontractive diseases, *Methods Achiev Exp Pathol* 1979; 9:187.

26. Wiseman, D. M.; Rovee, D. T.; and Alvarez, O. M., Wound dressing: Design and use. In I. K. Cohen, R. F. Diegelmann, W. J. Lindblad, eds; *Wound healing: Biochemical and Clinical Aspects,* Philadelphia: W. B. Saunders, 1992:562–580.

27. Weingarten, M. S., Obstacles to wound healing. *Wounds* 1993; 5(5):238–244.

28. Irvin, T. T., Effects of malnutrition and hyperalimentation on wound healing. *Surg Gynecol Obstet* 1978; 146:33.

29. Levenson, S. M., and Seifter, E., Dysnutrition, wound healing and resistance to infection, *Clin Plast Surg* 1977; 4:375.

30. National Diabetes Data Group, *Diabetes in America,* Diabetes data compiled 1984. U.S. De-

partment of Health and Human Services, NIH Publication NO. 85-1468.

31. Davidson, M. B., preface to *Diabetes Mellitus: Diagnosis and Treatment,* New York: John Wiley & Sons, 1981:v.

32. Rosenberg, L., In L. J. Greenfield, M. W. Mulholland, K. T., Oldham, G. B., Zelenock, *Surgery: Scientific Principles and Practice,* Philadelphia: J. B. Lippincott, 1993; 559–571.

33. Levin, M. E., and O'Neal, L. W., preface to *The Diabetic Foot,* 3rd ed., St. Louis, Mosby, 1983:xi.

34. Greenfield, L. J., Chronic venous insufficiency, In L. J. Greenfield, M. W. Mulholland, K. T., Oldham, G. B. Zelenock, *Surgery: Scientific Principles and Practice,* Philadelphia: J.B. Lippincott, 1993:1778–1784.

35. Ryan, T. J., and Copeman, P. M. W., Microvascular patterns and blood stasis in skin disease, *Brit J Dermatol* 1970; 8:563.

36. Browse, N. L.; Burnand, K. G., The cause of venous ulceration, *Lancet* 1982; 2:243–245.

37. Comptom, C. C., Wound healing potential of cultured epithelium, *Wounds* 1993; 5(2): 97–111.

38. Rheinwald, J. G.; Green, H., Serial cultivation of strains of human epidermal keratinocytes: The formation of keratinizing colonies from single cells, *Cell* 1975; 6:331–343.

39. McAree, K. G.; Klein, R. L.; and Boeckman, C. R., The use of cultured epithelial autographs in the wound care of severely burned patients, *J Pediatr Surg* 1993; 28(2): 166–168.

40. O'Conner, N.; Mulliken, J.; and Banks-Schlegel, S., Grafting of burns with cultured epithelium prepared from autologous epidermal cells, *Lancet* 1981; 1:75–78.

41. Compton, C. C., Current concepts in pediatric burn care: The biology of cultured epithelial autographs: An eight-year study in pediatric burn patients, *Eur J Pediatr Surg* 1992; 2:216–222.

42. Barbul, A., Immune aspects of wound repair, *Clin Plast Surg* 1990; 17 (3):433–441.

43. Rappolee, D. A.; Mark, D.; Banda, M. J., et al., Wound macrophages express TGF-α and other growth factors in vivo: Analysis by mRNA phenotyping. *Science* 1988; 241: 708–712.

44. Leibovich, S. J., and Ross, R., The role of the macrophage in wound repair. A study with hydrocortisone and antimacrophage serum, *Am J Pathol* 1975; 78:71–91.

45. Barbul, A., Role of the immune system, In I. K. Cohen, R. F. Diegelmann, W. J. Lindblad, eds; *Wound healing: Biochemical and Clinical Aspects,* Philadelphia: W. B. Saunders, 1992:282–291.

5

TOPICAL THERAPY OF CUTANEOUS ULCERS AND WOUNDS

James T. Evans, M.D.

TOPICAL THERAPY OF CUTANEOUS ULCERS AND WOUNDS

The selection of the appropriate topical therapy for cutaneous ulcers is dependent upon proper assessment of the lesion and the patient. The major areas of clinical concern are etiology, overall patient condition, lesion stage and status, and prior treatment of the lesion. The current emphasis on cost-effective therapy also impacts the clinician's therapeutic choices. The most commonly utilized aspects of topical therapy are (1) debridement, (2) cleansing, (3) dressing selection and application, and (4) adjunctive therapies.

CLASSIFICATION OF WOUNDS

LEVEL OF TISSUE INJURY

All wounds are visible evidence of disruption of the skin and underlying blood supply with or without associated injury of deeper underlying structures such as fascia, muscle, and bone. All wounds begin with an acute event, i.e., surgical incision, burn, trauma, prolonged pressure, or acute disease event. Following the acute event, the wound will be either open or closed. Many clinicians have traditionally utilized a classification that combines the type of wound closure with a proposed mechanism of repair. This classification is described in the following paragraphs.

Classic Wound Classification

The classification is as follows:

(a) **Primary intention.** The wound edges are held together by sutures, staples, tapes, dressings, etc., placed shortly after wounding. The mechanism of repair involves mainly connective tissue repair with minimal epithelization.

(b) **Secondary intention.** This type of wound is not closed mechanically but allowed to remain open. The mechanism of repair is by the process of contraction and epithelization.

(c) **Delayed primary intention.** The wound is left open following the wounding; after a delay to assure minimal bacterial presence in the wound depth, the wound is closed with sutures, staples, tapes, or dressings.

(d) **Partial thickness healing.** For wounds requiring only epithelization, such as burns. Residual epithelial cells, especially those from skin appendages and wound margins, migrate, proliferate, and resurface the skin.

Classification By Color

Another wound classification system used by many clinicians is the color code system: (1) red, (2) yellow, (3) black. This has generally been used for wounds healing by second intention. Red is used to describe wounds with healing red granulation tissue with associated epithelization. Yellow is used to describe a wound with exudate and bacterial contamination or infection. Black is used to describe wounds with necrotic tissue. The system has been expanded to a five level system by some clinicians with the use of combinations, i.e., (1) red, (2) red/yellow, (3) yellow, (4) yellow/black, (5) black. The color (red = best, black = worst) representative of wound status is used for therapy decision making.

"CHRONIC" ULCERATIVE WOUNDS

The term "chronic" has been misapplied to wounds. The proper reference terms are healed, healing, and nonhealing. The real problem is to determine when a wound is nonhealing especially as there are some wounds that are very slow healing. Only accurate assessment and measurement will decide if a wound is chronic or nonhealing. Generally, any wound treated with acceptable therapy for three or four weeks with no change in wound characteristics (less exudate, more granulation, etc.) or wound size (utilizing measurement or photography) can be said to be nonhealing. The objective of wound therapy is to provide an environment conducive to healing.

INFECTION AND WOUNDS

Normal intact human skin has a relatively constant environment of bacteria present on the surface. When there is a break in the normal skin barrier, the normal skin bacteria move into and colonize the wound. When wound conditions support of higher levels of bacteria growth, the wound is defined as contaminated. When the level of bacteria becomes very high (greater than 100,000 CFU/g of tissue) and invades the tissue, the wound is said to be infected. Only quantitative tissue microbiological testing from a wound biopsy can definitively estab-

lish the extent of wound bacterial contamination. Wound swabs for bacterial culture are a worthless expense. The use of cultures from needle aspirates have been advocated by some, but this method is not really useful for ulcerative lesions. Clinical signs have been thought to be associated with wound infection. Local signs include erythema, edema, induration, purulent or malodorous drainage, pain, crepitance. Systemic signs include fever and leukocytosis. Wounds treated with moist wound healing methods have been reported to have a lower incidence of wound infections. There is ample data that all open wounds are colonized with bacteria. This wound colonization is the reason that clinicians utilize microbial wound cleansers and silver sulfadiazine cream 1% in wound therapy.

WOUND THERAPY

When a patient presents with a cutaneous ulcer containing necrotic tissue, the initial therapy is debridement. The presence of necrotic, nonviable tissue is associated with an increased bacterial burden. This necrotic tissue and bacteria must be removed to allow the patient's defense system to combat infection. Healing epithelial tissue is delicate and must be treated gently. Healthy granulation tissue should not be debrided.

DEBRIDEMENT

The timing of debridement is relatively noncontroversial; it should be done as soon as the presence of necrotic tissue is identified. Debridement is performed to reduce the volume of tissue that will support bacterial growth; a retardant of healing. There has been some controversy surrounding the method of debridement. The literature most often mentions sharp, mechanical, enzymatic, and autolytic methods [Bergstrom, 1994]. When a patient presents with a cutaneous wound requiring urgent debridement, the preferred method is LASER scalpel or sharp scalpel debridement. The presence of cellulitis and/or sepsis are widely accepted indications for sharp debridement. Sharp debridement should be performed by a surgeon skilled in such techniques. Small wounds and those with diminished sensation may be debrided at the bedside when proper instruments and lighting are available. Extensive ulcers, including most stage III or IV pressure ulcers require debridement in the operating room. If contiguous osteomyelitis is suspected then a concurrent bone biopsy should be performed. Bone scans are an inadequate method for establishing the diagnosis of osteomyelitis and only add unnecessary expense. Adequate analgesia for pain control for patients with wounds is the standard of patient care.

The term mechanical debridement has been assigned to the following methods: (a) the use of wet to dry dressings at fixed intervals, (b) hydrotherapy, (c) high pressure, wound irrigation, (d) topical dextranomers. There are no well performed random studies of the benefits, risks, efficacy, or cost of any of the forms of mechanical debridement. The use of mechanical debridement relies on expert opinion and empirically demonstrated efficacy. Wet-to-dry dressings adhere to devitalized tissue which is forcibly removed with the dressing removal. The disadvantages of using wet-to-dry dressing are that it is (a) labor intensive, (b) nonselective and injures some vital tissue, (c) painful for the patients, often requiring analgesia. Hydrotherapy is really only useful for extremity lesions in ambulatory patients.

There is no reason to use enzymatic preparations for wound debridement, especially when considering the excessive cost of these agents. The enzymatic agents are ineffective at the usual wound pH. Similarly, the use of dextranomers (absorptive beads) is expensive and time consuming. The method of mechanical debridement reserved for those lacking access to sharp debridement is autolytic.

Autolytic debridement is the process of optimization of the wound environment for the liquification of the necrotic debris. This is achieved by selecting the proper dressings. Generally, a transparent adhesive film dressing is sufficient for autolysis of necrotic debris. Some available transparent films are:

Acu-derm	(Acme United Corp.)
Bioclusive	(Johnson & Johnson)
Blister Film	(Sherwood Medical)
Opsite	(Smith & Nephew)
Polyskin	(Kendall)
Tegaderm	(3M Health Care)

WOUND CLEANSING

The general principles of wound therapy include the cleansing of wounds at the appropriate interval. The usual times are as follows: (a) at the time of initial assessment and therapy, (b) after debridement, (c) at each dressing change. The traditional method of wound cleansing is to use normal saline delivered using a 30–60ml syringe and 19 gage needle. Recent reevaluation of this method has shown it to be more expensive and time consuming than the use of specifically formulated wound cleansers. Additionally, some clinicians prefer commercial wound cleansers containing microbial and surfactant ingredients. Some available wound cleansers are:

Micro-Klenz	(Carrington)
Puri-Clens	(Sween Corporation)
Septicare	(Sage Laboratories)
Techni-Care	(Care-Tech Laboratories)

TYPES OF WOUNDS PRESENTING AS CUTANEOUS ULCERS

VASCULAR

Venous Stasis Ulcers

The lower extremity venous stasis ulcer is the dominant venous lesion seen by wound therapy specialists. Approximately 1% of Western countries' populations are affected. Most venous stasis ulcers follow deep venous thrombosis with valve destruction. A second cause is communicating (perforator) vein incompetence, a result of congenital vein wall weakness or valve destruction from thrombosis. Both result in lower extremity venous hypertension, which must be controlled, along with the topical therapy that is applied. Each patient's venous insufficiency should be graded [Committee, 1988]. Most patients with stasis ulcers have grade

3 chronic venous insufficiency, but are ambulatory or in a wheelchair.

Guidelines for clinical management of venous stasis ulcers

(a) General evaluation
1. Review of all available old medical records
2. Complete patient history
3. Physical exam with full nutritional assessment
4. Careful exam of extremity pulses

(b) Vascular studies
1. Arterial Doppler for ankle/brachial ratio to rule out combined arterial-venous disease
2. Plethysmography
3. Duplex scan to evaluate venous system

(c) General treatments
1. Diet
   a. Weight reduction for obese patients is very important
   b. Adequate calories with vitamin supplements for most patients
   c. Special diets as needed [Lidowski, 1988]
2. Pharmacologic agents
   Pentoxifylline 400 mg p.o.t.i.d [Colgan, 1990, Evans, 1993]
3. Physical therapy
   a. upper and lower extremity muscle strength training
   b. crutch walking if needed
   c. Non-thermal Pulsed Electromagnetic Energy treatment daily for 30 minutes
4. Patient education
   a. Instructions regarding avoiding trauma
   b. Post healing compression therapy: stockings, pneumatic compression devices

(d) Surgical treatments
1. Linton Procedure: subfascial ligation of incompetent perforators, stripping of greater and lesser saphenous venous systems, excision of all visible varicosities, a full posterior fasciotomy, and excision of the ulcer with skin grafting [Cranley, 1961].
2. Perforator ligation: ligation of all mapped-out perforators to reduce the high venous pressure

3. Ulcer excision with skin graft
4. Ulcer excision with muscle transposition and skin graft

(e) Compression therapy

External compression is the most effective therapy to treat the underlying venous hypertension. Sufficient compression must be used to control the swelling. The compression therapy is accomplished by dressing therapy to the ulcer and surrounding skin accompanied by elastic wrappings, stockings, or pneumatic compression. The venous ulcer is treated with direct nonadherent dressing and pressure. The rationale for direct ulcer compression is that it disperses local edema, compresses the feeding veins, and levels the edges of the ulcer to facilitate epithelization. There is a clear relationship between a reduction in edema and healing [Myers, 1972]. The classic therapy is Unna's boot (a two layer system). The dressing to which his name is attached was described by Dr. Paul Gerson Unna in the late 1800s. Unna's boot consists of zinc-impregnated gauze wrapped from toe to knee with an elastic wrap applied over the zinc oxide treated gauze. The dressing is changed weekly in an outpatient or home care setting and at the time of dressing change, the wound and surrounding skin are thoroughly cleansed using a microbicidal agent. Silver sulfadiazine cream 1% is then applied to the ulcer and surrounding skin. Subsequently Unna's boot is applied. Additionally, the patient is urged to elevate the legs above the heart as much as possible during the day and at night. There are multiple variations of this basic Unna's boot including:

1. Impregnated gauze bandages; applied directly to the ulcer and skin.

a.	Dome Paste	(Miles)
b.	Gelocast Unna Boot	(Beiersdorf)
c.	Medicopaste Unna Boot	(WTS)
d.	Viscopaste	(Smith & Nephew)

2. Elastic compressive wraps; applied over the gauze bandage.

a.	ACE bandage	
b.	Coban	(3M)
c.	Elastoplast	(Beiersdorf)

d. Setopress   (Acme United)
e. Tubigrip   (Acme United)

More recently, numerous bandaging systems have been introduced which claim improved compression without the need for paste [Duby, 1993]. An example of the four layer bandage system is Profore by Smith & Nephew. Another non-paste venous ulcer compression system is a contact dressing such as Allevyn foam (Smith & Nephew) or Lyofoam (Acme United) covered by Tubigrip (Acme United Co.) and compression applied with Setopress (Acme United Co.).

When epithelization is complete, compression gradient stockings are required as daily therapy. This may be supplemented by external pneumatic compression. Patients with postphlebitic syndrome and venous stasis ulcers require lifelong follow-up therapy.

Arterial Ulcers

The etiology of ulcers associated with inadequate arterial perfusion is tissue trauma superimposed on the insufficient blood supply. The ankle/brachial index (ABI) will confirm the diagnosis and predict the patient's ability to heal. The ABI is obtained by dividing the ankle systolic pressure by the brachial systolic pressure ABI. The normal is 1.0 or greater. Patients with an ABI of 0.45 or less will generally not heal without revascularization. Patients with an ABI in the 0.5 to 0.75 range with or without revascularization will usually heal. Pentoxifylline is definitely indicated in these patients. The most effective therapy is surgery for revascularization of extremities with arterial ulcers. Common procedures include aorto-bifemoral, femoro-popliteal bypass, and distal bypass to dorsalis pedis or posterior tibial arteries. These latter two procedures are best performed as in-situ venous bypass. Every patient requires a full vascular study workup. The characteristics of arterial ulcers include moderate pain relieved by dependent leg position, minimal exudate, dry necrotic tissue, and shallow depth. The ulcers are irregular in shape and present almost anywhere, including the dorsum of the foot. The periulcer tissue is shiny, tight, and purpuric.

Guidelines for clinical management of arterial ulcers

(a) General therapy
All underlying disease conditions must be treated.
(b) Pharmacologic therapy
Pentoxifylline 400 mg. p.o.q.i.d. [Cherry, 1991]
(c) Patient education
1. counseling on smoking cessation
2. local foot care and proper shoe selection
(d) Wound therapy
1. Debridement
If necrotic tissue is present then debridement is needed. Autolytic debridement is usually sufficient due to the shallow depth of these ulcers.
2. Post autolytic debridement, several types of dressing may be used to achieve healing in arterial ulcers.
   a. Transparent adhesive film dressing (as in debridement section)
   b. Hydrocolloid or hydrogel wafer dressings
1. Elasto-Gel   (South West Technologies)
2. Replicare   (Smith & Nephew)
3. J&J Ulcer Dressing (Johnson & Johnson)
4. PanoGauze   (Sage Laboratories)
   c. Semipermeable foam dressings
1. Allevyn   (Smith & Nephew)
2. Cutinova   (Biersdorf)
3. Epigard   (Becton Dickinson)
4. Lyofoam   (Acme United)
5. Polymcm   (Ferris Corp.)

The author's personal preference is a semipermeable foam dressing. The patient's wound is followed until reepithelization occurs. If the wound develops a clean granulating base and shows little epithelization, then a skin graft may prove useful to achieve closure. If there are any signs of infection, systemic antibiotic therapy should be instituted promptly as arterial ulcers have little local tissue resistance. Some clinicians would add topical therapy such as silver sulfadiazine cream 1% or Iodosorb Gel (an iodophor containing topical wound therapy) distributed by Healthpoint Medical. Alternatively, some clinicians would use an antimicrobial cleanser such as those listed under the wound cleansing section combined with more frequent dressing changes.

Combined Arterial and Venous Ulcers

Some patients have both long-standing postphlebitic and arterial vascular insufficiency ulcers. These patients represent the most difficult challenge of wound care. If possible, these patients should undergo arterial revascularization for limb salvage. Subsequently, the venous ulcer guidelines should be used.

DIABETIC LESIONS

The frequency of morbidity and mortality in patients with diabetic ulcers is directly related to the pathophysiology of the disease. The most prominent etiologic factors of diabetic ulcers are neuropathy and ischemic vascular disease. Diabetics experience a neuropathy that affects the motor, sensory, and autonomic peripheral nerves. This leads to intrinsic changes in foot anatomy with distinctive pressure point deformities. Loss of sensation in the diabetic foot masks the response to minor trauma. Ulcers in the plantar region result from the deformed anatomy and nonfitting shoes. The altered gait and decreased fat pad lead to callous formation and eventual ulcer. Frequent sites for ulcers are submetatarsal head, distal digits, medial second and fifth metatarsal head, and the first metatarsophalangeal joint space. The characteristics of diabetic vascular disease remain controversial; however, LoGerfo and associates [LoGerfo, 1984] present a convincing argument that vascular reconstructive surgery should be done in diabetics. Additionally, diabetics can be spared amputations by the use of local reconstructive surgery, especially muscle transposition [Ger, 1985]. When the underlying diabetes and vascular disease have been treated, then local wound care for diabetic ulcers is successful.

Guidelines for Diabetic Ulcer Treatment

(a) Evaluation
  1. photograph for size, character, etc.
  2. grade of ulcer
  3. size
  4. appearance of ulcer base
  5. periwound skin condition
  6. evaluation for tracts, sinuses, and underlying osteomyelitis

(b) Treatment
  1. daily foot care, inspection, ointments
  2. orthotic devices to relieve pressure
  3. crutches for non-weight bearing
  4. Dressings
     Because of the predominance of ulcers in weight bearing areas many dressings are not useful. Preferred dressings are as follows:
     a. Unna's boot without elastic wrap
     b. Contact casts. These should be applied by those specially trained as they are different from standard fracture-type casts. Patient compliance is high because weight bearing is not a problem.
     c. conformable foam dressing (as listed under arterial)
  5. Adjunctive treatments
     a. Hyperbaric oxygen therapy
     b. Non-thermal Pulsed Electromagnetic Energy

PROBLEM SURGICAL WOUNDS

The surgeon or wound care specialist is often confronted with complex problem wounds including a) traumatic wounds with tissue loss, b) post-trauma and post-operative wounds which are infected, c) nosocomial pressure wounds in immunocompromised patients.

TRAUMATIC WOUNDS

Patients sometimes sustain traumatic wounds with accompanying tissue loss. Frequently, their associated injuries prohibit surgical closure. These wounds may be treated openly utilizing topical dressings. For most traumatic wounds, the dressings of choice are hydrogels which are easy to use for irregular wounds. The secondary dressing of choice is a transparent film dressing. For heavily exudating wounds a foam dressing may be utilized.

ABDOMINAL WOUNDS

Occasionally, patients undergoing abdominal surgeries may develop infected or dehised wounds. Often these wounds are large, irregular and cavitary. These wounds may be managed effectively using several regimens designed to fill the cavity and absorb the exudate; including hydrogel combined with a secondary transparent film dressing or impregnated gauzes combined with a transparent film dressing.

Examples of Hydrogels:

a. Cavity Wound Gel   (Carrington Laboratories)
b. Intrasite Gel   (Smith & Nephew)
c. NU-Gel   (Johnson & Johnson)
d. Panoplex   (Sage Laboratories)
e. Inerpan   (Sherwood)
f. Hypergel   (Scott Health Care)
g. Royl-Derm Hydrogel   (Acme United)
h. MPM Hydrogel   (MPM Medical)
i. Iamin Hydrating Gel (Procyte Corp.)

Examples of Impregnated Gauzes

a. Aquafor   (Beiersdorf)
b. Carrington Wound   (Carrington)
c. Dermagran   (Dermasciences)
d. Mesalt   (Scott Healthcare)
e. Scarlet Red   (Sherwood)
f. Xeroform   (Sherwood)

The secondary dressing which is most often used is a transparent film.

Groin Wounds

The possibility of a nonhealing groin wound follows aorto-femoral and femoro-popliteal bypass surgery. The development of postoperative bleeding or drainage can lead to morbidity or even mortality. The most important element in the management of these wounds is the assessment. The critical determination to be made is whether graft material is exposed. If graft material is exposed, then immediate reoperation and coverage with protective tissue is necessary. Otherwise, local wound therapy is indicated. The same dressing utilization as outlined for abdominal wounds is appropriate.

Pressure Ulcers

The occurrence of pressure ulcers is significant enough to require the attention of all health care professionals. The United States government Agency for Health Care Policy and Research has developed a Clinical Practice Guideline for Prediction and Prevention (AHCPR, 1992) as well as a therapy guideline (Bergstrom, 1994). A full and complete understanding of the etiology of pressure ulcers is still lacking. However, risk factors are well known (Abruzzese, 1985), assessment tools are available (Braden, 1989), management programs are described (Lidowski, 1988), and multiple surgical procedures are described for treatment (Lee, 1985; Wellisz, 1993). When an ulcer has developed, the shift in focus is towards treatment. However, a diligent program for the prevention of a second lesion should also assume a very high priority, especially in the patient with a projected prolonged institutional course. The three components of the treatment protocol become pressure relief, nutritional support, and topical wound therapy. Clinical experience has shown that optimal surgical and nursing care will not result in healing of pressure ulcers if the patient lacks sufficient nutritional support.

Ulcer Assessment

Pressure ulcers are graded as follows: "Stage I pressure ulcers are defined as nonblanchable erythema of intact skin—the heralding lesion of skin ulceration (reactive hyperemia should not be confused with Stage I pressure ulcers). Stage II is defined as partial thickness loss involving epidermis and/or dermis; Stage III as full thickness loss involving damage or necrosis of subcutaneous tissue that may extend down to, but not through, underlying fascia; and Stage IV as full thickness loss with extensive destruction, tissue necrosis or damage to muscle, bone, or supporting structures." [AHCPR, 1992].

Nutrition Assessment

Each patient with a pressure ulcer requires a nutritional assessment. A simple and useful method for nutritional assessment is the following 7-point checklist.

7-Point Nutritional Risk Assessment

1. Physical examination;   YES NO
    malnourished or obese
2. History of weight change   YES NO
3. Anemia   YES NO
4. Low total lymphocyte count   YES NO
5. Decreased serum albumin   YES NO
6. Decreased total protein   YES NO
7. Hypocholesterolemia   YES NO

A score of three yes answers is highly suggestive of malnutrition. The tests are done serially to reduce cost. Thus a history, physical, and complete blood count will often suffice to make the diagnosis of malnutrition. A well designed feeding plan should be developed based upon calculation of energy and protein requirements.

Guidelines for Therapy of Pressure Ulcers

Stage I   The treatment objectives are wound protection and provision of a moist wound healing environment. The wound dressing of choice for Stage I ulcers is a transparent film dressing, as listed in the section on debridement. These dressings are changed every two or five days. The surrounding skin is treated with a skin lubricant.

Stage II   The treatment objectives are to provide protection and provide a moist wound healing environment. The dressing of choice is a transparent film (as above); this may require more frequent changes if fluid leaks out. For Stage II pressure ulcers with significant drainage, the dressing of choice is a foam dressing—see product listing under arterial ulcers.

Stage III   The treatment objectives are protection, absorption, and moist wound healing. The dressing category of choice for wounds with moderate exudate is a foam dressing; examples are as previously listed. The second category of acceptable dressings, especially for wounds with minimal exudate, are the hydrogel dressings—see product listing under abdominal wounds. These dressings are changed every three to five days.

Stage IV   The treatment objectives of these wounds are protection, hydration, absorption, and proper moist wound healing environment. The wound dressing of choice for these Stage 4 pressure ulcers with exudate are the hydrogels as listed under abdominal wounds. These dressings require a secondary transparent film dressing. Another alternative for these wounds, especially those with heavy exudate, is a foam cavity dressing such as Allevyn (Smith & Nephew).

Debridement   The principles of debridement outlined earlier apply. The preferred methods are laser, scalpel, autolytic in that order. In infected wounds needing urgent debridement, scalpel debridement is used. For Stage IV pressure ulcers over tendon or bone with dry eschar, many clinicians will elect to avoid debridement. This has sometimes been accompanied with success and maximal tissue preservation.

Adjunctive therapy   The most useful adjunctive treatment in the author's opinion for pressure ulcers is non-thermal pulsed electromagnetic energy [Itoh, 1991]. The usual treatment is twice daily initially, then daily.

CONCLUSIONS

Careful assessment of the wound and the patient nutritional status, matched with proper therapy, will usually result in healing [Rolstad, 1991]. For those pressure ulcers that do not heal or have unusual circumstances, surgical flap coverage is often successful [Lee, 1991].

CHAPTER SUMMARY

This chapter has attempted to provide the reader with both general and specific guidelines for dressing selection. This area remains a constant challenge due to the advances in dressing technology and the ever dynamic status of wounds. Proper dressing selection follows only after accurate wound assessment and an estimate of the progress of healing. The most important factors in healing are minimizing bacteria and maintaining a moist healing environment.

REFERENCES

1. Bergstrom, N; Bennett, M. A.; Carlson, C. E.; et al., *Treatment of Pressure Ulcers,* Clinical Practice Guideline, no. 15, Rockville, MD: U.S. Department of Health and Human Services, Public Health Service, Agency for Health Care Policy and Research, AHCPR Publication No. 95-0652, December 1994.

2. *Reporting Standards in Venous Disease,* A report

of the ad hoc committee on venous standards, *J Vasc Surg* 1988; 8:172–181.

3. Lidowski, H., NAMP: A system for preventing and managing pressure ulcers, *Decubitus* 1988; 1(2): 28–37.

4. Colgan, M. P.; Dormandy, J. A.; Jones, P. W.; Schraibman, I. G.; Shanik, D. G.; and Young, R. A., Pentoxifylline treatment of venous ulcers of the leg, *Brith Med J* 1990; 300:972–975.

5. Evans, J. T.; Ger, R.; Badrinath, P.; and Calle, S., A meta-analysis of pentoxifylline treatment of leg ulcers, *Second Annual Wound Care Symposium,* Richmond, VA, 1993, (abstract), p. 136.

6. Cranley, J. J.; Krause, R. J.; and Strasser, E. S., Chronic venous insufficiency of the lower extremity, *Surgery* 1961; 49(1): 48–58.

7. Myers, M. B.; Rightor, M.; and Cherry, G., Relationship between edema and healing rate of stasis ulcers of the leg, *Am J Surg* 1972; 124:662–668.

8. Cherry, G. W.; Ryan, T. J.; and Cameron, J., Blueprint for the treatment of leg ulcers and the prevention of recurrence, *Wounds* 1991; 3(1): 1–15.

9. Logerfo, F. W., and Cottman, J. D., Vascular and microvascular disease of the foot in diabetes. Implications for foot care, *N Engl J Med* 1984; 311:1615–1619.

10. Ger, R., Prevention of major amputations in the diabetic patient, *Arch Surg* 1985; 120:1317–1320.

11. Panel for the Prediction and Prevention of Pressure Ulcers in Adults, *Pressure Ulcers in Adults: Prediction and Prevention.* Clinical Practice Guideline, no. 3, AHCPR Publication no. 92-0047, Rockville, MD: Agency for Health Care Policy and Research, Public Health Service, U.S. Department of Health and Human Services, May 1992.

12. Abruzzese, R. S., Early assessment and prevention of pressure sores, In B. Y. Lee, ed., *Chronic Ulcers of the Skin,* New York: McGraw-Hill, 1985:1–19.

13. Braden, B. J., Clinical utility of the Braden scale for predicting pressure sore risk, *Decubitus* 1989; 2(3):44–46, 50–51.

14. Lee, B. Y., and Thoden, W. R., Surgical management of pressure sores, In B. Y. Lee, ed., *Chronic Ulcers of the Skin,* New York: McGraw-Hill, 1985:147–170.

15. Wellisz, T.; Rubayi, S.; and Sherman, R., Management of pressure sores, *Surgical Rounds* 1993; 16(10): 755–764.

16. Fowler, E., and Papen, J. C., Evaluation of an alginate dressing for pressure ulcers, *Decubitus* 1991; 4(3):47–53.

17. Itoh, M.; Montemayor, J. S.; Matsumoto, E., Eason, A.; Lee, M. H. M.; and Folk, F. S., Accelerated wound healing of pressure ulcers by high peak power electromagnetic energy (diapulse), *Decubitus* 1991; 4(1): 24–25, 29–34.

18. Rolstad, B. S., Treatment objectives in chronic wound care, *Home Healthcare Nurse* 1991; 9(6):38–44.

19. Lee, B. Y., Plastic surgery for pressure sores, In B. Y. Lee, L. E. Ostrander, C. V. B. Cochran, W. W. Shaw, eds., *The Spinal Cord Injured Patient,* Philadelphia: W.B. Saunders, Co., 1991:223–230.

6

THE ROLE OF NUTRITION IN THE MANAGEMENT OF PRESSURE SORES

Nanakram Agarwal, M.D.

MALNUTRITION AND PRESSURE SORES

Malnutrition is an important factor, second only to excessive pressure, in the etiology, pathogenesis, and nonhealing of pressure sores. Nearly 150 years ago, Graves [1] wrote that "Want of a sufficiency of food or food of an unwholesome or an improper character predisposes the human frame to disease by its debilitating effects on the system." In 1930 Joseph [2] used insulin in the treatment of nondiabetic bedsores and noticed uniformly satisfactory results in the improvement of the general condition of the patient. In 1939 Robertson and Tisdall [1] demonstrated experimentally in rats that lack of almost any one of the 32 food elements essential for animal nutrition resulted in lowered resistance to infection. In 1941 McCormick [3] postulated that bedsores were caused by avitaminosis B. In 1943 Mulholland et al. [4] found that the extent and depth of the ulcers, as well as their multiplicity, were related to the level of hypoproteinemia. Ulcers failed to heal with a high-calorie and low-nitrogen diet, but signs of healing occurred on the fourth day and the ulcers healed rapidly after the nitrogen balance was made positive. Mulholland et al. postulated that protein malnutrition is important, as it results in tissues of "a changed character" that are

more vulnerable to tissue necrosis with smaller amounts of pressure, or the same amount of pressure for shorter periods of time.

Since then, several retrospective, cross-sectional, and prospective studies have shown that there exists a strong association between protein calorie malnutrition and pressure ulcers [5]. Of these, prospective studies in high-risk patients who are initially free of pressure ulcers provide the strongest evidence that malnutrition is a major risk factor in the development of pressure ulcers. In patients admitted to long-term geriatric wards [6] and chronic care hospitals [7], or those newly admitted to elderly nursing homes [8], it was found that patients who developed pressure ulcers had impaired nutritional intake, specifically dietary intake of protein, compared to patients without pressure sores. The recent clinical practice guidelines for the prediction and prevention of pressure ulcers in adults developed by the Agency for Health Care Policy and Research (AHCPR) [9] also emphasize the role of malnutrition as a risk factor in the multifactorial etiology of pressure ulcers (Figure 6-1).

Experimental studies have clearly demonstrated the detrimental effects of malnutrition on promoting the development and nonhealing of pressure ulcers. Mecray et al. [10], while studying the effect of hypoproteinemia on gastric emptying time in

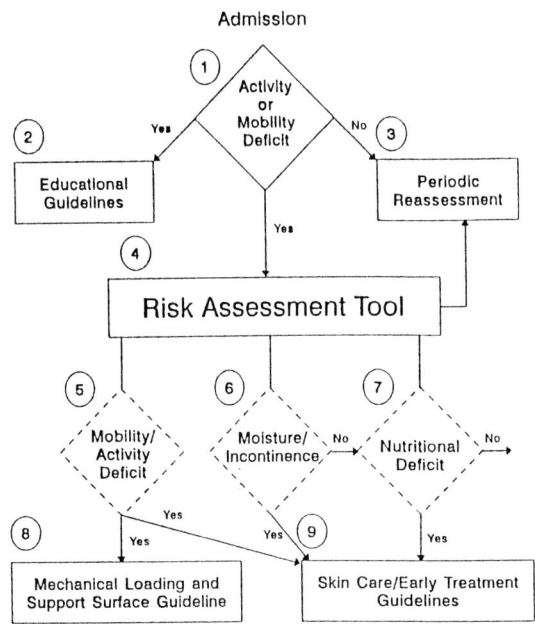

Admission

Figure 6-1. Role of malnutrition as risk factor in the multifactorial etiology of pressure ulcers. (Adapted from AHCPR [9].)

an experimental study in dogs, observed that all experimental animals rendered definitely hypoproteinemic developed ulcers over their forelegs and ankles. These ulcers increased in size as the protein intake was further reduced and healed rapidly as the protein intake was increased.

Recently, Takeda et al. [11] experimentally induced pressure sores by exposing the skin of normally fed and malnourished (no food, only water ad libitum for 20 days) rabbits to a balloon-produced compressive force of 120±10 mm Hg for four hours. Biopsies of skin were taken one, two, and three days after the pressure application. Malnourished rabbits who had a weight loss of approximately 30% exhibited significantly greater ischemic skin destruction on day 1. On day 2, normally fed rabbits demonstrated signs of healing as evidenced by proliferation of fibroblasts and macrophage infiltration, whereas signs of collagen fiber degeneration as well as microthrombi were seen in malnourished rabbits. On day 3, whereas the damaged epidermis was replaced by new epidermal cells in normal animals, massive necrosis of the epidermis was still recognized in the malnourished rabbits. Furthermore, im-

munocytological studies clearly indicated remarkable proliferation of epidermal cells after pressure-induced injury under normal nutritional conditions and significantly reduced proliferation in the presence of malnutrition.

The presence of decubitus ulcers results in a further deleterious metabolic drain in the already debilitated patient. Albumin elimination rates have been demonstrated to be significantly increased in paraplegics when compared to normal controls [12], and open wounds accentuate additional large protein losses [13]. Mulholland et al. [4] observed that discharge from an extensive ulcer contained 393 mg of nitrogen, corresponding to almost 5.56 g of protein, and losses up to 30 g of protein or more daily can occur through large open wounds.

The ulcer also causes considerable morbidity and mortality. Acting as a persistent source of inflammation or serving as an uncontrolled septic focus when infected, it can trigger the systematic inflammatory response syndrome (SIRS) and the multiple organ dysfunction syndrome (MODS). Although the cause of SIRS/MODS is complex and not fully understood at present, the release of multiple circulating mediators from the ulcer and stimulated macrophages are important components [14].

NUTRITION AND HEALING

Wound healing is a series of complex physiochemical interactions that require macronutrients and various micronutrients (Figure 6-2) at every step [15]. As defined by Moore [16] in 1959, the wound has a high biological priority for available nutrients. The metabolic response to injury or infection characterized by gluconeogenesis, lipolysis, and skeletal muscle proteolysis enriches the substrate pool available to the wound. In essence, the net balance in the wound, although positive, is negative overall, particularly in the muscle (Figure 6-3). Thus, it is not surprising that even in patients who are frequently malnourished wounds generally heal rather than not [17]. However, any element of malnutrition retards the healing process [18].

Protein is essential for normal wound healing. As early as 1938, Thompson et al. [19] demonstrated experimentally that wound healing was de-

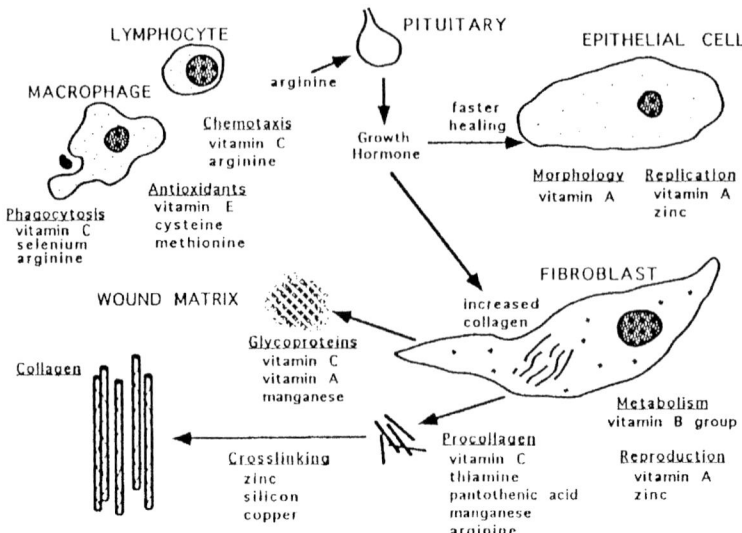

Figure 6-2.   Summary of micronutrient influence on wound healing. (Reproduced, with permission, from Meyer et al. [15].

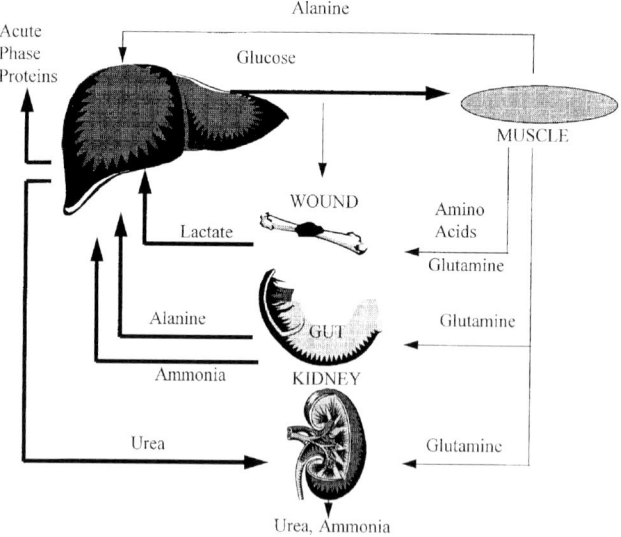

Figure 6-3.   Substrate exchange between major organ systems and wound. Proteolysis of skeletal muscle serves as the main source of amino acids, primarily alanine and glutamine. The metabolism of these amino acids by visceral organs results in the generation of glucose, acute phase proteins' urea and ammonia, and increased urinary loss of nitrogen. The net balance in the wound, although positive, is negative overall, particularly in the muscle. Adapted, with permission, from Bessey, P.Q., Parenteral nutrition and trauma, John L. Rombeau and Michael D. Caldwell, eds., *Clinical Nutrition Parenteral Nutrition,* 2nd edition, Philadelphia: W. B. Saunders, 1993:546.

layed in hypoproteinemic dogs. Macroscopically, tissues appeared unhealthy and edematous, with no apparent union. The microscopic picture was characterized by a marked delay in fibroblastic regeneration. Wound healing returned to normal following correction of the hypoproteinemic state by administration of lyophilized dog plasma. Other investigators using protein-deficient or protein-free diets in rats have also shown significant decreases in the bursting strength of colonic anastomoses [20, 21] and abdominal wall wounds [21]. Impaired wound healing results from reduced fibroblast proliferation, collagen synthesis, and angiogenesis [22].

In adult surgical patients, Haydock and Hill [23] assessed wound healing response by measuring the collagen content (hydroxyproline) in fine Gore-Tex tubes inserted subcutaneously in the arms. On the seventh postoperative day, hydroxyproline content in the tubing of the normally nourished patients (0.49 mg/cm) was significantly greater than that observed in the mildly malnourished (0.27 mg/cm) or moderately-to-severely malnourished (0.21 mg/cm). Contrary to the normal belief that mild-to-moderate nutritional deficiencies do not affect healing, Haydock and Hill observed that impaired wound healing occurs even in the presence of mild malnutrition. Nutritional support, either parenteral [24] or enteral [25], significantly increased hydroxyprolline accumulation in the tubes.

Of the various amino acids, arginine, a conditionally essential amino acid, appears to have a major role in the wound healing process [17]. In animal studies, deficiencies of arginine have decreased collagen deposition and wound breaking strength, whereas increased amounts of arginine have increased collagen deposition and wound breaking strength. In humans, arginine supplementation of the diet in the young [26] or the elderly [27] resulted in an increase in the hydroxyproline content of Gore-Tex tubes. Arginine appears to have multiple biological effects. It is a precursor of proline, the essential component of collagen. Second, it stimulates secretion of insulin, glucagon, prolactin, and growth hormone. Third, it has a thymotropic effect and appears to stimulate lymphocyte proliferation in response to stimulation by mitogens or cytokines [15].

VITAMINS

Several water- and fat-soluble vitamins serve as important cofactors in the wound healing process. Vitamin A stimulates epithelialization, collagen synthesis, and cross-linking. Supplemental vitamin A increases fibroplasia and collagen accumulation in wounds and reverses the deleterious effects of steroids on wound healing. Vitamin C is needed for the hydroxylation of both proline and lysine in collagen synthesis. Ascorbic acid is also necessary for neutrophil superoxide production and bacterial destruction. Vitamin C, like vitamin E, also serves as an antioxidant and counteracts oxidative changes induced by oxygen free radicals. Although all the B vitamins function as coenzymes in various energy metabolic pathways and are important in wound healing, riboflavin (B_2), pyridoxine (B_6), and pantothenic acid (B_5) appear to be crucial.

TRACE ELEMENTS

Zinc is a cofactor of various metalloenzymes, including RNA and DNA polymerases. Zinc deficiency appears to retard wound healing through impaired amino acid utilization. Copper, a cofactor of lysyl oxidase, is essential for the maturation or cross-linking of collagen fibrils. Manganese influences glycosylation of procollagen fibers through *o*-lysyl galactosyltransferase. It also plays a significant role in the production of mucopolysaccharides like hyaluronic acid, chondroitin sulfate, and heparin, which constitute the ground substance of a healing wound. Selenium, a cofactor of glutathione peroxidase, functions as a protein endogenous antioxidant.

NUTRITIONAL ASSESSMENT

Malnutrition, defined as depletion of an essential nutrient or tissue compartment, can develop rapidly without adequate nutrient intake in the presence of an acute stress or injury [28]. Protein-calorie malnutrition (PCM) is the most common nutritional deficiency, seen in approximately 40% to 50% of hospitalized patients [29]. Some patients are in poor nutritional condition when admitted, but others

(25% to 30%) who are admitted to the hospital without malnutrition become nutritionally depleted during their hospital stay. Weinsier et al. [30] reported that 75% of patients hospitalized for two weeks or longer showed deteriorating nutritional status. It is now well recognized that undetected and untreated PCM results in decrease of physiologic function of all organs (Table 6-1). This in turn leads to increased morbidity and mortality. The only organ that seems to be spared from the effects of malnutrition is the brain [31].

Controversy still exists about methods for identifying or classifying PCM [32]. Currently, available methods range from a simple bedside assessment based on nutritional history and physical examination (subjective global assessment), anthropometric measurements, plasma proteins, immunocompetence, and muscle function to highly sophisticated and expensive direct measurements of body composition. Of these, nutritional history and serum albumin appear to have the best predictive ability for the development of pressure sores.

Table 6-1.   End Organ Responses in Malnutrition

Organ	Anatomic	Physiologic
Heart	4-chamber dilatation Wall thinning	QT prolongation, low voltage, bradycardia Decreased cardiac output, stroke volume, and contractility Preload intolerance Diminished responsiveness to inotropic agents
Lung	Emphysematous changes Pulmonary infarcts Reduced bacterial clearance Muscle atrophy	Pneumonia Decreases in functional capacity, vital capacity, and maximum breathing capacity Depressed hypoxic/hypercarbic drives Reduced efficiency
Hematologic	Stem cell failure Depressed erythropoietin synthesis	Anemia
Renal	Epithelial swelling Atrophy Mild cortical calcification	Reduced glomerular filtration rate and inability to handle sodium loads Polyuria Metabolic acidosis
Gut	Disproportionate mass loss Hypoplastic and atrophic changes Decrease in total mucosal height	Depressed enzymatic activity Shortened transit time Impaired motility Propensity for bacterial overgrowth Maldigestion and malabsorption
Liver	Mass loss Periportal fat accumulation	Decreased visceral protein synthesis Depressed microsomal activity Eventual hepatic insufficiency
WBC	Decreased PMN chemotaxis Decreased lymphocyte count with reduced T helper and increased T suppressor and killer cells Decreased blastogenesis to PHA and MLC	Anergy Decreased granuloma formation Impaired response to chemotherapy Increased infection rate

Source: Cerra [31].

NUTRITIONAL HISTORY

A thorough nutritional history, specifically determining if there has been reduction in dietary intake, appears to be an important predictor for the development of pressure sores. In a prospective study of 185 patients admitted to a chronic care hospital without a pressure ulcer, Berlowitz and Wilking [7] observed that 20 patients developed a pressure ulcer during a three-week period. Impaired nutritional intake, history of cerebrovascular accident, and being bedridden or chairbound were the only factors significantly associated with the development of a pressure ulcer. Similarly, in another prospective study of 200 newly admitted, elderly nursing home patients at risk for development of pressure sores (Braden scale score < 17), Bergstrom and Braden [8] observed that dietary intake of all nutrients was lower in the 147 patients (73.5%) who developed pressure sores. Using logistic regression, the best predictors for pressure sore development were the Braden scale score, diastolic blood pressure, temperature, dietary protein intake, and age.

SERUM ALBUMIN

Visceral protein mass, the second largest component of body cell mass, accounts for about 2 kg of the total protein in a healthy male adult. It is generally measured by albumin, transferrin, and retinol-binding prealbumin. The levels of these plasma proteins are more sensitive tests for PCM than anthropometric measurements. In the presence of stress secondary to surgery, trauma, or sepsis, profound deficiencies in visceral proteins occur before any significant decrease in anthropometric measurements is seen [33]. Their fall represents decreased liver biosynthesis and turnover, and their rise parallels nutritional recovery [34].

Serum albumin, although easily measured, has some drawbacks: (1) relatively long serum half-life (approximately 20 days), (2) large pool size, and (3) low sensitivity. Furthermore, various nonnutritional factors may cause hypoalbuminemia [35]. Nevertheless, serum albumin still remains perhaps the most widely studied objective measurement and is considered the most useful marker for malnutrition. The magnitude of hypoalbuminemia is proportional to the degree of stress and malnutrition. An albumin level of 3.0 to 3.5 g/dl is suggestive of mild malnutrition; between 2.1 and 2.9 g/dl, of moderate malnutrition; and 2.0 g/dl or less, of severe malnutrition [33].

Several studies now demonstrate that low serum albumin concentration is positively associated with the presence, development, and stage of pressure ulcers, as well as their failure to heal. In a prospective study of 36 patients at risk for pressure ulcers (Norton score $\geq$ 10), Holmes and colleagues [36] observed that 20 developed ulcers. Seventy-five percent of patients with serum albumin levels less than 3.5 g/dl developed ulcers, as compared to only 17% of patients who had levels 3.5 g/dl or greater ($p<0.01$). Furthermore, in elderly hospitalized patients, serum albumin level within 24 hours of admission was the best single predictor of mortality [37]. When serum albumin was controlled for, logit regression analysis demonstrated that the impact of other nutritional indices; e.g., percentage ideal body weight, serum transferrin, total lymphocyte count, and delayed cutaneous hypersensitivity, on death was insignificant. The effect of serum albumin remained significant ($p<0.05$ to <0.01) even when age and physician's diagnosis were held constant. Thus, serum albumin levels can provide early identification of patients at increased risk for development of pressure sores, septic complications, and even death.

NUTRITIONAL SUPPORT

The goal of nutritional support is to prevent the development of malnutrition. As outlined in the clinical practice guidelines developed by the AHCPR [9], it is necessary to monitor the dietary intake of apparently well-nourished persons also. Nutritional support is unlikely to benefit a healthy patient who will be able to start oral intake within four to five days of an illness. In contrast, nutritional support is indicated in: (a) well-nourished patients at risk of developing pressure ulcers who are unlikely to resume oral intake in less than five days or whose dietary intake remains inadequate for longer than seven days; (b) patients exhibiting compromised nutritional status.

NUTRITIONAL REQUIREMENTS

Hypermetabolism following illness or sepsis is a graded response. For optimal nutritional therapy, it is therefore absolutely necessary to understand the character and magnitude of the metabolic stress in order to estimate the requirements of each patient. Table 6-2 outlines a staging system and lists the approximate nutritional requirements based on the stress level [31]. In general, total caloric needs for the majority of institutionalized patients range between 25 to 30 kcal/kg/day. Increasing amounts of protein, approaching 1.5 to 2 g/kg/day, are required to support protein synthesis, wound healing and maintenance of skeletal mass [38].

Both carbohydrates and fat should be used as nonprotein sources of energy following injury. The maximal rate of glucose oxidation is around 6 to 7 mg/kg/min, and higher infusion rates stimulate lipogenesis. As such, glucose infusion should not exceed 4 to 5 mg/kg/min, equivalent to 400–500 g/day of glucose in a 70-kg person, and providing approximately 50% to 60% of the total caloric requirement. Excess carbohydrate has been associated with hyperglycemia, hypercarbia, increased ventilatory drive, inability to wean from the ventilator, and a fatty liver. Blood glucose levels greater than 220 mg/dl have been shown to be associated with a significantly greater incidence of severe infection, bacteremia, or pneumonia. Insulin should be administered to maintain blood glucose levels below 200 mg/dl, as far as possible [39].

The balance of the 40% to 50% of the total caloric requirement should be 20% to 30% from lipids (not to exceed 2.5 g/kg/day) and 20% to 30% from protein. At least 3% of the total calories should be provided as fat to prevent essential fatty acid deficiency. Increasing fat calories up to 50% of total calories may be helpful in weaning patients off ventilators, and achieving a better blood glucose control in diabetics and patients receiving high doses of steroids [38]. However, increased fat administration has been associated with hyperlipidemia, hypoxia, cholestasis, and an increased rate of infection [39].

Overfeeding is deleterious and should be avoided. Overfeeding cannot reverse tissue catabolism until the acute metabolic stress response has resolved [40]. In effect, overfeeding increases the risk of mortality. Postoperative patients receiving calories equal to 150% of measured energy expenditure (MEE), when compared to patients given calories equal to MEE, had a significantly greater mortality (40% versus 28%) [41]. Therefore, it is suggested that during the acute stress period the best goal is "moderation." Caloric intake should be reduced to 80% of caloric needs with adequate protein supplements provided [38] (Table 6-3).

In addition, daily requirements of electrolytes, vitamins, and trace elements should be provided. It has been recommended that 25,000 IU of vitamin A per day be given to patients receiving steroids [42]. A few studies have shown increased healing of pressure ulcers with megadoses of vitamin C (1 gram per day) [43, 44] and zinc (200 mg two to three times daily) [45]. The results of megadose therapy are not always consistent [46]. Their safe levels and the risk of potential detrimental effects remain less defined. However, it is generally agreed that there is an increased need for vitamins (especially A, C, and E) and minerals (zinc, selenium, and magnesium).

TIMING AND ROUTE OF NUTRITIONAL SUPPORT

Several studies have shown that pressure sores develop within the first several days following ad-

Table 6-2.   Categories of Metabolic Stress and Metabolic Requirements

Stress level	Clinical example	Urinary nitrogen loss/day	Nonprotein caloric need (kcal/kg/day)	Protein (g/kg/day)	Nonprotein calorie/ nitrogen ratio
0	Starvation	5	25	1	150:1
1	Elective general	5–10	25	1.5	100:1
2	Polytrauma	10–15	30	2.0	100:1
3	Sepsis	15	35	2.5	80:1

Source: Cerra [31].

Table 6-3. Optimal Nutritional Requirements

Calories
  Amount: At least 80% of requirements
  Type: 70% carbohydrate/30% fat; ≥3% as essential fatty
    acids
Protein
  1.5 g/kg/day for most patients
  2.0 g/kg/day for severely catabolic patients; should include
    glutamine (about one-third of amino acids)
Vitamins
  Increased doses of A, C, and E; usually requirements can
    only be met by enteral administration
Minerals
  Increased needs for zinc, selenium, and magnesium
Route of feeding
  Enteral, enteral-parenteral, parenteral (in order of
    preference)
Method of feeding
  Institute nutrient administration early in the catabolic
    course, attending to administration of glucose, sodium,
    potassium, and vitamin and mineral needs; over time,
    add amino acids and increase calories until full
    nutritional support is achieved

Source: DeBiasse and Wilmore [38].

mission. The critical times for nutritional assessment are on admission and whenever the patient condition or mobility is compromised. If a deficit in dietary intake or nutritional status is identified, nutrient intake needs to be increased by dietary modification, supplementation, or spoon feeding.

Tube feeding should be considered if oral intake is compromised. Current evidence suggests that besides the advantages of safety, convenience, and cost, enteral feeding preserves gut mucosal mass and normal gut flora, prevents increased gut permeability to bacteria and other toxins, maintains mucosal immunity and gut-associated lymphoid tissue, and attenuates the hypermetabolic response to injury [47]. When compared to total parenteral nutrition, institution of early enteral nutrition significantly lowers the incidence of septic morbidity. Parenteral nutrition should be administered only when enteral access cannot be obtained, when enteral nutrition support fails to meet nutritional requirements, or when feeding into the gastrointestinal tract is contraindicated. Subsequent transition to oral feeding should be implemented as soon as enteral access is obtained or gastrointestinal function improves.

Although provision of nutrients by tube feeding is beneficial, there are also inherent disadvantages. In the individual more prone to development of pressure sores, fecal incontinence, diarrhea, and moisture can increase the likelihood of the sores occurring or worsen their conditions. Second, the use of restraints after the insertion of tubes can possibly limit mobility. Third, there is a significant risk of aspiration. Fourth, although they are difficult to estimate, adverse effects can result from loss of mealtime socialization and interaction with staff, including loss of self-esteem [48].

PHYSICAL ACTIVITY AND NUTRITIONAL SUPPORT

A positive nitrogen balance is often not achieved in patients despite the provision of sufficient amounts of both calories and amino acids. An important factor contributing to this may be immobility. In their classical studies, Deitrick et al. [49] have shown that immobilization of normal men with adequate nutrient intake resulted in a net loss of nitrogen, potassium, phosphorous, calcium, and sulfur. These deleterious effects were significantly reduced by the use of an oscillating bed [50].

As early as 1932, Cutbertson [51], in a study of patients recuperating from lower extremity fractures or osteotomy of long bones, demonstrated that massage, "an ancient therapeutic adjunct," supplemented by passive movement of the affected extremity, resulted in increased retention of nitrogen, sulfur, and phosphorus. Recently, Gibson et al. [52], in their study of patients with long leg casts for fracture of tibia, observed that short periods of low voltage percutaneous electrical stimulation of muscles improved muscle-protein synthesis and prevented disuse muscle atrophy.

GROWTH FACTORS AND WOUND HEALING

Over the last decade, the availability of various growth factors has fostered considerable interest in their use for wound healing. These peptide growth factors, or "wound hormones," by their action on specific larger cells are directly involved in cell growth, cell differentiation, embryogenesis, inflammation, the immune response, and tissue repair. Although normal wound healing fluid contains an abundance of peptide growth factors, lower levels of growth factors are seen in chronic wounds. Supplementing chronic wounds with growth factors may possibly dramatically improve the wound healing process. In early clinical trials, recombinant basic fibroblast growth factor, when topically applied to chronic pressure sores, reduced ulcer size and increased the numbers of fibroblasts and capillaries [53]. Similarly, Mustoe et al. [54] have shown that recombinant platelet-derived growth factor-BB appears to increase the healing rate of stages III and IV pressure ulcers. Further randomized controlled clinical trials on growth factors are needed to determine their overall benefit and role.

CONCLUSION

The treatment of pressure sores requires a multidisciplinary approach. The results of local care and surgical repair are generally unsatisfactory unless the nutritional status and general condition of the patient are optimized from the onset and maintained throughout. The goal of nutritional therapy should be to provide adequate amounts of protein, calories, macronutrients, and micronutrients.

REFERENCES

1. Robertson, E. C., and Tisdall, F., Nutrition and resistance to disease, *Canad Med Assoc J* 1939; 40:282–284.

2. Joseph, B., Insulin in the treatment of non-diabetic bed sores, *Ann Surg* 1930; 92:318–319.

3. McCormick, W. J., The nutritional aspects of bed sores, *Med Rec* 1941; 154:389.

4. Mulholland, J. H.; Tui, C.; Wright, A. M.; Vinci, V.; and Shafiroff, B., Protein metabolism and bed sores, *Ann Surg* 1943; 118:1015–1023.

5. Breslow, R. A., and Bergstrom, N., Nutritional prediction of pressure ulcers, *J Am Diet Assoc* 1994; 96:1301–1304.

6. Ek, A.; Unosson, M.; Larsson, J.; Von Schenck, H.; and Bjurulf, P., The development and healing of pressure sores related to the nutritional state, *Clin Nutr* 1991; 10:245–250.

7. Berlowitz, D. R., and Wilking, S. V., Risk factors for pressure sores. A comparison of cross-sectional and cohort-derived data, *J Am Geriatr Soc* 1989; 37:1043–1050.

8. Bergstrom, N., and Braden, B., A prospective study of pressure sore risk among instituionalized elderly, *J Am Geriatr Soc* 1992; 40:747–758.

9. *Pressure Ulcers in Adults: Prediction and Prevention,* Clinical Practice Guideline no. 3, AHCPR Publication no. 92-0047, Rockville, MD: Agency for Health Care Policy and Research, Public Health Service, U.S. Department of Health and Human Services, May 1992.

10. Mecray, P. M.; Barden, R. P.; and Ravdin, I. S., Nutritional edema: Its effect on the gastric emptying time before and after gastric operations, *Surgery* 1937; 1:53–64.

11. Takeda, T.; Koyama, T.; Izawa, Y.; et al., Effect of malnutrition on development of experimental pressure sores, *J Dermatol* 1992; 19:602–609.

12. Ring, J.; Seifert, J.; Lob, G.; Stephan, W.; Probst, J.; and Brendel, W., Elimination rate of human serum albumin in paraplegic patients, *Paraplegia* 1974; 12:139–144.

13. Tui, C.; Wright, A. M.; Mulholland, J. H.; Breed, E. S.; Barcham, I.; and Gould, D., Studies in surgical convalescence, II: A preliminary study in the nitrogen loss in exudates in surgical condition, *Ann Surg* 1945; 121:223–230.

14. Beal, A. L., and Cerra, F. B., Multiple organ failure syndrome in the 1990's. Systems inflammation response and organ dysfunction, *JAMA* 1994; 271:226–233.

15. Meyer, N.; Muller, M.; and Herndon, D., Nutrient support of the healing wound, *New Horizons* 1994; 2:202–214.

16. Moore, F. D., *Metabolic Care of the Surgical Patient,* Philadelphia: W. B. Saunders, 1959.

17. Albina, J. E., Nutrition and wound healing, *JPEN* 1994; 18:367–376.

18. Orgill, D., and Demling, R. H., Current concepts and approaches to wound healing, *Crit Care Med* 1988; 16:899–908.

19. Thompson, W. D.; Ravdin, I. S.; Rhoads, J. E.; and Frank, I. L., Use of lyophile plasma in correction of hypoproteinemia and prevention of wound disruption, *Arch Surg* 1938; 36:509–518.

20. Daly, J. M.; Vars, H. M.; and Dudrick, S. J., Effects

of protein depletion on strength of colonic anastomoses, *Surg Gynecol Obstet* 1972; 13(4):15–21.

21. Irvin, T. T., and Hunt, T. K., Effect of malnutrition on colonic healing, *Ann Surg* 1972; 180:765–772.

22. Irvin, T. T.; Effects of malnutrition and hyperalimentation on wound healing, *Surg Gynecol Obstet* 1978; 146:33–37.

23. Haydock, D. A., and Hill, G. L.; Impaired wound healing in surgical patients with varying degrees of malnutrition, *JPEN* 1986; 10:550–554.

24. Haydock, D. A., and Hill, G. L., Improved wound healing response in surgical patients receiving intravenous nutrition, *Brit J Surg* 1987; 74:320–323.

25. Schroeder, D.; Gillanders, L.; Mahr, K.; et al., Effect of immediate postoperative enteral nutrition on body composition, muscle function and wound healing, *JPEN* 1991; 15:376–383.

26. Barbul, A.; Laazarou, S. A.; Efron, D. T.; et al., Arginine enhances wound healing and lymphocyte immune response in humans, *Surgery* 1990; 108:331–337.

27. Kirk, S. J., Hurson, M.; Regan, M. C.; et al., Arginine stimulates wound healing and immune function in elderly human beings, *Surgery* 1993; 114:155–160.

28. Rationale for adult nutrition support guidelines, In *Guidelines for the use of Parenteral and Enteral Nutrition in Adult and Pediatric Patients,* ASPEN Board of Directors, JPEN 17, no. 4 Supplement, 5SA–6SA, 1993.

29. Bistrian B. R.; Blackburn, G. L.; Vitale, I., et al., Prevalence of malnutrition in general medical patients, *JAMA* 1976; 235:1567.

30. Weinsier, R. L.; Hunker, E. M.; Krumdieck, C. L.; et al., Hospital malnutrition, *Am J Clin Nutr* 1979; 32:418–426.

31. Cerra, F. B., Nutrition in the critically ill. Modern metabolic support in the intensive care unit, In B. Chernow, W. C. Shoemaker, eds., *Critical Care: State of the Art,* Fullerton, CA: Society of Critical Care Medicine, 1986: 1–19.

32. Jeejeebhoy, K. N., How should we monitor nutritional support: Structure or function? *New Horizons* 1994; 2:131–138.

33. Blackburn, G. L., and Harvey, K. B., Nutritional assessment as a routine in clinical medicine, *Postgrad Med.* 1982; 71:46–63.

34. Goldan, M. H. N.; Waterlow, J.C.; and Picun, D., Protein turnover, synthesis and breakdown before and after recovery from protein-energy malnutrition, *Clin Sci Mol Med* 1977; 53:473–477.

35. Rothschild, M. A.; Oratz, M.; and Schreiber, S. S., Albumin synthesis, *N Engl J Med* 1972; 286:748–757.

36. Holmes, R.; Macchianok; Jhangiani, S.; Agarwal, N.; and Savino, J., Combating pressure sores nutritionally, *Am J Nursing* 1987; 87:1301–1303.

37. Agarwal, N.; Acevedo, F.; Leighton, L. S.; Cayten, C. G.; and Pitchumoni, C. S., Predictive ability of various nutritional variables for mortality in elderly people, *Am J Clin Nutr* 1988; 48:1173–8.

38. DeBiasse, M. A., and Wilmore, D. W., What is optimal nutritional support? *New Horizons* 1994; 2:122–130.

39. Frankel, W. L.; Evans, N. J.; and Rombeau, J. L., Scientific rationale and clinical application of parenteral nutrition in critically ill patients, In John L. Rombeau and Michael D. Caldwell, eds., *Clinical Nutrition Parenteral Nutrition,* 2nd edition, Philadelphia: W. B. Saunders, 1993: 597–616.

40. Chwals, W. J., Overfeeding the critically ill child: Fact or fantasy? *New Horizons* 1994; 2:147–155.

41. Vo, N. M.; Wayscaster, M.; Acuff, R. V.; et al., Effect of postoperative carbohydrate overfeeding, *Am Surg* 1987; 53:632–635.

42. Levenson, S. M., and Demetriou, A. A., Metabolic factors, In I. K. Cohen, R. F. Diegelmann, W. J. Lindblad, eds., *Wound Healing: Biochemical and Chemical Aspects,* Philadelphia: W. B. Saunders, 1992: 248–273.

43. Hunter, T., and Rajan, K. T., The role of ascorbic acid in the pathogenesis and treatment of pressure sores, *Paraplegia* 1971; 8:211–215.

44. Taylor, T. V.; Rimmer, S.; Day, B.; Butcher, J.; and Dymock, I. W., Ascorbic acid supplementation in the treatment of pressure sores, *Lancet* 1974; 1:544.

45. Cohen, C., Zinc sulphate and bed sores, *Brit Med J* 1968; 2:561.

46. Breslow, R., Nutritional status and dietary intake of patients with pressure ulcers: Review of research literature 1943 to 1989, *Decubitus* 1991; 4:16–21.

47. Minard, G., and Kudsk, K. A., Is early feeding beneficial? How early is early? *New Horizons* 1994; 2:156–163.

48. Finucane, T. E., Malnutrition, tube feeding and pressure sores: Data are incomplete, *J Am Geriatr Soc* 1995; 43:447–451.

49. Deitrick, J. E.; Wheldon, G. D.; and Shorr, E., The effects of immobilization upon various metabolic and physiologic functions of normal men, *Am J Med* 1948; 4:3–36.

50. Wheldon, G. D.; Deitrick, J. E.; and Shorr, E., Modifications of the effects of immobilization upon metabolic and physiologic functions of normal men by the use of an oscillating bed, *Am J Med* 1949; 6:684–711.

51. Cutbertson, D. P., Certain effects of massage on the metabolism of convalescing fracture cases, *O J Med* 1932; 25:401–408.

52. Gibson, J. N. A.; Smith, K.; and Rennie, M. J., Prevention of disuse muscle atrophy by means of electrical stimulation: Maintenance of protein synthesis, *Lancet,* 1988; 2:767–771.

53. Robson, M.; Phillips, L.; Lawrence, T.; et al., The safety and effect of topically applied recombinant basic fibroblast growth factor on the healing of chronic pressure sores, *Ann Surg* 1992; 216:401–408.

54. Mustoe, T. M.; Cutler, N. R.; Allman, R. M.; et al., A phase II study to evaluate recombinant platelet-derived growth factor-BB in the treatment of stage 3 and 4 pressure ulcers, *Arch Surg* 1994; 129:213–219.

7

SKIN ULCERS SECONDARY TO ARTERIAL AND VENOUS DISEASE

E. A. Husni, M.D.

Ulceration of the skin in peripheral vascular disease is invariably preceded by trauma. The chronic pathologic changes incident to vascular insufficiency render the skin extremely vulnerable to injury, no matter how trivial. Trauma associated with ulcers can take one of five basic forms: mechanical, thermal, chemical, surgical, and prolonged external pressure.

Mechanical trauma, probably the leading cause of ulcers, can be anything from a simple scratch to actual laceration.

Thermal injuries, primarily exposure to heat or cold, especially in patients with arteriosclerosis obliterans, account for a good percentage of ulcerations of the feet and toes. The patient with ischemic pain of the foot unwittingly invites ulceration, even gangrene, by applying heat to a cold, painful foot in an effort to warm it up and relieve the discomfort. Blisters often result and these may turn to ulcers.

In a similar situation, chemicals and medicated ointments applied to the skin of a postphlebitic or ischemic limb may cause blister formation, especially when allergic reaction occurs. In addition, that may invite irresistible scratching that eventually breaks the skin surface.

Surgical procedures undertaken on limbs with vascular insufficiency may result in a nonhealing incision, especially in patients with arteriosclerosis obliterans.

Finally, prolonged external pressure applied over bony prominences, such as the sacrum and the heel, during long surgical procedures, invariably leads to breakdown of the skin if special precautions are not taken.

Vascular insufficiency takes one of two clinical pictures, that of venous insufficiency, as in postphlebitic disease, and arteriosclerosis obliterans with ischemia of the skin.

VENOUS STASIS

It has long been established that venous stasis is directly linked to incompetent perforating veins. Perforators, mostly located along the course of the medial cutaneous veins of the leg, become incompetent as a result of the phlebitic process or the excessive venous pressure of the regurgitant blood [5, 9]. The clinical entities associated with venous stasis, (1) postphlebitic disease, (2) long-standing primary varicose veins, (3) arteriovenous communications, and (4) extraluminal compression of veins, have one common denominator: *ambulatory venous hypertension*. The mechanism by which this pathologic physiology brings about tissue change that are identified with venous stasis has been the subject of considerable research and speculation. Stagnation with tissue anoxia was a popular explanation until several clinical studies demonstrated that the oxygen tension in the venous blood of postphlebitic skin was actually higher than normal [3].

The more recent studies of Browse and his colleagues relative to venous hypertension offer a more plausible working hypothesis for the genesis of the skin changes in venous stasis [2, 4]. They demonstrated that venous hypertension is associated with a remarkable proliferation of capillaries in the dependent part of the limb. They further established that the ground substance, long observed to surround the capillaries of the postphlebitic skin reaction, is actually fibrin. It is entirely reasonable to assume that the high venous pressure that is transmitted to the venules and capillaries may explain the pathologic changes. The vessels become dilated, and the intercellular capillary pores increase in size, thus allowing the escape of fibrinogen and formed elements into the pericapillary areas (diapedesis). The fibrinogen is converted to fibrin, and the fibrin surrounds the capillaries as a collar, acting as a barrier to the diffusion of oxygen from said capillaries to the cells in the area, thus rendering them easy prey to the slightest injury. In addition, the high resistance posed by the recanalized veins to the return of blood may cause the opening of A-V shunts proximal to the diseased skin, thereby diverting arterial inflow from the capillaries and further depriving the skin of more needed oxygen and nutrients.

MANAGEMENT

There are two principal aims in the management of venous stasis: (1) reducing the ambulatory venous hypertension, and (2) restoring the skin changes to normal. Although ambulatory venous hypertension can only be alleviated by venous reconstruction, nonoperative management in the form of good hygiene, elevation, and elastic compression can provide definite beneficial effects in most instances. The judicious use of anabolic steroids has

also been shown to be beneficial [2]. Whenever conservative means suffice, surgery is not indicated.

PRIMARY VARICOSE VEINS

Primary varicose veins of long standing may be associated with venous stasis in at least 10% of patients. Mild to moderate cases should probably be managed with good hygiene and elastic support. The saphenous systems have come to be recognized as very precious "spare parts" to be utilized in arterial and venous reconstructive procedures. However, in advanced cases of venous stasis and in those cases where repeated episodes of superficial phlebitis have rendered these veins unsuitable as vascular substitutes, aggressive surgical management is indicated [7, 12]. Every case of venous stasis has to be looked upon as possibly related to postphlebitic disease, and therefore phlebography and pressure studies should precede any surgical procedure. These examinations will evaluate the peripheral venous pressure and demonstrate the incompetent perforators, presence of thrombus, and the morphology of the deep venous system. Once it is established that the case is indeed one of primary varicose veins, the surgical procedure must include removal of all of the incompetent saphenous system with all incompetent communicators, including the medial cutaneous veins of the leg, and the routine ligation of the perforators [10].

POST PHLEBITIC DISEASE

Ambulatory venous hypertension and stasis are prominent features of postphlebitic disease, the degree varying directly with the extent of deep venous incompetence and the paucity of collaterals. Here again, surgical intervention is reserved to those cases that are refractory to conservative management. As stated earlier, conservative management includes: good hygiene and the use of elastic support, pneumatic compression, fibrinolysis, anticoagulants, antibiotics, and diuretics. In cases where no significant improvement is derived from these measures over a period of six to twelve months, surgical intervention may be entertained. Here the primary aim of the surgical approach is the reconstruction of the deep veins and the restoration of the venous hemodynamics to normal. When venous reconstruction is undertaken, the procedure must include ligation of the perforators, removal of the secondary varicose veins, and skin grafting when indicated.

Prerequisites for venous reconstruction are: (1) segmental venous disease, (2) poor collaterals, and (3) marked ambulatory venous hypertension. The ideal candidates for this modality are those with extraluminal compression [10]. For pathology of the iliac and common femoral veins, the cross-pubis bypass graft as devised by Palma and Esperon [15] is the procedure of choice. In this procedure the contralateral saphenous vein is utilized as the bypass graft. For a successful outcome in this endeavor, the bypass should be more than 3 mm in diameter and free of disease, and the site of anastomosis should be free of thrombus and excessive recanalization webs. In cases where the pathology involves the femoral and popliteal veins, the in situ saphenopopliteal vein bypass procedure [11] has yielded reasonable benefits.

Clinical results of venous reconstruction appear to be enhanced by ligation of incompetent perforators and removal of secondary varicose veins [9]. In addition, no matter what surgical treatment is instituted, knee-high elastic support will be necessary in at least 50% of patients.

Data provided by numerous reports of reconstructive procedures show a success rate in over 66% of the cases, with a 50% reduction of venous hypertension and satisfactory clinical results in most cases. The patency rate of venous repair could also be further enhanced by employing the adjuvant arteriovenous fistula for a period of three to eight weeks [9, 11].

EXTRALUMINAL COMPRESSION

Extraluminal compression of major veins of the limbs will invite development of collateral venous channels, as in any case of venous occlusion. Relief may be obtained by removing the cause of the occlusion—such as tumor, aneurysm, scar tissue, etc. However, in instances where such procedures are not feasible, venous reconstruction may be indicated. The outcome of such an endeavor is invariably successful because, in this instance, the integrity of the venous anatomy is preserved.

ARTERIOVENOUS COMMUNICATIONS

When congenital or acquired arteriovenous communication presents a classical picture of venous hypertension and stasis, the treatment is directed at the repair of the fistula, and that should normally alleviate the pathology. However, certain cases of multiple communications of the congenital type pose a very difficult problem. Treatment in these instances is symptomatic; no cure is possible short of amputation of the limb.

ARTERIAL INSUFFICIENCY

Ulcerations of the skin occurring in arterial disease are usually incident to trauma as in the case of venous disease, except perhaps in the hypertensive patient, where the hypertensive ischemic ulcer may occur spontaneously. All arterial diseases that feature peripheral ischemia have one thing in common—a reduction in the flow of blood to the skin. This reduction is due to acute or subacute arterial occlusion or arteritis. Under normal conditions, blood flow to the skin is controlled by neurogenic as well as metabolic factors. The sympathetic vasoconstrictor tone supervenes in muscular arteries and arterioles, whereas the metabolites predominantly influence the metarterioles and precapillary sphincters. The balance between those factors determines the amount of blood reaching the skin. To maintain blood flow, the perfusing pressure must be high enough to overcome (1) viscosity, (2) luminal irregularities, and (3) external pressures applied to the skin. Normally, the higher the blood pressure, the greater the flow, provided the peripheral resistance is unchanged, and conversely, the lower the pressure, the smaller the rate of blood flow. In arterial disease, the blood flow through the vessel is not significantly altered until the occlusive lesion exceeds 20% of the lumen [14]. At 50% narrowing, the flow is reduced precipitously from normal levels [17], as flow is directly proportional to the fourth power of the radius (Poiseuille's law). However, even at 50% narrowing of an artery, the tissue may not experience a great reduction in the flow of blood because of two factors: (1) local vasodilatation effected by the metabolites will lower the peripheral resistance, thus attracting more blood, and (2) the reduced blood flow across the stenotic arterial segment will diminish the hydrostatic pressure in the arterial bed distal to the stenosis, thereby creating a pressure gradient that will open up preexisting collateral channels. The gradient will be much greater in total occlusion and the flow through collaterals will greatly increase. The flow through collaterals is determined by both the pressure gradient and the length and diameter of these collaterals, as the resistance to blood flow is directly proportional to the length and the diameter of a vessel.

In cases where the occluded arterial segment is long and the collateral channels are poor, the flow of blood to the skin may be critically reduced. The blood pressure at the ankle may drop to such low levels that the arterioles do not stay open [14]. The critical closing pressure for arterioles is approximately 20 mm Hg, and that for capillaries is 5 mm Hg [6]. When the capillary pressure drops below normal, tissue perfusion may actually cease, and necrosis may ensue. In these critical situations, any trauma to the ischemic area may precipitate the formation of ulcers because blood is not available to heal the traumatized tissue. In clinical practice most ulcers of the skin are encountered in arteriosclerosis obliterans, thromboangiitis obliterans, diabetes mellitus, Raynaud's disease, hypertension, and chronic pernio.

In arteriosclerosis obliterans, the large arteries are involved, notably the femoral artery. The most common location for occlusion starts at the level of the adductor hiatus. The common femoral and iliac arteries are also involved in many cases. Occasionally the popliteal artery may be the seat of significant disease. In the diabetic patient, the occlusive disease may also extend to involve the smaller arteries, as instances of traumatic gangrene of the toes are commonly seen in the presence of satisfactory pedal pulses. In cases of inflammatory arterial occlusive disease, small-to-medium-size arteries are involved, such as the digital and plantar arteries. Occasionally the inflammatory occlusive disease may involve the tibial and peroneal arteries. The inflammatory process is usually segmental, and, concomitant with the arterial problem, phlebitis is a common manifestation. Thromboangiitis obliterans is predominantly a disease of males. Raynaud's disease, on the other hand, is seen mostly in females under age fifty.

Unlike arteriosclerosis obliterans or thromboangiitis obliterans, Raynaud's disease has a symmetrical distribution in the extremities, and the patient continues to experience severe attacks of Raynaud's phenomenon. Scleroderma is a disease that can be confused with Raynaud's disease in the early stages. In patients with arteriosclerosis obliterans, Raynaud's phenomenon is rare, and Raynaud's disease among female patients is seldom seen after the age of fifty. Most ulcers in these preceding conditions involve the toes and occasionally the dorsum of the foot and heel. The hypertensive ischemic ulcer is located on the lateral or extensor surfaces of the lower leg and ankle. Here again, lesions are precipitated by trauma, but spontaneous ulcerations have been observed to start as a small, painful red spot in the skin. This becomes hemorrhagic and breaks down into a superficial ulcer. The ulcer is typically superficial and very sharply demarcated. Extension of the ulcer is preceded by a purpuric, hemorrhagic zone in the surrounding skin. The patient is usually a long-term hypertensive.

Ulcers of the skin can also occur in infectious diseases, cold injuries, livedo reticularis, chronic ergot poisoning, rheumatoid arthritis, and embolization of atherosclerotic vegetations from the large arteries (trash feet).

A patient history and physical examination should be the primary tools for diagnosing the underlying conditions. Noninvasive methods for evaluating the peripheral blood flow by plethysmography, Doppler studies, and blood pressure ankle/brachial indices are useful screening tools. Arteriography remains the prerequisite study to arterial reconstruction.

The treatment of ischemic ulcers is aimed at increasing the peripheral circulation. Peripheral vasodilators and sympatholytic drugs have been used for decades, but have provided little objective evidence of improvement except in vasospastic conditions. Arterial reconstruction is, to date, the operative treatment of choice. The autogenous saphenous vein remains the best material for arterial replacement in the lower limb. The umbilical vein (biograft) and the PTFE graft have also been used successfully in the absence of suitable autogenous veins. Intraluminal balloon dilatation and atherectomy have yielded lasting satisfactory results in lesions of the iliac arteries, but have not proven as successful below the level of the inguinal ligament [1]. Laboratory research continues in the pursuit of the ideal prosthesis that will yield long-term patency comparable to that of the autogenous vein.

When arterial reconstruction is not feasible, lumbar sympathectomy may be considered in selected cases of arteriosclerosis and thromboangiitis obliterans. Lumbar sympathectomy increases blood flow through collateral channels to the skin of the foot and toes, especially in vasospastic conditions, and may help prevent or limit the extent of amputation [8]. Prior to any surgical procedure, however, evaluation of the cardiopulmonary status is mandatory, because the presence of significant coronary artery disease in these patients is not uncommon.

Finally, whatever treatment is administered in these conditions, certain fundamental precautionary measures must also be observed, especially good hygiene and the avoidance of mechanical, chemical, or thermal trauma to the lower extremities.

PRESSURE ULCERS

Pressure applied to bony prominences for long periods can severely compromise the circulation to the overlying skin. This is commonly seen in immobilized patients and in those undergoing long operative procedures. These decubitus ulcers are simply a matter of the external pressure exceeding the internal tissue perfusion pressure.

For normal capillary flow at the cellular level, the residual hydrostatic arterial pressure should be at least 25 mm Hg. This is normally augmented by the interstitial osmotic and the negative interstitial fluid pressures (a total of approximately 11 mm Hg), resulting in an effective infiltration pressure from the capillaries of 36 mm Hg. Working in the opposite direction is the plasma colloid osmotic pressure of 28 mm Hg, yielding a net perfusion

pressure of about 8 mm Hg. In the elderly patient, the incidence of ASO of the terminal aorta, iliac, and femoral arteries is very significant, especially in those undergoing coronary reconstruction. In studying the transcutaneous oxygen tension in the lower extremity in health and in occlusive disease, Lee found that in patients with claudication of the limb, the cutaneous PO_2 level was reduced to 20%, and in those with ischemic changes, that level was further reduced to 5% from normal control levels of 86%. These changes are the result of, and directly proportional to, the severity of the arteriosclerosis obliterans. These severely reduced levels were greatly improved by successful arterial reconstruction [13].

Utilizing the same methodology, Salisbury [16] studied the changes in the skin oxygen tension over the greater trochanter in healthy adults in the supine position (no external pressure) and in the lateral decubitus position (pressure of the body weight). For interface, he used the regular hospital mattress, a sheepskin, a water mattress, an air-fluidized bed, and an alternating air mattress. Within 30 minutes in the decubitus position, the PO_2 dropped precipitously from a control level of 76.3 to 4.6 when the regular mattress and the sheepskin were used, and the PO_2 dropped further with time. When the water mattress and the air-fluidized bed were used, the drop was only 16–17% from the control level and the value did not change significantly after one hour. The results for the alternating air mattress were not comparable to other interfaces because of the alternating cycle.

It is therefore not unreasonable to deduct from these studies that the skin of extremities with a precarious circulation or as a result of ASO [13] can be easily devitalized by external pressure. With the steadily increasing lifespan of our population, the number of patients immobilized by CVA and of those requiring extensive operative procedures for ASO and/or cancer is also increasing proportionately. This is the segment of our population that is prone to decubitus ulcerations.

The management here should be one of prevention. Every one of these patients, especially the diabetics, should undergo a thorough evaluation of their peripheral circulation. In those demonstrating significantly diminished parameters, precautionary measures should be undertaken in an effort to neutralize the deleterious effects of external pressure.

REFERENCES

1. Bergan, J. J., Introduction to the symposium on transluminal angioplasty, *Arch Surg* 1981; 116:804.

2. Browse, N. L., Venous insufficiency: Nonoperative management, in N. U. Ban, J. L. Glover, R. W. Holden, D. A. Triplett, eds., *Thrombosis and Atherosclerosis: Prevention, Diagnosis and Management,* Chicago: Year Book Medical Publishers, 1982: 275.

3. Burnand, K. G.; Whimster, I.; et al., Relationship between the number of capillaries in the skin of venous ulcer-bearing area of the lower leg and the fall in foot vein pressure during exercise, *Brit J Surg* 1981; 68:297.

4. Cockett, F. B., Pathology and treatment of varicose ulcers of the leg, *Brit J Surg* 1955; 43:260.

5. Fontaine, R., Remarks concerning venous thrombosis and its sequelae, *Surgery* 1957; 41:6.

6. Guyton, A. C., *Textbook of Medical Physiology,* 5th ed., Philadelphia: W. B. Saunders, 1976.

7. Husni, E. A., Venous stasis: Surgical management, In N. U. Ban, J. L. Glover, R. W. Holden, D. A. Triplett, eds., *Thrombosis and Atherosclerosis:* Chicago: Year Book Medical Publishers, 1982: 283–300.

8. Husni, E. A., and Simeone, F. A., Results of lumbar sympathectomy in peripheral vascular disease: An evaluation of preoperative laboratory tests, *Arch Surg* 1957; 75:530.

9. Husni, E. A., Venous reconstruction, in John L. Cameron, ed., *Current Surgical Therapy—3,* D. C. Decker, 1989: 619–624.

10. Husni, E. A., Reconstruction of veins: The need for objectivity, *J Cardiovasc Surg* 1983; 24:525–528.

11. Husni, E. A., Venous reconstruction procedures; in Rob and Smith's *Operative Surgery,* London: Butterworth, 1985: 334–341.

12. Husni, E. A., and Williams, W. A., Superficial phlebitis of the lower limbs, *Surg* 1982; 91:70–74.

13. Lee, B. Y., and Thoden, W. R., Noninvasive evaluation of the cutaneous circulation in chronic sores of the skin, in Bok Y. Lee, ed., *Chronic Ulcers of the Skin,* New York: McGraw-Hill, 1985: 77–91.

14. May, A. G.; Van deBerg, L.; DeWeese, J. A.; and Rob, C. E., Critical arterial stenosis, *Surgery* 1963; 54:250.

15. Palma, E. C., and Esperon, R., Vein transplants and grafts in the surgical treatment of postphlebitic syndrome, *J Cardiovasc Surg* 1960; 1:94.

16. Salisbury, R. E., Transcutaneous PO_2 monitoring in bedridden burn patients: A physiological analysis of four methods to prevent pressure sores, in Bok Y. Lee, ed., *Chronic Ulcers of the Skin,* New York: McGraw-Hill, 1985; 189–195.

17. Shipley, R. E., and Gregg, D. E., The effect of external constriction of blood vessel on blood flow, *Am J Physiol* 1994; 141:289.

18. Yao, J. S. T., and Bergan, J. J., Predictability of vascular reactivity relative to sympathetic ablation, *Arch Surg* 1973; 107:676.

8

ADVANCES IN THE DIAGNOSIS AND TREATMENT OF CHRONIC VENOUS ULCERATION

Ralph G. DePalma, M.D.

INTRODUCTION

Cutaneous ulceration due to chronic venous insufficiency (CVI) has been recognized as a serious problem for over two millennia. Bergan [1] recently provided a historical account of venous disease and leg ulcers. Important relationships were inferred from the initial understanding of the direction of venous blood flow, pressure dynamics, and ultimately the discovery by Harvey in 1628 of the circulatory system itself. Crucial to this revolutionary understanding was the recognition of the structure and function of venous valves by Fabricius in 1603 at Padua. Fabricius, a prominent Renaissance surgeon, had been a teacher of Harvey, who later left for England.

Venous ulceration had long been known to relate to the effects of venous pressure exacerbated by gravity. Hippocrates [2], in the fourth century B.C., wrote, "In the case of an ulcer it is expedient not to stand, more especially if the ulcer be situated in the leg." Nullifying gravitational effects to promote healing of venous ulceration remains today one of the most important means of treatment.

Compression therapy can be viewed as a method to overcome gravitational effects, although exactly how compression accomplishes this effect is not completely clear. The efficacy of lower limb compression was mentioned by Hippocrates and Celsus and culminated in the development of *Unna's boot* by a dermatologist in 1896 [3]. This medicated support bandage is still in use. In the seventeenth century, Wiseman, surgeon to Charles the II, developed a lace-up leather support [4] to treat venous ulceration; this appliance was remarkably similar to modern elastic supports, which are equipped, with a posterior zipper.

Although venous ulceration is viewed by some as a vexing, unglamorous problem, many prominent surgeons in the past, including Pare', Vicary, John, Hunter, Brodie, Trendelenburg [5], and, more recently, Linton [6] and Homans [7] of Boston, concerned themselves with venous ulceration. In 1946 Homans linked venous ulceration to prior thrombophlebitis, leading to a concept that venous ulceration occurs in a "post-phlebitic leg." It is now recognized, however, that venous ulceration quite often relates to valvular incompetence and superficial venous disease, processes which are amenable to surgical intervention. Both Linton [8] and Homans [9] were aware of valvular insufficiency and, in certain cases, recommended ligation of incompetent superficial femoral veins to overcome gravitational reflux.

The modern understanding of venous disease is characterized by concerns with the pathophysiology of CVI and related skin changes, rather than the waste basket diagnosis of "postphlebitic leg." CVI, as pointed out by Browse and Burnand [10] and Bergan and Kistner [11], now demands precise anatomic and physiologic definition for each individual. This concept of CVI, combined with the use of modern diagnostic methods [12], medical treatment [13], and surgical techniques [11], promises better outcomes for patients suffering from venous ulceration.

PATHOGENESIS

The skin and its subcutaneous tissues are the ultimate targets of venous hypertension. In the early stages of stasis dermatitis, skin pigmentation is caused by hemosiderin deposition in the lower third of the leg, usually on its medial aspect. Initial staining is followed by itching, then a weeping dermatitis, which untreated progresses to chronic ulceration. Cellular changes in the skin and subcutis ultimately cause zones of regional hypoxemia characterized by lipodermatosclerosis and skin breakdown. Untreated, this process is inexorable, in spite of what seems to be a regional superabundance of blood. One theory of venous ulceration invoked accumulation of a pericapillary fibrin cuff, which interferes with the diffusion of oxygen and other metabolites [14].

Newer theories of tissue damage relate to unique findings of lower extremity white blood cell trapping after limb dependency in CVI [15]. When lipodermatosclerosis and ulceration are present, up to 30% of circulating white blood cells are trapped in the limb after one hour of dependency. Tissue destruction can then be induced by leukocyte activation, proteolytic enzyme release, and free radical activity. Alternatively, peripheral resistance might increase as white cells obstruct the capillaries [16]. With repeated episodes of dependency, repeated reperfusion phenomena are thought to inflict continued damage as white cells (WBC) are activated and continue to escape into the tissues. Biopsies from the skin of patients with CVI including varicose veins, lipodermatosclerosis, and ulceration [17] show increasing white counts from 6 WBC/mm^2 in varicose veins, 45 WBC/mm^2 in lipodermatosclerosis, to 211 WBC/mm^2 with ulceration. T lymphocytes and macrophages are the predominating WBC in afflicted skin areas; an increase in capillaries also occurs in the papillary dermis. Whether white cell infiltration is the cause or effect of ulcerative change remains uncertain; clearly progressive skin infiltration is associated with progressively more severe CVI.

PATHOPHYSIOLOGY

Venous hypertension underlies the skin changes that progress to ulceration. This can be due to several mechanisms. Skin changes are related in an approximate manner to increased venous pressure [17], but a linear relationship cannot be unequivocally assumed. Nicolaides et al. [18] reiterated recently that venous ulceration did not occur with ambulatory venous pressures (AVP) below 30 mm Hg, but was always present when AVP exceeded 90 mm Hg. Ulceration was also associated with a short recovery time; i.e., the time needed to recover to 90% of standing resting pressure. However, there is considerable overlap in other types of physiologic measurements; for example, air plethysmography [19]. Thus, the magnitude of cutaneous pathology may not always depend on linear pressure or volume relationships. The variable and complex anatomy of the venous system and its valves, as well as the importance of the muscular calf pump, contribute to variable expressions of venous hypertension. Altered lymphatic drainage might also play a role in ulceration.

Three sources of venous hypertension impacting the skin of the lower leg should be considered. These are:

1. **Hydrostatic.** Caused by weight of the blood column from the right atrium to the ankle area [20]. The weight of this column is normally mitigated by venous valves and muscles, including the plantar muscles when standing.

2. **Dynamic.** Caused by the force of calf muscular contraction, which normally aids in pumping blood proximally within the deep compartments [21].

3. **Distal.** Caused by increased venous flow into the distal saphenous vein from communicating foot and ankle veins [22].

Abnormally high hydrostatic pressures are generated either by incompetent valves or proximal obstruction or a combination of both. Vena caval obstruction combined with distal disease cause inexorably severe lower limb venous hypertension. Obstruction due to any cause is more often associated with refractory ulceration. Failed perforator check valves in the posterior leg venous arcade are thought to contribute to increased pressure on ambulation. Characteristic perforator leg veins that transmit pressure have been named for Cockett [23]. Others more proximal in the calf and thigh have been named for Boyd, Dodd, and Hunter, respectively. Identification of these perforating veins as they contribute to the transmission of venous hypertension is needed for individualizing surgical treatment. Finally, *distal flow* from the foot, as previously mentioned, is an important factor in recurrent ulceration [22]. Other mechanisms contributing to venous hypertension are congenital arteriovenous fistulae. In these cases, venous ulceration, often in unusual sites, is a presenting symptom. Venous ulceration in the upper leg can also occur with large perforators related to Klippel-Trenaunay's syndrome. Stasis ulceration is associated with obesity, rheumatoid and other arthritides, and calf or foot pump muscular failure due to muscular wasting. The role of the lymphatics in clearing the overflow from excess venous pressure has recently been reemphasized [24].

In the past, ulceration was most commonly attributed to CVI due predominantly to deep venous disease. The author's clinical experience [25, 26] and recent reports indicate that the source of CVI in over half the cases seen is mainly superficial venous insufficiency [27]. Superficial insufficiency can be associated with deep venous reflux in the absence of obstruction. When superficial venous reflux is clearly demonstrated, elimination of this factor is the most effective treatment. In some in-stances, distal deep reflux improves after superficial stripping [28], implying a need for a staged approach.

DIAGNOSIS OF CVI

A careful physical examination in slender subjects may suffice to delineate incompetent superficial varicosities. A large dilated saphenous vein is visible and palpable; physical signs of greater or lesser saphenous reflux can be detected by palpation or Doppler insonation in the groin or popliteal fossa. Disturbing the blood column by percussion can start pressure transmission through the static column of blood contained with the incompetent dilated vessel. Although Doppler insonation is useful in slender subjects, when the subcutaneous tissue thickness is greater than 2.5 cm, duplex sonography is much more accurate in delineating sites of reflux, incompetency, and valvular insufficiency [29]. The duplex scan is invaluable for estimating the rate of deep reflux and for ruling out obstruction. This is the most important single study to be obtained to guide treatment. Although classic tests using tourniquets; e.g., the Trendelenburg test [5], are useful clinically, duplex scanning is recommended before axial vein stripping.

In examining the lower leg and sites of venous ulceration, the clinician must rule out arterial insufficiency by palpation and Doppler insonation of foot pulses. Edema or cellulitis can make arterial palpation difficult, but Doppler-verified ankle-to-arm pressure ratios make clear the cases where arterial and venous disease coexist. The venous ulcer has a characteristic appearance and location, as does lipodermatosclerosis. These changes involve the lower limb in the "gaiter area." This zone comprises the lower one-third of the limb and near the ankle is often posterior to the medial malleolus. Lateral involvement occurs with lesser saphenous incompetence. Occasionally, Kaposi's sarcoma lesions mimic venous ulcers when these become confluent or ulcerated in areas of limb dependency. The unilateral occurrence of Kaposi's lesions can be deceptive and must be kept in mind.

Although the diagnosis of venous ulceration is usually apparent, the examiner must seek to accurately define its underlying anatomic bases. These include superficial or deep incompetence or obstruction. Local perforators contributing to ulcers sometimes can be palpated as fascial defects. However, abnormal flow patterns from deep to superficial compartments are difficult to assess even by duplex scanning [30]. Direct venous reconstructive surgery for intractable ulcers must be planned using ascending and descending venography [31]. The former delineates sites of obstruction; the latter delineates sites of valvular insufficiency.

TREATMENT

The mainstay of treatment for venous ulceration is compression; it is used first. A review of conservative treatment and pathophysiology of cutaneous ulceration was published as a consensus statement in 1992 [13]. Compression is achieved by graded elastic supports that cause compression of interstitial tissues, rather than a reduction in pressure in the veins themselves. During acute phases of venous ulceration with cellulitis and infection, bed rest and limb elevation above the level of the atrium are critical. This usually also requires hospitalization and aggressive wound care with plain gauze dressing changes and ulcer cleansing. Tetracycline is an effective antibiotic in venous ulcers, possibly because of nonspecific antiinflammatory effects. However, the ulcer bed should be cultured and specific antibiotics used intravenously to control local infection and surrounding cellulitis.

Once acute inflammatory changes are controlled, limb compression devices are applied. These include Unna's paste boot, short and long stretch elastic bandages, and semirigid Velcro supports; i.e., the Circaid appliance. When healing has been achieved, *below-knee* gradient stockings are prescribed to deliver 30–40 mm Hg pressure at the ankles. Rarely do patients require higher ankle pressures or above-knee compression. In the elderly or in patients with an element of arterial insufficiency, support stockings delivering 20 mm Hg at the ankle are advised. The patient must not wear compression stockings at night; instead elevation of the foot of the bed on 12-inch blocks should be arranged. Triamcinolone cream, .025%, is applied nightly to control itching and surrounding areas of dermatitis.

Medication with ointments and poultices must be avoided, as well as misguided overexposure to water, strong detergents, and soap.

New drug treatment options for venous ulcers and lipodermatosclerosis are based upon current theories of pathogenesis and prospective trials recently reviewed [13]. None of these agents has been widely used in the United States. They have been studied on the Continent and will require familiarity as they become used in the United States. These drugs include fibrinolytics, hydroxyrutosides, prostaglandins, methylxanthines, and antioxidants. Fibrinolytic treatment has yielded conflicting results; hydroxyrutosides have been used on the continent for many years to treat the symptoms of CVI. These agents are not particularly effective for venous ulcers. Intravenous prostaglandins have been reported to promote ulcer healing, and methylxanthines, which improve both red and white cell deformability, have also been described as effective [32] when combined with compression therapy. Antioxidants and free radical scavengers such as allopurinol and dimethyl sulfoxide have also been shown to promote healing. Allopurinol and xanthine oxidase may act by ameliorating reperfusion effects and the toxic effects of oxygen metabolites and free radicals.

SURGICAL TREATMENT

Surgical interventions must be based on an accurate anatomic and physiologic diagnosis. When superficial venous incompetence is the main contributing factor to ulceration, an operation should be performed sooner rather than later in fit candidates. In all cases, duplex scanning and a physical examination are essential to assess the status of the deep venous system. With deep venous incompetence or occlusion, operative intervention is recommended if a trial of compression and medical therapy fails. Surgical procedures include saphenous or axial stripping to control gravitational reflux, excision of varicose clusters and perforators, perforator interruption, either extra or subfascial, venous bypass, and valvular reconstructions.

Figure 8-1 demonstrates the healing of an ulcer by saphenous vein stripping and ligation of the indicated perforator and communicators. This

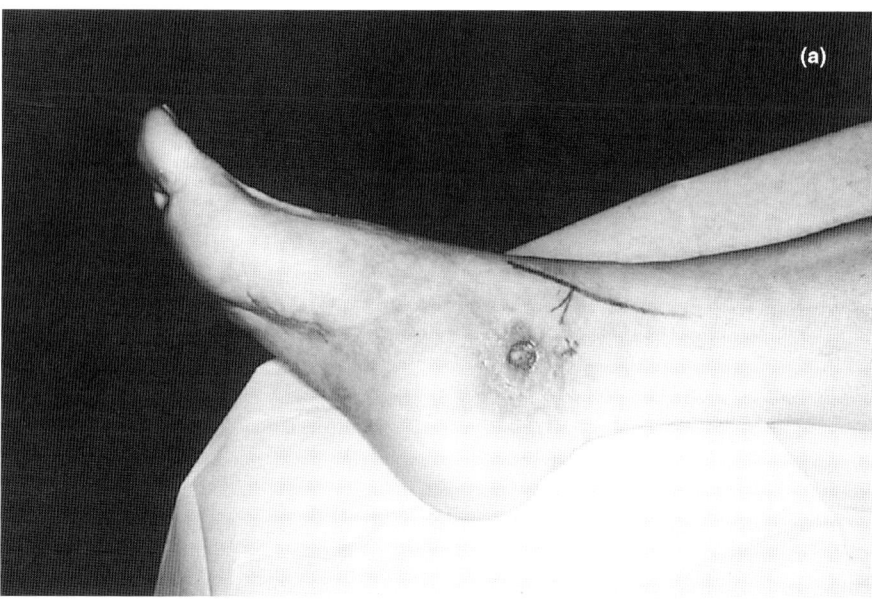

Figure 8-1(a).   Chronic venous ulcer in a forty-year-old woman due to saphenous incompetence with one perforator and communicators as indicated.

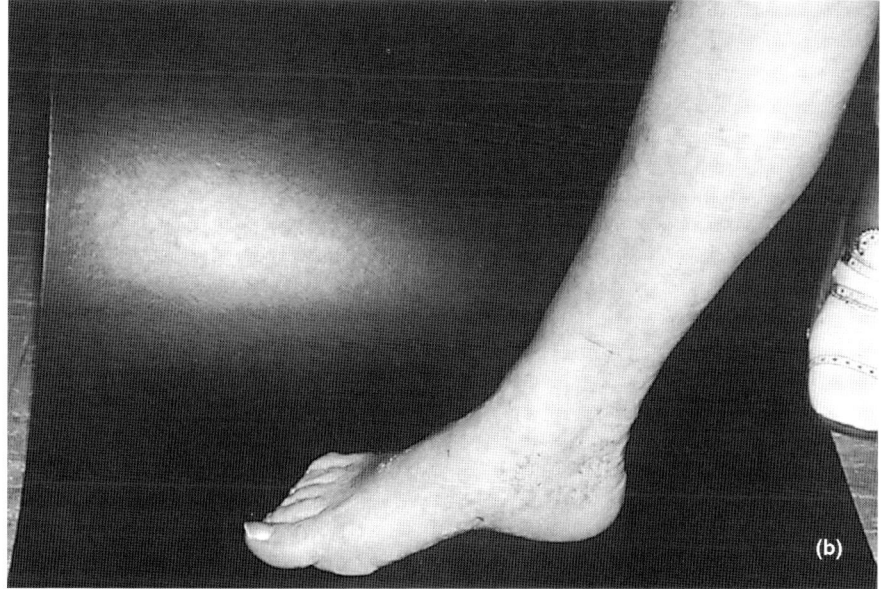

Figure 8-1(b).   Result at one year after stripping and skin grafting.

forty-year-old female twin had minimal deep involvement. She remained healed using only light cosmetic compression, as did her identical twin, who suffered from a mirror image lesion of the opposite leg.

For perforator incompetence, DePalma [33] modified Linton's principles [6] to interrupt perforating and communicating veins. This procedure aimed to minimize transmission of venous hypertension to the skin and subcutaneous tissues. Complete interruption of incompetent perforating and communicating veins and grafting of ulcers were achieved in one operation. This differed from the traditional operation in that, rather than creating a longitudinal incision notorious for its poor healing, the procedure used a series of bipedicled flaps with incisions in the skin lines. A follow-up report detailed experience in fifty-three patients observed for up to twelve years [25]. Four recurrences in this period related to failure to wear postoperative support, lateral recurrence treated by a "modified Cockett" procedure, and caval occlusion.

More recently, an extrafascial shearing operation through a proximal skin line incision over Boyd's perforator is employed [34]. A shearing phlebotome [35] is passed from above to the malleolus along the posterior arcade, severing perforators subcutaneously. The only subfascial dissection is done near the leg ulcer retromalleolar area. This achieves precise ligation of perforators originating from the posterior tibial vein. Removal of saphenous veins, external femoral valvuloplasty, and crossover femoral procedures have been combined as staged or simultaneous procedures when needed to relieve severe incompetence or obstruction. The preoperative and postoperative appearances following femoral crossover graft and staged shearing perforator interruption are shown in Figure 8-2. Preoperative ascending and descending venography are required for planning these procedures.

Using the shearing extrafascial approach, hospitalization time has been reduced from 14 days to 3–4 days, as skin grafting is not required for ulcers less than 3 cm in diameter. When skin grafting is done, 7 or more hospital days are needed, as the leg must be kept elevated. Generally, in a ten-year follow-up of over 80 limbs, recurrences again related to caval occlusion, lateral malleolar lesions,

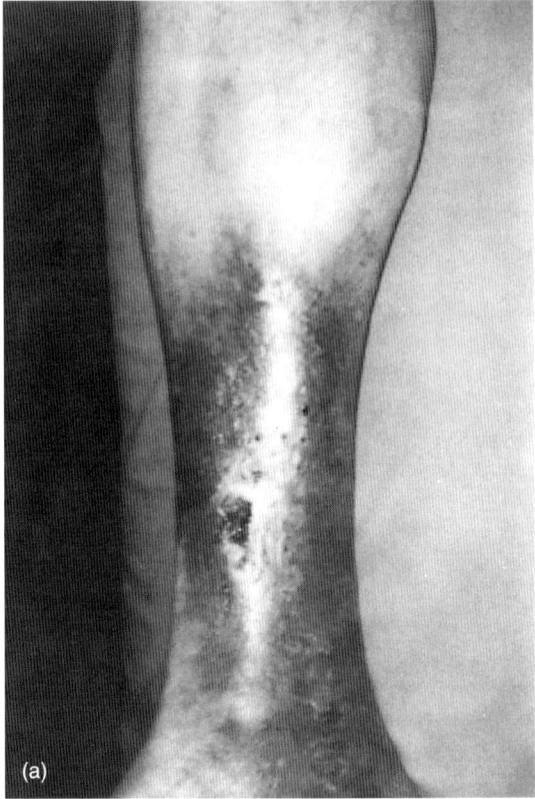

(a)

Figure 8-2(a).   Extensive lipodermatosclerosis and ulceration in a sixty-year-old man with iliac vein occlusion and perforator incompetence.

and failure to wear support. Proximal occlusion is the main problem contributing to recurrent ulceration; it is imperative that individuals with proximal occlusion continue to wear firm, graded support after operation.

A sequence of management of venous ulceration includes outpatient care to promote ulcer healing, graded elastic compression, meticulous treatment of dermatitis, and avoidance of local treatment with "wound healing" poultices. Based on duplex scanning, if CVI involves mainly saphenous incompetence, axial stripping should be recommended. This procedure can be combined with interruption of calf perforator veins. The author's preference is extrafascial division of perforating veins; recently, subfascial ligation of perforating veins within the deep compartments using a laparoscopic approach [36] has yielded initially favorable results.

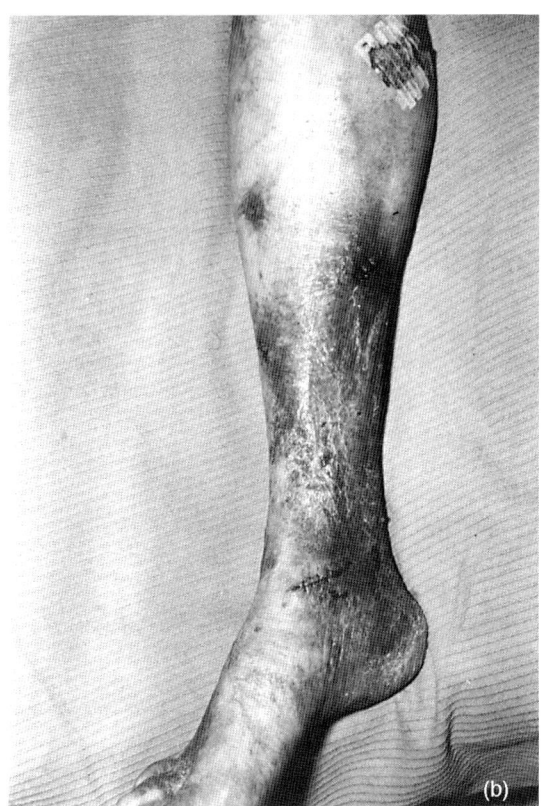

Figure 8-2(b). Immediate appearance after Palma saphenous vein crossover graft and perforator shearing operation at a second stage.

Direct venous reconstruction was first performed by Palma [37, 38]. This procedure, which is practical and durable, uses a crossover saphenous vein graft from the opposite limb for unilateral iliac occlusion. Sapheno-popliteal bypass grafts for superficial femoral vein occlusive disease, first used by Warren [39], have not been as successful and are now rarely done. Kistner [40–42] pioneered open valveplasty as early as 1968 as well as venous transfer operations to provide direct flow through competent valvular segments in the groin. In evaluating long-term results, Kistner emphasized [42] perforator interruption in addition to femoral valve reconstruction for incompetence. This combined approach was used in the case seen in Figure 8-2, because caval or proximal iliac occlusion presage a poor prognosis for healing of venous ulcerations. Large vein reconstruction in the abdominal position

requires arteriovenous fistulae to maintain patency [1, 43]. Short expanded polytetrafluoroethylene grafts with a large diameter can be considered for intractable venous hypertension and ulceration in selected patients. Few long-term follow-ups exist to document the efficacy of caval reconstruction for this troublesome subset of patients. In the author's experience, caval obstruction is most recalcitrant to perforator ligation as well as to aggressive conservative therapy.

SUMMARY

Within the last decade, a more rational view of CVI has developed. Patients with venous ulceration are no longer relegated to a waste basket diagnosis of "postphlebitic limb." Duplex scanning and venography now provide roadmaps for diagnosis. Improved surgical interventions exist when conservative therapy fails. The recognition of superficial venous incompetence as an important contributor to ulceration deserves reemphasis. A more sophisticated understanding of skin alterations subjected to venous hypertension promises more effective future medical interventions.

REFERENCES

1. Bergan, J. J., Historical highlights in treating venous insufficiency, in J. J. Bergan, J. S. T. Yao, eds., *Venous Disorders,* Philadelphia: W. B. Saunders, 1991:3.

2. Hippocrates, *The Genuine Works of Hippocrates,* E. F. Adarns, Transl., vol. 2, New York: W. M. Wood & Co., 1886:305.

3. Unna, P. G., Über paraplaste eine naue form medicamentöse pflaster, *Wein Med Wochenschrift* 1896; 43:1854.

4. Wiseman, R., *Several Chirurgical Treatises,* London: Rogston & Took, 1676.

5. Trendelenburg, J., Über die Unterbinding der Vena saphena magna bei Unterschekelvaricen, *Beitr Klin Chir* 1890–1891; 195.

6. Linton, R. R., The communicating veins of the lower leg and the operative technique for their ligation, *Ann Surg* 1938; 107:582.

7. Homans, J., The late results of femoral thrombophlebitis and their treatment, *N Engl J Med* 1946; 235:249.

8. Linton, R. R., Post thrombotic ulcerations of the lower extremity: Its etiology and surgical treatment, *Ann Surg* 1953; 138:582.

9. Homans, J., The etiology and treatment of varicose ulcers of the leg, *Surg Gynecol Obstet* 1917; 24:300.

10. Browse, N. L., and Burnand, K. G., The postphlebitic syndrome: A new look, in J. J. Bergan, J. S. T. Yao, ed., *Venous Problems,* Chicago: Year Book Medical Publishers, 1979:395.

11. Bergan, J. J., and Kistner, R. L., *Atlas of Venous Surgery,* Philadelphia: W. B. Saunders.

12. Van Bemmelen, P. S., and Bergan, J. J., eds., Photoplethysmography and light reflection rheography, in *Quantitative Measurement of Venous Incompetence,* Austin, TX and New York: R. G. Landes, 1992:37.

13. The consensus paper on venous leg ulcers, The Alexander House Group, *Phlebology* 1992; 7:48.

14. Browse, N. L., and Burnand, K. G., The cause of venous ulceration, *Lancet* 1982; 2:243.

15. Thomas, P. R. S.; Nash, G. P.; and Dormandy, J. A., White cell accumulation in the dependent legs of patients with venous hypertension: A possible mechanism for trophic changes in the skin, *Brit Med J* 1988; 296:1693.

16. Schmid-Schonbein, G. W., Granulocyte: Friend or foe, *Nips* 1988; 3:6.

17. Scott, H. J.; Coleridge-Smith, P. D.; and Scurr, J. H., Histological study of white blood cells and their association with lipodermatosclerosis and venous ulceration, *Brit J Surg* 1991; 78:212.

18. Nicolaides, A. N.; Hussaein, M. K.; Szendro, G.; et al., The relation of venous ulceration with ambulatory venous pressure measurements, *J Vasc Surg* 1993; 17:414.

19. Cordts, P. R.; Hartono, C.; LaMorte, W. W.; et al., Physiologic similarities between extremities with varicose veins and with chronic venous insufficiency utilizing air plethysmography, *Ann J Surg* 1992; 164:260.

20. Bjordal, R. I., Haemodynamic studies of varicose veins and the post thrombotic syndrome, in J. T. Hobbs, ed., *The Treatment of Venous Disorders,* MTP Press Ltd, 1977:37.

21. Arnoldi, C. C., Venous pressure in patients with valvular incompetence of the veins of the lower limb, *Acta Chir Scand* 1996; 132:628.

22. Negus, D. The distal long saphenous vein in recurrent venous ulceration, in P. Raymond-Martinbeau, R. Prescott, M. Zummo, eds., *Phlebologie,* John Libbey Eurotext 1992: 1291.

23. Cockett, F. B., and Elgan-Jones, D. E., The ankle blow out syndrome, *Lancet* 1953; 1:17.

24. Meade, F. W., and Mueller, C. B., Lymphatic and venous examination of the ulcerated leg: A preliminary report, *Surgery* 1992; 112:872.

25. DePalma, R. G., Surgical therapy for venous stasis: Results of a modified Linton operation, *Am J Surg* 1979; 137:810.

26. DePalma, R. G., Surgical treatment of chronic venous ulceration, In P. Raymond-Martinbeau, R. Prescott, M. Zummo, ed., *Phlebologie* 92 John Libbey Eurotext, 1992: 1235.

27. Shami, S. K.; Sarin, S.; Cheatle, T. R.; Scurr, J. H.; and Coleridge-Smith, P. D.; Venous ulcers and the superficial venous system, *J Vasc Surg* 1993; 17:487.

28. Walsh, J.; Bergan, J. J.; Beeman, S.; and Moulton, S. L., Femoral vein reflux is abolished by saphenous vein stripping, *Ann Vasc Surg* 1994; 8:566.

29. DePalma, R. G.; Hart, M. T.; Zanin, L.; and Massarin, E. H., Physical examination, Doppler ultrasound and colour flow duplex scanning: Guides to therapy for primary varicose veins, *Phlebology* 1993; 8:7.

30. Sarin, S., Scurr, J. H.; and Smith, P. D. C., Medial calf perforators in venous disease: The significance of outward flow, *J. Vasc Surg* 1992; 16:40.

31. Kamida, C. B., and Kistner, R. L., Descending phlebology: The Straub technique, in J. J. Bergan, R. L. Kistner, eds., *Atlas of Venous Surgery,* Philadelphia: W. B. Saunders, 1992:105.

32. Weitgasser, H., The use of pentoxifylline (Trental 400) in the treatment of leg ulcers: Results of a double-blind trial, *Pharmatherapeutica* 1983; 3:143.

33. DePalma, R. G., Surgical therapy for venous stasis, *Surgery* 1975; 76:910.

34. DePalma, R. G., Surgical treatment of chronic venous ulceration in J. J. Bergan, J. S. T. Yao, eds., *Venous Disorders,* Philadelphia: W. B. Saunders, 1991:396.

35. Simpson, C. J., and Smellie, G. D., The phlebotome

in the management of incompetent perforating veins and venous ulcers, *J Cardiovasc Surg* 1987; 28:274.

36. O'Donnell, T. F., Surgical treatment of incompetent communicating veins, in Bergan, J. J., R. L. Kistner, eds., *Atlas of Venous Surgery,* Philadelphia: W. B. Saunders, 1992:111.

37. Palma, E. C., and Esperon, R., Vein transplants and grafts in the surgical treatment of the postphlebitic syndrome, *J Cardiovasc Surg* 1960; 1:94.

38. Palma, E. C., et al., Tratamiento de los trastornos postflebiticos mediante anastomosis venosa safeno-femoral controlateral, *Bull Soc Surg Uruguay* 1958; 29:135.

39. Warren, R., and Thayer, T. R., Transplantation of the saphenous vein for postphlebitic stasis, *Surgery* 1954; 35:867.

40. Kistner, R. L., Surgical repair of a venous valve, *Straub Clin Proc* 1968; 34:41.

41. Kistner, R. L., Surgical repair of the incompetent femoral vein valve, *Arch Surg* 1975; 110:1336.

42. Kistner, R. L., Late results of venous valve repair, in J. S. T. Yao, W. L. Pearce, ed., *Long-Term Results of Vascular Surgery,* Philadelphia: W. B. Saunders, 1993:451.

43. Gloviczki, P.; Pairolero, P. C.; Toomey, B. J.; et al., Reconstruction of large veins for nonmalignant venous occlusive disease, *J Vasc Surg* 1992; 16:750.

9

PRESSURE ULCERS: AN OVERVIEW

Bok Y. Lee, M.D.
Milon G. Karmakar, M.D.

INTRODUCTION

Pressure ulcers are a serious concern in patients with spinal cord injury (SCI) and in residents of nursing homes and geriatric care facilities. Pressure ulcers have a tremendous impact on overall well-being as well as an adverse impact on morbidity and mortality. They increase the overall cost of the patient care by prolonging hospital stay and by escalating nursing costs and time. Additional losses may be incurred from consequent litigation. Of central import is the fact that, although the estimated costs of healing a single pressure ulcer range from $2,000 to $40,000 [1], up to 95% of pressure ulcers are preventable. Judicious and prudent resource allocation is best directed towards this goal.

The Agency for Health Care Policy and Research (AHCPR) [73] has identified pressure ulcers as one of the seven conditions affecting large number of patients involving relatively expensive treatment and urgently needing strategies for prevention and cost containment. This view assumes ever-increasing importance in the context of increasing age of the population and the use of life support technologies to prolong the life of severely ill patients.

DEFINITION

Pressure ulcers are areas of tissue necrosis that occur in susceptible individuals secondary to external physical compression, friction, shear force, moisture, or a combination of these factors. An individual susceptibility to develop pressure ulcers may also exist. Pressure ulcers have been variously referred to as bed sores, decubitus ulcers, and pressure sores. The term *decubitus,* derived from the latin *decumbere* (to lie down), is restrictive and inaccurate, implying as it does that the ulcer is produced only as a result of prolonged recumbency. It fails to recognize that ulcers that can result from a combination of shear and friction, as seen over nonbony prominences, occur particularly in patients with spinal cord injury. Therefore, the term *pressure ulcer* is preferable.

HISTORICAL ASPECTS

Pressure ulcers as a clinical problem have been noted throughout history. Thompson [2] reported pressure ulcers in Egyptian mummies, and Fabricius (according to a citation by Vasconez) attributed the formation of pressure sores to a "pneuma" that resulted from severed nerves and loss of blood supply [3]. The most important contribution, however, was made by Ambrose Pare, one of the founding fathers of modern medicine, who documented in an autobiographical work entitled *The Apology and Treatise* (circa 1585) a detailed description of the successful cure of a pressure ulcer in a wounded French aristocrat [4]. In his tract, *Of ulcers, fistula, and hemorrhoides* [5], he presented an extensive discussion on the treatment of this condition, laying down principles of management that are valid even today. He emphasized first the removal of the cause, "which unless it be taken away, the ulcer cannot be healed." Pain relief was addressed, followed by recommendations for diet, sleep, rest, and moderate exercise. He went on to emphasize that if cure did not follow these steps, then it was mandatory to consider debridement, using the phrases: "the rottenesse of the bone . . . and you shall cut away the callous hardnesse." The final task was attention to rebuilding of the tissue, "For the generation of the flesh, (one must induce) an attraction, digestion, apposition, and assimilation of the laudable juices to the part affected" [5].

In 1852 Brown-Sequard [6] suggested that moisture, along with skin pressure, was important in pressure ulcer development. He based this on the observation of the absence of pressure ulcers in animals with experimentally induced transections of the spinal cord, who were kept dry. In 1873, Sir James Paget [7] defined pressure sores as "sloughing and mortification or death of a part due to pressure" and called these lesions "bed sores." In 1879, Charcot [8] observed that pressure ulcers developed in paraplegic and debilitated patients, and that it was an inevitable and natural complication seen in anesthetic skin. He believed that an injury to a nerve released a neurotrophic factor that led to tissue necrosis. This theory was the forerunner of an era of "therapeutic nihilism" [3], that was evident as late as 1940 by Munro's suggestion (reported by Vasconez) that a disturbance in the autonomic nervous system altered the peripheral reflexes of the skin and predisposed the patient to ulceration. Munro reportedly was opposed to any form of surgical intervention because he believed that progressive ulceration was a natural consequence of the condition [3]. Although disturbance in the autonomic nervous system does occur in some SCI patients, the direct role of such disturbances in the development of pressure ulcers has not been substantiated [9]. Observation and treatments conducted during World War I showed that both paraplegic and debilitated patients developed pressure sores and that these lesions could be prevented and effectively treated.

The history of the surgical management of pressure ulcers can be attributed to Davis (1938) who used flap replacement of scarred epithelium to heal ulcers in order to provide bulky and well-padded skin coverage over bony prominences [10]. In 1940, Brooks and Duncan [11] demonstrated that both the duration of pressure application and the magnitude of pressure were important in etiology and noted that the time of pressure application required to produce necrosis was inversely proportional to the magnitude of applied pressure. Scoville in 1944 [3] and Lamon and Alexander in 1945 [12] reported the first successful excision of a sacral ulcer and primary closure in patients receiving parenteral penicillin. In 1945, White et al. reported favorable outcomes in patients with sacral ulcers treated by rotation flaps [13]. Cronway and Griffith [14] in 1946 published the results of their five-year experience in the surgical treatment of 374 patients with 600 lesions. Their findings suggested the need for long hospitalizations and for both multiple and staged surgical procedures to attain successful healing. In 1947 Kostrubola and Greeley [15] advised the removal of bony prominences underlying the ulcers and the use of muscle flaps to provide mechanical padding. Traditional surgical management encompassed primary closure and the use of conventional rotational flaps with suboptimal results. The use of myocutaneous flaps provided an excellent alternative to these conventional methods. Tansini reportedly developed a latissimus dorsi myocutaneous flap in 1894 to close a chest defect resulting from wide surgical resection of a breast [16]. In 1955 Owens [17] used a myocutaneous rotation flap to repair a massive facial defect. In 1972 the vascular basis of the procedure was described by Orticochea [18], and in 1977 McGraw and associates [19] described a systematic approach for devising a variety of myocutaneous flaps to accommodate a variety of surgical needs.

The period following World War II saw the

elucidation of the biomechanics of pressure in the development of pressure ulcers. Prevention emerged as the cornerstone in the management of these patients, reducing both morbidity and cost. Unfortunately, medical education on this topic has heretofore been generally deficient [20], but it is expected that the U.S. Department of Health and Human Services will shortly release updated treatment guidelines for predicting, preventing, and treating pressure ulcers.

EPIDEMIOLOGY

It is difficult to generalize the incidence and prevalence of pressure ulcers because there is a wide variation in data acquisition and analyses from diverse care facilities such as acute care hospitals, long-term facilities, and home care settings. The incidence and prevalence are, however, high enough to be a serious concern.

INCIDENCE

Rudman et al. reported an incidence rate of 4.2% to 10.3% in the Veterans Administration (VA) system over a six-month period [21]. Oot-Giromini [22] reported an incidence rate of 16.5%. Guralnik [29] reported an incidence of 3.3% over ten years based on a population aged seventy to seventy-five years. Allman [30, 31] reported incidence ranging from 7.7% to 25% over several weeks in an acute care hospital. In another report of critical care populations, Bergstrom and associates [141] reported an incidence of 33%. Berlowitz [32] reported an incidence of 10.5% over a thirteen-month period in a chronic care hospital. In nursing home patients, Michocki [33] and Reed [34] reported an incidence of 24% and 26%, respectively, developing over a six-month period. Brandeis and associates [23] found that, at the end of one year, the incidence of pressure ulcers for new residents admitted to the nursing homes was 13.2%, and the incidence was 9.5% for people already residing in the nursing homes. He also found that, for these groups, at the end of two years the incidences had risen to 21.6% and 20.4%, respectively. The Royal London Hospi-

tal prevalence study in the United Kingdom reported an incidence of 5% to 8.8%. Versluysen [35] reported an incidence of 66% in elderly orthopedic patients with hip fracture. It has been noted that more than half of the patients had more than one sore and that multiple pressure ulcers are more common in the elderly [35, 36].

PREVALENCE

The prevalence of pressure ulcers shows variations between different institutions as well as between different countries. A recent publication shows that in the United States, the VA medical system reported a prevalence rate of 2% to 16% [21]. Oot-Giromini [22] reported a higher prevalence of 29% in the community within the United States. Brandeis and associates [23] reported a prevalence rate of 17.4% for new residents following admission to nursing homes, which decreased to 8.1% by the end of two years; the prevalence for residents already present in the nursing homes at the start of the study was 8.9% and remained more or less constant over a two-year period. In various other studies, the prevalence for hospitalized patients has been reported to be between 3% to 11% [24–26]. The National Nursing Home Survey reported a 2.6% prevalence rate [27]. This low rate may be attributed to the fact that the survey was conducted by interviews and encompassed all levels of care, including boarding homes (which have a more ambulatory population). Richardson and Meyer [142] reported a high prevalence rate of 60% in a high-risk SCI population. The 1971 study conducted in Denmark [25] showed a prevalence of 3% of pressure ulcers in inpatients and a 0.01% prevalence in the community. In Scotland 8.8% of hospital patients and 8.7% of community patients were found to have pressure ulcers [28].

MORTALITY

Berlowitz and Wilking [32] found a mortality of 24% at 6 weeks among patients admitted to nursing homes with a pressure ulcer and a 21% mortality among those patients who subsequently developed pressure ulcers while in the facility. Reed [34] reported a 64% mortality within six months

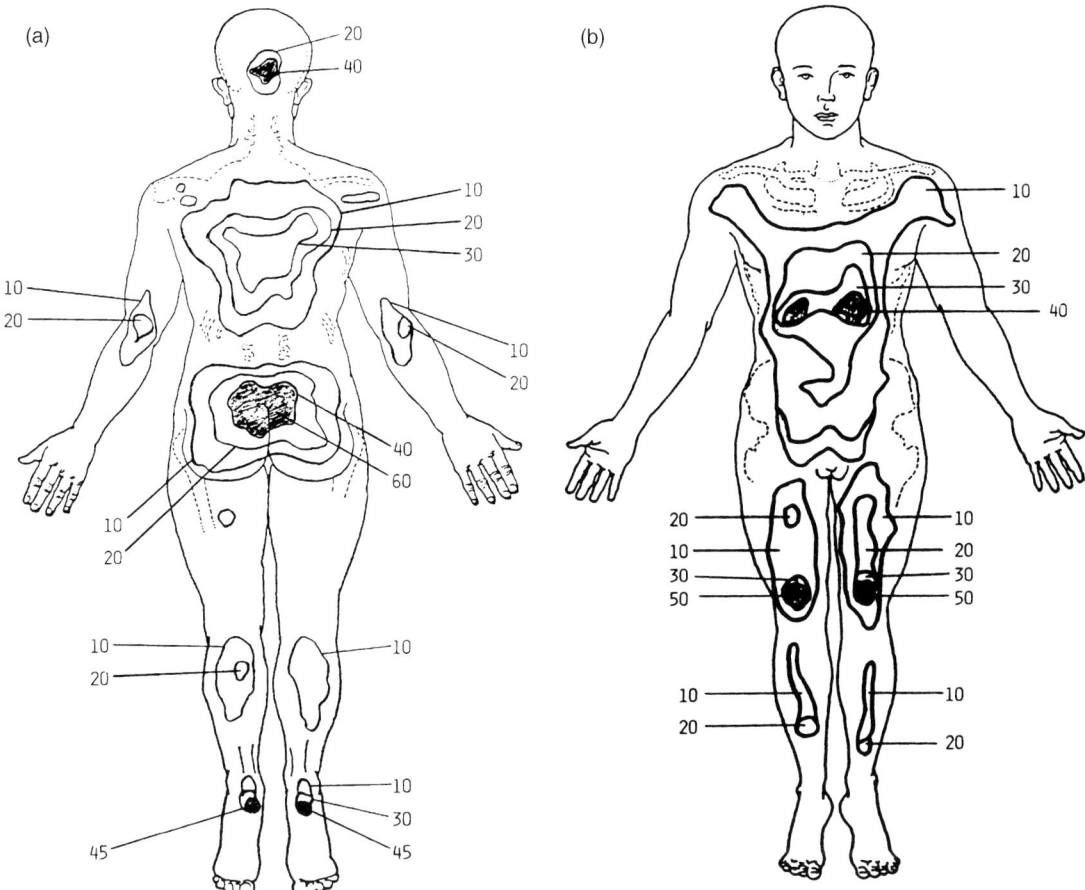

Figure 9-1. (a) The regions of highest pressure in a supine patient, (b) The regions of highest pressure in a patient who is in a prone position. (From chap. 18 figs 18-1)

for patients whose pressure ulcers had not healed. Brandeis and associates [23] reported an overall increased mortality in patients with pressure ulcers compared to those who did not have them. Those patients admitted with pressure ulcers had an 88.1% greater death rate at the end of one year, which decreased to 50.6% at the end of two years. The resident group with pressure ulcers had a 129% greater death rate by the first year, which decreased to 31.2% by the end of two years. Brandeis also showed increased mortality in both groups of patients who developed new pressure ulcers during their stay in the nursing homes [23].

SITES OF PRESSURE ULCER FORMATION

The distribution of pressure points in humans in recumbent and seated positions has been documented [37]. (See Figures 9-1 and 9-2.) The regions of highest pressure in the supine position include the sacrum, buttocks, heel and occiput (40 to 60 mm Hg of pressure). The knees and chest receive the most pressure in the prone position (approximately 50 mm Hg). In the seated position a hard surface provides for decreased distribution and resultant higher point pressure. Seated pressures of

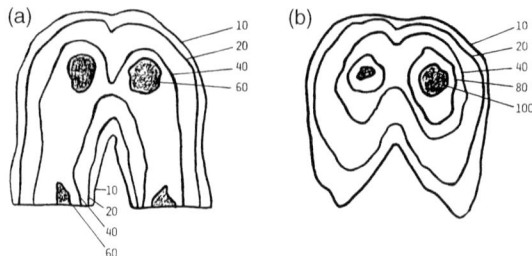

Figure 9-2.   Examples of pressure distribution in the seated position. (From chap. 18 figs 18-2)

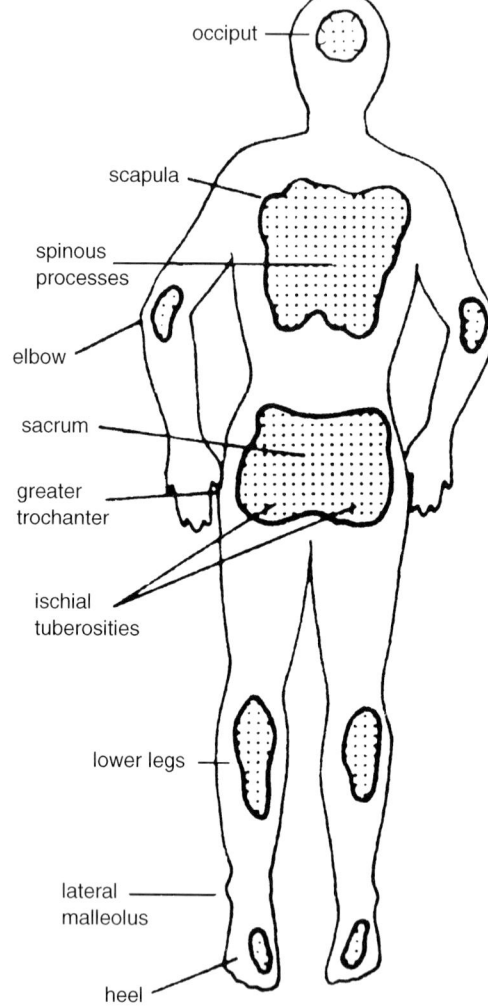

Location of pressure sores

Figure 9-3.   Areas at risk for the development of pressure ulcers. (From chap. 18 figs 18-3)

40 to 60 mm Hg are seen at the ischial tuberosities and the thigh when the feet are dangling free; pressure at the ischial tuberosity rises to approximately 100 mm Hg when the feet are supported [147].

Most pressure ulcers (96%) occur in the lower part of the body; the hips and buttocks account for 67% of these pressure ulcers, and the lower limbs account for 29% [25]. However, these pressure ulcers can occur at any part of the body (Figure 9-3). Dansereau and Conway [38] reviewed 1604 pressure sores in 649 patients in the VA hospitals and found that the ischial tuberosity pressure ulcers had the highest occurrence rate (28%) followed by ulcers of the trochanters (19%), sacrum (17%), heel (9%), malleolus and pretibial area (5% each), and the patella (4%); other miscellaneous sites accounting for the remaining 13%. Lee et al. [39] reporting on 142 surgical repairs of pressure ulcers in 70 patients, found that the majority of the pressure ulcers (45.6%) were located at the ischium, and the sacrum and trochanters were the next two common sites, accounting for 26.5% and 23.1%, respectively. Other areas included the calcaneus and hip with 1.4% each, and the ribs, thorax, and thighs with 0.7% each. Leigh [40], however, reported the sacrum as being the most common site for pressure ulcers (60%), followed by the ischial tuberosity.

ETIOLOGY AND RISK FACTORS

Factors that have been identified as being critical for the formation of pressure ulcers are pressure, shearing force, friction, and moisture [41]. Other important factors include impairments in ambulation, feeding, and grooming, incontinence of urine or feces, and associated debilitating diseases such as diabetes, Parkinson's disease, paraplegia, and malnutrition [42, 43]. Additional adverse factors identified are male gender [42, 43] and inadequate numbers of nursing personnel [21]. Patients with orthopedic problems and patients with SCI are at a much higher risk of developing pressure ulcers [35, 40]. Although smoking has not been unequivocally implicated as a risk factor, 36% of smokers develop pressure ulcers, compared to 26% of non-smokers [31]. Mattress quality and positioning are frequently overlooked, but recent studies have identified poor skin cushion support and positioning as being important risk factors [44–46]. Many studies have identified increasing age as a risk factor, particularly age greater than seventy years [36, 42, 47, 48].

Meijer et al. [49] reported a significant relationship between the risk of developing pressure ulcers secondary to external factors such as pressure, shear forces, and immobility and the susceptibility of the patient to develop pressure ulcers. He termed factors such as cardiovascular status and elastic tissue properties *intrinsic factors*. He quantitated the susceptibility to form pressure ulcers by utilizing a pressure-temperature-time method [50], which measured the blood flow recovery time after a constant pressure was applied for 10 minutes. The recovery time in susceptible persons was significantly longer than in nonsusceptible patients. To score external determinants, Meijer constructed a pressure index using three parameters: mental state, activity, and mobility. Each parameter was scored from 0 to 3, which produced a scale ranging from 0 to 9 for the pressure index. (See Table 9-1.)

Meijer found that a significant relationship existed between a higher pressure index score and the risk of developing pressure ulcers. He showed that patients who were highly susceptible (as shown by an increase in blood flow recovery time) but had a low pressure index score were at low risk for developing pressure ulcers. Similarly, a high pressure index, but low susceptibility score, also resulted in a low incidence of occurrence for pressure ulcers. However, for those patients who had an increased susceptibility score as well as an increased pressure index score, the incidence of pressure ulcers was the greatest.

Meijer postulated that individual susceptibility score is as important as external determinants, such as pressure and shear forces, and he suggested that nursing homes and hospital staff plan to incorporate quantitation of individual susceptibility as part of their evaluative process in formulating strategies to prevent pressure ulcers.

It is generally acknowledged that pressure is the primary causative factor in the formation of pressure ulcers. The prolonged application of pressure leads to local ischemia, which precipitates mechanical damage, ultimately leading to tissue necrosis. It is clear that the cutaneous circulation plays an important role in maintaining the integrity of the skin, and its interruption is crucial to the formation of pressure ulcers. It is appropriate to briefly review the anatomy and physiology of the cutaneous microcirculation to provide an understanding of the pathophysiology of pressure ulcers.

ANATOMY AND PHYSIOLOGY

The cutaneous microcirculation is composed of microvascular beds that contain vessels less than 100 μm in diameter. Terminal arteries (50 μm in diameter) have vessel walls composed of an inner layer of epithelium, an internal elastic lamina, and a surrounding sheath of at least two continuous layers of vascular smooth muscle cells. Arising from the terminal arteries are arterioles (20–50 μm in diameter), which have a single continuous layer of vascular smooth muscle. The arterioles give rise to metarterioles (10–15 μm in diameter), which have a single discontinuous layer of vascular smooth muscle cells. A band of vascular smooth muscle cells, referred to as the precapillary sphincter, is frequently found at the origin of the metarterioles. The metarterioles gives rise to arterial capillaries (5 μm in diameter), which consist of a single layer of endothelial cells and a basement membrane surrounded by a finely reinforced network of reticular collagen fibers. The arterial capillaries anasto-

Table 9-1. Meijer's Pressure Index for Scoring External Determinants

Mental state	Score	Activity	Score	Mobility	Score
Alert	0	Ambulant	0	Full	0
Apathetic		Walks with		Slightly	
	1	help	1	limited	1
Confused				Very	
	2	Chairbound	2	limited	2
Stuporous	3	Bedbound	3	Immobile	3

Source: Meijer et al. [49].

Note: The pressure index was used to score the external determinants of the risk to develop decubitus; i.e., the intensity and duration of pressure and shear force.

mose with the venous capillaries (8 µm in diameter), which drain into the venules. The capillary walls function as a selective permeable membrane. The single layer of endothelial cells that makes up the wall of the capillaries ranges from 0.1 to 3 µm in thickness, and where two endothelial cells meet, there is an intercellular space, or cleft, approximately 100 Å wide. Most clefts have a constricted area about 40 Å wide. In general, the lumen sizes of the metarterioles and precapillary sphincters are influenced by tissue waste products and oxygen deprivation and usually show rhythmically alternating vasodilation and vasoconstriction.

Peripheral arteriolar vasoconstriction or vasodilation controls the diameter of the arterioles and therefore influences the amount of blood that enters the capillaries. Vasoconstriction and dilation are regulated by both sympathetic and parasympathetic fibers, as well as by catecholamines, such as epinephrine and norepinephrine. In many tissues, the presence of arteriovenous shunts may cause a complete bypass of the capillary bed. Increased cardiac output, which elevates arterial blood pressure, will increase arterial blood flow, whereas elevation of arterial blood pressure due to arteriolar constriction decreases capillary blood flow. The presence of capillary sphincters, which open and close due to intensive contractability of capillary endothelial cells, also influences the amount of blood reaching the capillaries. The capillary constriction and dilation is independent of the action of the arterioles, but may be sensitive to anoxia and histamine production.

Blood viscosity is also an important factor in capillary blood flow; it is influenced by plasmaprotein concentration, hematocrit, and other factors such as capillary size. The capillary size (4–10 µm) is frequently smaller than the diameter of red blood cells (7 µm). The red blood cells therefore may need to deform themselves to pass through a capillary. Blood viscosity decreases as capillary size diminishes, promoting capillary blood flow. At a critical diameter, however, capillary blood flow dramatically decreases as blood viscosity sharply increases, perhaps due to the sticking together of red blood cells in the capillaries. The deformation of red blood cells can be adversely affected by bacterial endotoxins, swelling of the cells by fluid absorption, and low pH.

Severe increase in tissue pressure, such as may be seen in immobilized patients, can virtually shut off capillary blood flow. The total tissue pressure is typically zero. External pressure increases the interstitial fluid pressure, which, at approximately 12 mm Hg, causes a substantial increase in total tissue pressure. This increases capillary arteriolar pressure, leading to filtration of fluid from the capillaries, edema formation, and autolysis. The amount of pressure applied is inversely related to the length of time of application in the production of pressure sores.

The plasma volume and volume of the interstitial space are controlled by factors at the capillary level: plasma oncotic pressure, hydrostatic pressure, oncotic pressure of interstitial fluid, and hydrostatic pressure of interstitial space. Plasma oncotic pressure develops because of the restricted passage of large molecules such as proteins. Albumin comprises up to 51% of plasma proteins. Albumin, with its high concentration and relatively low molecular weight, is primarily responsible for determining oncotic pressure. Other proteins include globulin (17%), fibrinogen (4%), and other miscellaneous proteins (28%). The plasma oncotic pressure is approximately 25 mm Hg, and the capillary hydrostatic pressure ranges from 32 mm Hg at the arterial capillaries to approximately 15 mm Hg at the venous capillaries. The hydrostatic pressure at midcapillary is about 25 mm Hg. The interstitial fluid oncotic pressure is unknown but is assumed to be very small; the tissue hydrostatic pressure is approximately 1.8 mm Hg.

PATHOPHYSIOLOGY

Most work on the pathophysiology of pressure ulcers centers around three factors: ischemia, pressure, and shear. Dinsdale [51] has shown pathologic changes to be associated with friction. Although moisture has also been associated with pressure ulcer development, few studies have addressed this factor.

The application of a constant pressure of 70 mm Hg for more than two hours has been shown to produce irreversible tissue damage [51]. If pressure is relieved intermittently, however, minimal tissue damage is seen, even at pressures up to 240 mm Hg. Brooks and Duncan [11] demonstrated that the duration of pressure application and the magnitude of pressure are critical; the greater the magnitude of pressure, the shorter is the duration of application required to produce necrosis. Kosiak [52] has confirmed Dinsdale's work [51] by showing that a pressure of 70 mm Hg applied constantly for two hours causes irreversible changes. Kosiak also found, however, that if pressure was relieved every 5 minutes, few changes were noted [53]. These studies suggest that a period of 1–2 hours of pressure application is critical; after that time of constant pressure application, irreversible tissue changes are noted to occur.

The work of Lindan [54] strongly suggests that the etiology of pressure ulcers is pressure occluding blood flow, causing necrosis. Nola and Vistnes [55] have shown that muscle fibers are more sensitive to the ischemic effects of prolonged pressure than skin by itself. Daniel et al. [56] confirmed this and also showed that the initial pathologic changes in response to pressure first occur in the muscle layer overlying the bony prominence and spread outward.

Shear forces [57, 58] come into play, for example, when the head of the bed is raised, causing the torso to slide down and transmit pressure to the sacrum and deep fascia [41]. In this scenario, the posterior sacral skin is fixed secondary to friction with the bed, and shear forces in the deep part of the superficial fascia lead to stretching and angulation of vessels, causing thrombosis and undermining of the dermis [57]. The vessels particularly affected are the posterior branches of the superior gluteal artery. Subcutaneous fat, which lacks tensile strength, is also particularly vulnerable to mechanical forces accentuating the shear phenomenon [41]. The addition of shear forces to pressure can lead to pressure ulcer formation at lower pressures. Goossens and associates, in their recent article [59], measured the cutoff pressure (defined as the level of external pressure exerted on the skin at which oxygen tension is 1.3 kPa when skin ischemia can be expected) by measuring oxygen tension at the sacrum of young healthy volunteers. He found that

the mean cutoff pressure was 11.6 kPa when no shear stress was applied but decreased to 8.7 kPa when shear stress was applied.

Work by Bennett et al. [60–62] has shown that, in normal subjects, shear is roughly half as effective as pressure in driving the skin over the thenar eminence towards occlusion. When seated on a hard, slick seat, paraplegic, geriatric, and ill patients develop three times the median shear load experienced by normal subjects in skin lateral to the ischial tuberosities, and normal subjects reflect roughly three times the median pulsatile blood volume flow rate developed by paraplegic, geriatric, and ill patients.

Friction plays a role in the formation of pressure ulcers as it removes the outer protective layer of the stratum corneum [41]. Dinsdale has studied the role of friction in the etiology of pressure ulcers [51] and found that a direct application of 160 mm Hg pressure did not cause pressure ulcers, but that same pressure, dragged across the skin, created friction force that produced an ulcer. It should be noted, however, that although friction can cause surface lesions, pressure ulcers develop subepidermally [56, 63].

Other etiologic factors in the formation of pressure ulcers include aging skin, nutrition, and moisture. Poor nutrition has been correlated to pressure ulcers by Pinchafsky-Devin [64]. Allman et al. [30] have shown the importance of hypoalbuminemia. Other investigators have shown that vitamin C has a preventive and healing effect on pressure ulcers [65, 66]. Aging skin has altered barrier properties, diminished pain perception, reduced immunity, and slow wound healing ability, all of which may contribute to the breakdown of the skin [67]. The role of moisture has been demonstrated by Allman and Desforges [24] and Witkowski and Parish [63]. Witkowski and Parish have also studied the histopathology of pressure ulcers [63]. They divided the dermatologic changes seen in pressure ulcers into the following sequence: blanchable erythema, nonblanchable erythema, decubitus dermatitis, early ulcer, healing ulcer, chronic ulcer, and black eschar. The initial sign of damage occurs in the upper epidermis and in particular, at the capillaries and venules. Edema of the papillary dermis follows. Epidermal changes, however, appear to occur late in the development process and are apparently the results of ischemia and anoxia.

CLASSIFICATION SYSTEMS

The most commonly used classification to describe pressure ulcers is the one proposed by Shea in 1975 [68] (see Table 9-2). Some of the other classifications in use are the ones proposed by Johnson [69], Lowthian [70], and Yarkony [71]. The United Kingdom consensus classification of pressure sores [72] (Table 9-3) and the classification proposed by the Agency for Health Care Policy and Research (AHCPR) [73] (Table 9-4) have attempted to meet the need for a standardized, widely adopted classification system in order to achieve uniformity in epidemiological studies, clinical trials, teaching,

Table 9-2. Shea's System For Grading Pressure Ulcers

Grade I	The pressure ulcer is noted to be an acute inflammatory response involving the epidermis. Soft tissue erythema of an irregular and ill-defined area is accompanied by induration, and heat persists for more than 24 hours; the epidermis remains intact and the ulcer is reversible.
Grade II	The pressure ulcer involves a break in or a blistering of the epidermis surrounded by erythema and induration and is potentially reversible.
Grade III	The pressure ulcer is an inflammatory fibroblastic response that extends through the dermis to the junction with subcutaneous fat. It is seen as an irregular, shallow ulcer that has subcutaneous fat at its base and is surrounded by erythema, induration, and heat.
Grade IV	The pressure ulcer extends through the full thickness of the skin into the deep fascia and/or muscle. The draining necrotic base is often foul smelling, and undermining of the surface tissue may be excessive.
Grade V	The pressure ulcer penetrates to the underlying bone causing osteomyelitis, has no anatomic limit, and is surrounded by erythema and induration. The sore is seen as an extensive ulcer with exposed bone, joint, muscle, and/or fascia at its base.

Source: Shea [68].

Table 9-3. The U.K. Consensus Classification of Pressure Sores

Stage 0:	*No clinical evidence of a pressure sore.*
0.0	Normal appearance, intact skin
0.1	Healed with scarring
0.2	Tissue damage, but not assessed as a pressure sore
Stage 1:	*Discoloration of intact skin—light finger pressure applied to the site does not alter the discoloration.*
1.1	Nonblanchable erythema with increased local heat
1.2	Blue/purple/black discoloration. The sore is at least stage 1
Stage 2:	*Partial-thickness skin loss or damage involving epidermis and/or dermis.*
2.1	Blister
2.2	Abrasion
2.3	Shallow ulcer, without undermining of adjacent tissue
2.4	Any of these with underlying blue/purple/black discoloration or induration. The sore is at least stage 2.
Stage 3:	*Full-thickness skin loss involving damage or necrosis of subcutaneous tissue but not extending to underlying bone, tendon, or joint capsule.*
3.1	Crater, without undermining of adjacent tissue
3.2	Crater, with undermining of adjacent tissue
3.3	Sinus, the full extent of which is not certain
3.4	Full-thickness skin loss, but wound bed covered with necrotic tissue (hard or leathery black/brown tissue or soft tissue or softer yellow/cream/gray slough) which masks the true extent of tissue damage. The sore is at least stage 3. Until debrided it is not possible to observe whether damage extends into the muscle or involves damage to bone or supporting structures
Stage 4:	*Full-thickness skin loss with extensive destruction and tissue necrosis extending to underlying bone, tendon, and capsule.*
4.1	Visible exposure of bone, tendon, or joint capsule
4.2	Sinus assessed as extended to bone, tendon, or capsule
	Third-digit classification for the nature of the wound bed
x.x0	Not applicable, intact skin
x.x1	Clean, with partial epithelization
x.x2	Clean, with or without granulation, but no obvious epithelization
x.x3	Soft slough, cream/yellow/green in color
x.x4	Hard or leathery black/brown necrotic (dead/avascular) tissue
	Fourth-digit classification for the infective complications
x.xx0	No inflammation surrounding the wound bed
x.xx1	Inflammation surrounding the wound bed
x.xx2	Cellulitis bacteriologically confirmed

Source: Reid and Morison [72].

Table 9-4. AHCPR Staging of Pressure Ulcers

Stage I	Nonblanchable erythema of intact skin; the heralding lesion of skin ulceration.
Stage II	Partial-thickness skin loss involving epidermis and/or dermis. The ulcer is superficial and presents clinically as an abrasion, blister, or shallow crater.
Stage III	Full-thickness skin loss involving damage or necrosis of subcutaneous tissue that may extend down to, but not through, underlying fascia. The ulcer presents clinically as a crater with or without undermining of adjacent tissue.
Stage IV	Full-thickness skin loss with extensive destruction, tissue necrosis, or damage to muscle, bone, or supporting structures (for example, tendon or joint capsule). Note: Undermining and sinus tracts may be associated with Stage IV pressure ulcers.

Source: Agency for Health Care Policy and Research [73].

Note: Staging definitions recognize these assessment limitations: (1) Identification of stage I pressure ulcers may be difficult in patients with darkly pigmented skin; (2) When eschar is present, accurate staging of the pressure ulcer is not possible until the eschar has sloughed or the wound has been debrided [73].

and evaluation of patient care settings. The ultimate usefulness of a system will depend on demonstrating its reliability, reproducibility, and utility in different settings.

The United Kingdom consensus classification grades pressure sores in four stages. A fifth stage (stage 0) records skin conditions in the absence of pressure sores. The full classification uses four digits for documentation. It has been recommended that at least the first two digits be applied when using this classification. The third digit relates to the nature of the ulcer bed, and the fourth digit allows for coding of infective complications. This classification depends upon visual observations except at the fourth-digit level. The classification proposes to include all clinical presentations of pressure ulcers, giving the user the option to choose the degree of precision needed in documentation by using either two-, three-, or four-digit codes.

The AHCPR classification [73] stages pressure ulcers into four stages to classify the degree of tissue damage. The staging of pressure ulcers recommended for use was consistent with the recommendations of the National Pressure Ulcer Advisory Panel (NPUAP, 1989 Consensus Conference) [143], as derived from previous staging systems proposed by Shea [68] and the International Association for Enterostomal Therapy [144].

RISK ASSESSMENT

The first step in the prevention of pressure ulcers is the identification of those patients at high risk. The Norton scale [74] (Table 9-5), introduced in 1962, was the first formal risk assessment scale. It graded patients into four categories, including physical condition, mental state, and activity, mobility, and incontinence levels. This scale is most popular with nurses because it is simple, expeditious, and widely known. The Braden scale [75] (Table 9-6) grades patients on six levels including sensory perception, moisture, activity, mobility, nutrition, and friction and shear. The other assessment scales are the Medley scale [76] (Table 9-7) and the Waterlow scale [77] (Table 9-8). Assessment and identification of patients at risk is critical for appropriate prospective allocation of resources.

Table 9-5. The Norton Score

A score of 14 or below = at risk	
Physical condition	**Score**
Good	4
Fair	3
Poor	2
Very bad	1
Mental condition	
Alert	4
Apathetic	3
Confused	2
Stuporous	1
Activity	
Ambulant	4
Walk with help	3
Chairbound	2
Bedfast	1
Mobility	
Full	4
Slightly limited	3
Very limited	2
Immobile	1
Incontinence	
Not	4
Occasionally	3
Usually urine	2
Doubly	1

Source: Goldstone and Goldstone [74].

Table 9-6   The Braden Scale for Predicting Pressure Sore Risk

1. Sensory perception Ability to respond meaningfully to pressure-related discomfort	**Score**
Completely limited: Unresponsive (does not moan, flinch or gasp) to painful stimuli, due to diminished level of consciousness or sedation **OR** limited ability to feel pain over most of body surface.	1
Very limited: Responds only to painful stimuli. Cannot communicate discomfort except by moaning or restlessness **OR** has a sensory impairment which limits the ability to feel pain or discomfort over ½ of the body.	2
Slightly limited: Responds to verbal commands but cannot always communicate discomfort or need to be turned **OR** has some sensory impairment which limits ability to feel pain or discomfort in 1 or 2 extremities.	3
No impairment: Responds to verbal commands. Has no sensory deficit which would limit ability to feel or voice pain or discomfort.	4

2. Moisture Degree to which skin is exposed to moisture.	**Score**
Constantly moist: Skin is kept moist almost constantly by perspiration, urine, etc. Dampness is detected every time the patient is moved or turned.	1
Often moist: Skin is often but not always moist. Linen must be changed at least once a shift.	2
Occasionally moist: Skin is occasionally moist, requiring an extra linen change approximately once a day.	3
Rarely moist: Skin is usually dry; linen requires changing only at routine intervals.	4

3. Activity Degree of physical activity	**Score**
Bedfast: Confined to bed.	1
Chairfast: Ability to walk severely limited or nonexistent. Cannot bear own weight and/or must be assisted into chair or wheel chair.	2
Walks occasionally: Walks occasionally during day but for very short distance, with or without assistance. Spends majority of each shift in bed or chair.	3
Walks frequently: Walks outside the room at least twice a day and inside room at least every 2 hours during waking hours.	4

4. Nutrition Usual food intake pattern	**Score**
Very poor: Never eats a complete meal. Rarely eats more than ⅓ of any food offered. Eats 2 servings or less of protein (meat or dairy products) per day. Takes fluids poorly. Does not take a liquid dietary supplement **OR** is NPO[a] and/or maintained on clear liquids or IV[b] for more than 5 days.	1
Probably inadequate: Rarely eats a complete meal and generally eats about ½ of any food offered. Protein intake includes only 3 servings of meat or dairy products per day. Occasionally will take a dietary supplement **OR** receives less than optimal amount of liquid diet or tube feeding.	2
Adequate: Eats over ½ of most meals. Eats a total of 4 servings of protein (meat or dairy products) each day. Occasionally will refuse a meal, but will usually take a supplement if offered **OR** is on tube feeding or TPN[c] regime, which probably meets most of nutritional needs.	3
Excellent: Eats most of every meal. Never refuses a meal. Usually eats a total of 4 or more servings of meat and dairy products. Occasionally eats in between meals. Does not require supplementation.	4

5. Mobility Ability to change and control body position.	**Score**
Completely immobile: Does not make even slight changes in body or extremity position without assistance.	1
Very limited mobility: Makes occasional slight changes in body or extremity position but unable to make frequent or significant changes independently.	2
Slightly limited mobility: Makes frequent though slight changes in body or extremity position independently.	3
No limitation in mobility: Makes major or frequent changes in position without assistance.	4

Continued

Table 9-6 *Continued*

6. Friction and Shear	Score
Problem: Requires moderate to maximum assistance in moving. Complete lifting without sliding against sheets is impossible. Frequently slides down in bed or chair, requiring frequent repositioning with maximum assistance. Spasticity, contractures or agitation leads to almost constant friction.	**1**
Potential problem: Moves feebly or requires minimum assistance. During a move skin probably slides to some extent against sheets, chair, restraints or other devices. Maintains relatively good position in chair or bed most of the time but occasionally slides down.	**2**
No apparent problem: Moves in bed and in chair independently and has sufficient muscle strength to lift up completely during move. Maintains good position in bed or chair at all times.	**3**

Source: Berystrom et al. [n5].

[a]NPO: Nothing by mouth; [b]IV: Intravenously; [c]TPN: Total parenteral nutrition.

Table 9-7. The Medley Score

Patient risk score: 0–9 = low risk; 10–19 = medium risk; 20–36 = high risk

Activity—ambulation	Score	Nutritional status	Score
Ambulant without assistance	0	Good (eats/drinks/or naso-gastric feeds)	0
Ambulant with assistance	2	Fair (insufficient intake to maintain weight)	1
Chairfast (longer than 12 hours)	4	Poor (eats/drinks very little)	2
Bedfast (longer than 12 hours)	6	Very poor (unable or refuses to eat; emaciated)	3
Skin condition		**Incontinence—bladder**	
Healthy (clear and moist)	0	None or catheterized	0
Rashes or abrasions	2	Occasional (less than two per 24 hours)	1
Decreased turgor, dry skin, advanced age	4	Usually (more than two per 24 hours)	2
Edema and/or (redness)	6	Total (no control)	3
Pressure sore involved	6		
Predisposing disease		**Incontinence—bowel**	
No involvement	0	None	0
Chronic stable state	1	Occasional (formed stool)	1
Acute or chronic unstable	2	Usually (with semiformed stools)	2
Terminal or grave	3	Total (no control)	3
Mobility—range of motion		**Pain**	
Full active range of motion	0	None	0
Moves with limited assistance	2	Mild	1
Moves only with assistance	4	Intermittent	2
Immobile	6	Severe	3
Level of consciousness (to commands)			
Alert	0		
Lethargic/confusion	1		
Semicomatose (absence of response to stimuli)	2		
Comatose (absence of response to stimuli)	3		

Source: Williams [76].

Table 9-8.   The Waterlow Pressure Sore Assessment/Treatment Policy

Score: 10+ at risk, 15+ high risk, 20+ very high risk

Build, weight for height	Score	Mobility	Score
Average	0	Fully	0
Above average	1	Restless/fidgety	1
Obese	2	Apathetic	2
Below average	3	Restricted	3
Skin type, visual risk areas		Inert	4
Healthy	0	Chairbound	5
Tissue paper	1	**Appetite**	
Dry	1	Average	0
Edematous	1	Poor	1
Clammy (temperature up)	1	Naso-gastric tube	2
Discolored	2	Fluids only	2
Broken/spot	3	Anorectic	3
Age and sex		**Medications**	
Male	1	Steroids	4
Female	2	Cytotoxics	4
14–49	1	High dosages	4
50–64	2	Anti-inflammatory	4
65–74	3	**Special risk factors**	
75–80	4	*Tissue malnutrition*	
81+	5	Cachexia	8
Continence		Cardiac failure	5
Catheterized or continent	0	Peripheral vascular disease	5
Occasionally incontinent	1	Anemia	2
Catheterized but incontinent of feces	2	Smoking	1
Doubly incontinent	3	*Neurological defect*	
		Diabetes/MS/paraplegia	4/6
		Major surgery/trauma	
		Below waist spinal	5
		Over two hrs	5

Source: Waterlow [77].

MANAGEMENT

Pressure ulcers affect approximately 10% of patients in developed countries, but because of a widespread perception that it represents a nursing concern, most physicians are unaware of their responsibility for this condition [78], and receive little formal education in this regard [20]. Medical research is directed toward the development of new and ingenious methods to treat pressure ulcers once they occur, rather than strategies for prevention. The challenge lies in identifying and implementing new and effective policies and principles of prevention and care.

NONSURGICAL MANAGEMENT

Recognition of increased occurrence of pressure ulcers within an institution is the first step. This requires a multidisciplinary approach. It involves the various caregivers who are directly in contact with the patients, but also the hospital management, the policy makers, and the insurance companies, which may not be directly associated with patient care.

Formation of resource groups like the Pressure Sore Resource Group (PSRG) and the Wound Care Group (WCG), as undertaken at the Churchill John Radcliffe Hospital in London [79] or the wound unit at the University of Maryland School of Medicine

[80], can help in improving the quality of patient care by identifying those at high risk and by implementing effective education programs and directing more efficient use of resources. This can reduce the incidence of pressure ulcers to about 2.63% and also provide savings in treatment costs [79].

Turning the patient every two hours may make pressure ulcers totally preventable, but this regimen is frequently not sustainable in a busy hospital [68]. Gel pads, sheepskin, plastic casts, and specialty beds are helpful adjuncts. Specialty beds such as mechanical oscillating beds and mattresses and air-filled, floating-bead, and water mattresses may be of particular benefit to the patient in providing relief from pressure.

Eighty percent of pressure ulcers can be healed conservatively [81]; grades III, IV, and V pressure ulcers usually require surgery. Conservative measures for treating pressure ulcers include good nutrition, especially adequate intake of protein, vitamins, especially vitamin C, and the trace element zinc. Relief of pressure, adequate rehydration, relief of pain, and the treatment of underlying medical conditions, particularly diabetes mellitus, are also crucial.

Local care involves wound cleaning with normal saline and the use of moist wound dressings. Most wounds of grade II or less will heal in one to two weeks if treated with moist dressings [82, 83]; the healing time for grades III and IV wounds is six weeks to three months. Various dressing materials have been specifically designed to manage pressure ulcers; these are documented in studies to be superior to standard saline dressings. When copolymer moisture dressings were compared to saline wet-to-dry dressings, a statistically significant difference of 64% in ulcer improvement or healing was found, as compared to 22% with saline dressings [84]. Oleske and associates [85] compared a polyurethane dressing to normal saline and concluded that those patients treated with polyurethane dressings demonstrated a statistically significant decrease in size of the total surface area of the wound. Recently, Kraft [86] compared the Epi-Lock dressing (a nonadherent, semiocclusive polyurethane foam wound dressing) with saline dressing and reached the same conclusion. The general consensus has been that these dressing materials are better and more cost effective, and require less frequent changes, thereby reducing nursing time, when compared to saline dressings [84–86]. Another recent article by Poteete [87] reported that when 0.75% of metronidazole gel was used as the dressing material, malodor from the wounds was substantially reduced. It is important to recognize that if deep wound size does not decrease by 30% in approximately two weeks with the previously described treatment, then a reevaluation is justified so that a change in management may be initiated [88].

A number of exogenous growth factors are currently being used in the management of deep pressure ulcers. These include recombinant growth factors like recombinant platelet-derived growth factor-BB (rPDGF-BB), transforming growth factor (TGF) b, basic fibroblast growth factor (FGF), and epidermal growth factor (EGF). These growth factors are small peptides that regulate the growth of different cell types promoting either the formation of granulation tissue or reepithelization [89–95].

Recently, Pierce and associates [96] concluded a small phase 2 trial evaluating rPDGF-BB in the treatment of grades III and IV pressure ulcers and found significant reduction in ulcer volume when rPDGF-BB was used at a dose of 100 m/dl. This beneficial effect was however not seen beyond 28 days. The use of laboratory-cultured epidermal keratinocytes forming living skin equivalents may be another promising product to prove beneficial in the management of pressure ulcers [145, 146].

INFECTION AND ANTIBIOTICS

Most pressure ulcers are colonized by surface microbes and therefore do not warrant routine culture and sensitivity studies. Routine use of antibiotics for the prevention of infection is not recommended. If, however, there is evidence of systemic infection, proper antibiotic coverage after obtaining culture and sensitivity samples is recommended [97]. Deep tissue biopsy cultures are superior to superficial swab cultures and needle aspiration cultures in identifying infecting organisms. Superficial cultures taken by swabs reflect surface colonization, and the yield by needle aspiration does not give the true nature of the infection [97].

The most common organisms are the Gram-negative rods, accounting for 50–70% of infections. These include *Proteus mirabilis, Pseudomonas, Klebsiella,* and *Escherichia coli.* Gram-positive organisms account for 20–40% of the infections. These include *Staphylococcus aureus, Streptococcus* A, and other streptococci. Anaerobes account for 16–50% of the infections and include *Bacteroides fragilis* [98–100].

Rudensky et al. showed that patients receiving antibiotics had a high percentage of positive biopsy cultures, which frequently included organisms that were resistant to the antibiotics in use. The findings indicated that antibiotics used routinely do not lower the incidence of colonization in pressure ulcers, but merely change the ecology of the wound [97]. Indeed the pressure ulcer may serve as a reservoir of resistant organisms [101] and, in these patients, may be the etiologic factor contributing to septicemia and poor prognosis [99, 100].

NUTRITION AND PRESSURE ULCERS

Malnutrition has long been recognized as a major contributing factor in the formation of pressure ulcers [102–104]. Mulholland et al. [105] postulated that protein malnutrition makes tissues more vulnerable to necrosis. They found that none of their 35 random cases of pressure ulcers, whether on the fracture, surgical, or psychiatric ward, had a plasma protein concentration over 6.35 g/dl. Clauss-Walker et al. [106, 107] and Daniel et al. [108] have shown by biochemical and histological studies that paralysis is associated with skin changes that make it highly susceptible to pressure ulcer formation. Clauss-Walker found increased cutaneous collagen catabolism, as evidenced by an increased excretion of skin collagen degradation products such as glycosyl galactosyl hydroxylysine in the urine, and decreased amounts of collagen-related amino acid and hydroxyproline in skin biopsy specimens [106, 107]. Perkash [109] found that anemic SCI patients had a significantly higher incidence of pressure ulcers and that these patients had significant decreases

in visceral protein status as evidenced by a decreased serum iron binding capacity.

Malnutrition causes significant retardation in wound healing, marked delay in fibroblastic regeneration [110], and a reduction in the skin breaking tension of wounds [111]. It also adversely affects immunity [112–116], pulmonary [117, 118], and cardiac functions [119, 120]. Vitamin C, administered at a dose of 500 mg orally, twice daily, has been shown to reduce pressure ulcer surface area by 84% as compared to 43% in a placebo group [121]. Zinc sulfate has been shown to improve wound healing and to restore immunocompetence in patients with zinc deficiency [122, 123]. It is therefore important in the prevention and management of pressure ulcers to recognize malnutrition as a significant contributing factor [124]. Simply employing measures for relief of pressure, without diagnosing and correcting nutritional deficiencies, will result in delayed wound healing [124, 110, 125], decreased resistance to infection [126–128], increased length of hospitalization, and increased mortality [127, 129, 130, 131].

Recently, Lee et al. [132] have used anthropometric, biochemical, immunologic, and indirect calorimetric measurements in an attempt to define the nutritional and metabolic status of 17 healthy SCI patients. Significant deficiencies in energy expenditure were found: 29% of patients were normometabolic and 35% of patients were either hyper- or hypometabolic. Obesity was found to be maximum in hypometabolic patients because of the imbalance between caloric intake and energy expenditure. No patient had normal values on all objective measurements of nutritional assessments. Forty-seven percent of patients had mild and 53% of patients had evidence of moderate malnutrition. The author suggested that nutritional therapy based on measurement of energy expenditure instead of predictive equations could be of benefit to SCI patients.

AHCPR GUIDELINES FOR PREDICTION AND PREVENTION OF PRESSURE ULCERS IN ADULTS

The AHCPR [73] published the clinical practice guidelines for the prediction and prevention of pressure ulcers in adults in 1992. The purpose was to help identify adults at risk of pressure ulcers, to define early interventions for prevention, which is a primary goal, and to manage stage I pressure ulcers.

Excerpts from the clinical practice guideline are included in the following sections.

RISK ASSESSMENT TOOLS AND RISK FACTORS

The goal is to identify at-risk individuals needing prevention and the special factors placing them at risk [73].

Bed- and chairbound individuals or those with impaired ability to reposition should be reassessed for additional factors that increase risk for developing pressure ulcers. These factors include immobility, incontinence, nutritional factors such as inadequate dietary intake and impaired nutritional status, and altered level of consciousness. The individual should be assessed on admission to acute care and rehabilitation hospitals, nursing homes, home care programs, and other health care facilities. A systematic risk assessment can be accomplished by using a validated risk assessment tool such as the Braden or Norton scale. The pressure ulcer risk should be reassessed at periodic intervals and documented [73].

SKIN CARE AND EARLY TREATMENT

The goal is to maintain and improve tissue tolerance to pressure in order to prevent injury [73].

1. All individuals at risk should have a systematic skin inspection at least once a day, with particular attention paid to the bony prominences. Results of skin inspection should be documented.

2. Skin cleaning should occur at the time of soiling and at routine intervals. The frequency of skin cleaning should be individualized according to need and/or patient preference. Avoid hot water, and use a mild cleansing agent that minimizes irritation and dryness of the skin. During the cleansing process, care should be utilized to minimize the force and friction applied to the skin.

3. Minimize environmental factors leading to skin drying, such as low humidity (less than 40%) and exposure to cold. Dry skin should be treated with moisturizer.

4. Avoid massage over bony prominences.

5. Minimize skin exposure to moisture due to incontinence, perspiration, or wound drainage. When these sources of moisture cannot be controlled, underpads or briefs can be used that are made of materials that absorb moisture and present a quick-drying surface to the skin. Topical agents that act as a barrier to moisture can also be used.

6. Skin injury due to friction and shear forces should be minimized through proper positioning, transferring, and turning techniques. In addition, friction injury should be reduced by the use of lubricants (such as corn starch and creams), protective films (such as transplant film dressings and skin sealants), protective dressings (such as hydrocolloids), and protective padding.

7. When an apparently healthy individual develops an inadequate dietary intake of protein or calories, caregivers should first attempt to discover the factors compromising intake and offer support with eating. Other nutritional supplements or support may be needed. If dietary intake remains inadequate and if consistent with overall goal of therapy, more aggressive nutritional intervention such as enteral or parenteral feedings should be considered. For nutritionally compromised individuals, a plan of nutritional support and/or supplementation should be implemented that meets individual needs and is consistent with the overall goal of therapy.

8. If potential for improving mobility and activity exists, rehabilitation efforts should be instituted if consistent with overall goal of therapy. Maintaining current activity level, mobility, and range of motion is an appropriate goal for most individuals.

9. Interventions and outcomes should be monitored and documented.

MECHANICAL LOADING AND SUPPORT SURFACES

The goal is to protect against the adverse effect of external mechanical forces: pressure, friction, and shear [73].

1. Any individual in bed who is assessed to be at risk for developing pressure ulcers should be repositioned at least every two hours if consistent with overall patient goal. A written schedule

for systematically turning and repositioning the individual should be used.

2. For individuals in bed, positioning devices such as pillows or foam wedges should be used to keep bony prominences (for example, knees or ankles) from direct contact with one another, according to a written plan.

3. Individuals in bed who are completely immobile should have a care plan that includes the use of devices that totally relieve pressure on the heels, most commonly by raising the heels off the bed. Do not use donut-type devices.

4. When side-lying position is used in bed, avoid positioning directly on the trochanter.

5. Maintain the head of the bed at the lowest degree of elevation consistent with medical conditions and other restrictions. Limit the amount of time the head of the bed is elevated.

6. Use lifting devices such as trapeze or bed linen to move (rather than drag) individuals in bed who cannot assist during transfers and position changes.

7. Any individual assessed to be at risk of developing pressure ulcers should be placed, when lying in bed, on a pressure-reducing device, such as foam, static air, alternating air, gel, or water mattress.

8. Any patient at risk for developing a pressure ulcer should avoid uninterrupted sitting on a chair or wheelchair. The individual should be repositioned, shifting the point under the pressure at least every hour, or be put back to bed if consistent with overall patient management goals. Individuals who are able should be taught to shift every 15 minutes.

9. For chairbound individuals, the use of pressure-reducing devices such as those made of foam, gel, air, or a combination is indicated. Do not use donut-type devices.

10. Positioning of chairbound individuals in chairs or wheelchairs should include consideration of postural alignment, distribution of weight, balance and stability, and pressure relief.

11. A written plan for the use of positioning devices and schedules may be helpful for chairbound individuals.

EDUCATION

The goal is to reduce the incidence of pressure ulcers through educational programs [73].

1. Educational programs for the prevention of pressure ulcers should be structured, organized, and comprehensive, and directed at all levels of health care providers, patients, and family caregivers.

2. The educational programs for prevention of pressure ulcers should include information on the following items: Etiology and risk factors for pressure ulcers. Risk assessment tools and their application. Skin assessment. Selection and/or use of support surfaces. Development and implementation of an individualized program of skin care. Demonstration of positioning for decreased risk of tissue breakdown. Instruction on accurate documentation of pertinent data.

3. The educational program should identify those responsible for pressure ulcer prevention, describe each person's role, and be appropriate to the audience in terms of level of information presented and expected participation. The educational program should be updated on a regular basis to incorporate new and existing techniques or technologies.

4. The educational program should be developed, implemented, and evaluated using principles of adult learning.

SURGICAL TREATMENT

Stage I pressure ulcers do not require surgical intervention but their presence should alert physicians and nursing staff to the need for mobilizing resources to prevent progression of the lesion. The patient ought to be reevaluated by the wound care or pressure ulcer prevention team with special attention toward identifying and eliminating (if possible) various extrinsic and intrinsic factors that may be present. Frequent repositioning of the patient, maintaining hygiene, and improving nutrition are important. This should also include treatment of any underlying medical problem, particularly diabetes mellitus and ischemic vascular disease, provision for adequate pain relief, and maintenance of adequate hydration. Stage I lesions generally heal by institution of conservative measures alone.

Patients with stage II pressure ulcers require debridement to remove all dead and necrotic tissue and require daily dressing changes to help the wound to heal. The newer dressing materials are better and more cost effective. It is important to identify the occurrence of epithelization, as its absence may indicate more serious underlying problems requiring special attention [98]. At the end of two weeks, in the presence of good epithelization and absence of infection, a meshed split-thickness skin graft will help in prompt closure of large defects.

The initial management of stage III ulcers is similar to that of stage II pressure ulcers, which includes thorough debridement and daily dressing changes. A sonogram to delineate the true extent of the ulcer and radiographic evaluation to identify the presence of bony spurs and osteomyelitis are important. If these problems are identified, bony ostectomy to remove all involved bone may be required. These pressure ulcers may be closed with rotational or transposition random pattern flaps. For recurrent pressure ulcers, an arterialized myocutaneous flap or a combination of a muscle flap followed by an overlying skin flap may be employed.

Stage IV pressure ulcers are treated as stage III ulcers, with inclusion of bony ostectomy to remove all underlying involved bone.

The following basic principles of pressure ulcer surgery have been outlined by Linder [98].

1. There should be no evidence of ongoing infection at the site of the pressure ulcer or elsewhere.

2. Inflammation at the site of pressure ulcers should be minimal prior to removal of all nonviable tissue.

3. During the actual surgical procedure, in positioning the patient, an attempt should be made to mimic the position in which the closure will be in the greatest tension. For example, when closing ischial pressure ulcers, the patient should be placed in a prone jackknife position in order to flex the hip maximally. If the closure is loose in this position, the wound will be in even less tension when the patient is back in bed after surgery.

4. All contaminated tissue should be removed by totally excising the ulcer.

5. All scar tissue surrounding the ulcer should be removed.

6. Bony ostectomy is indicated to remove contaminated bone and to decrease underlying bony protuberance.

7. Incisions taken, particularly flap incisions, must not cross over bony prominences.

8. Following ulcer excision, all residual defects should be filled with unscarred vascularized tissue such as muscle or fasciocutaneous flaps.

9. To collapse dead space and to prevent postoperative seroma, closed drainage systems must be employed after all flap procedures.

10. In the postoperative period, pressure necrosis must be prevented by proper patient positioning and by the use of low-pressure beds.

11. Antibiotics must be used in the perioperative period.

The spontaneous healing of pressure ulcers occurs in only a small percentage of patients, frequently with unsatisfactory results. Inappropriate surgical intervention can result in even larger areas of ulceration. Much patient morbidity could be avoided through the use of any technique capable of assessing the healing potential of various surgical procedures for pressure ulcer management. One such method available is to determine the status of the cutaneous circulation preoperatively. The cutaneous pressure plethysmograph (Figure 9-4) is a noninvasive vascular assessment instrument that detects the blood flow in the skin at various skin bearing pressures using a hand-held probe. The probe can be applied to any skin surface for recording cutaneous blood flow waveforms (Figure 9-5). With the application of incrementally increased pressure, the blood flow waveform is gradually reduced and at a critical pressure it is obliterated.

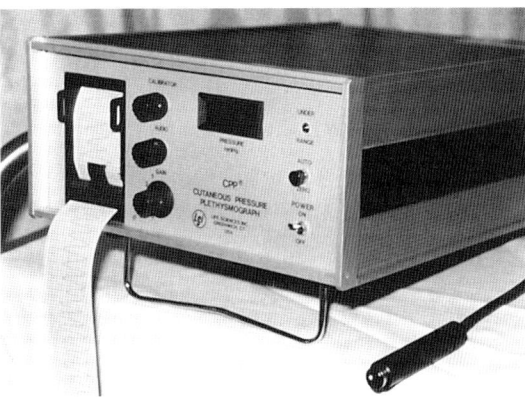

Figure 9-4. The cutaneous pressure plethysmograph.

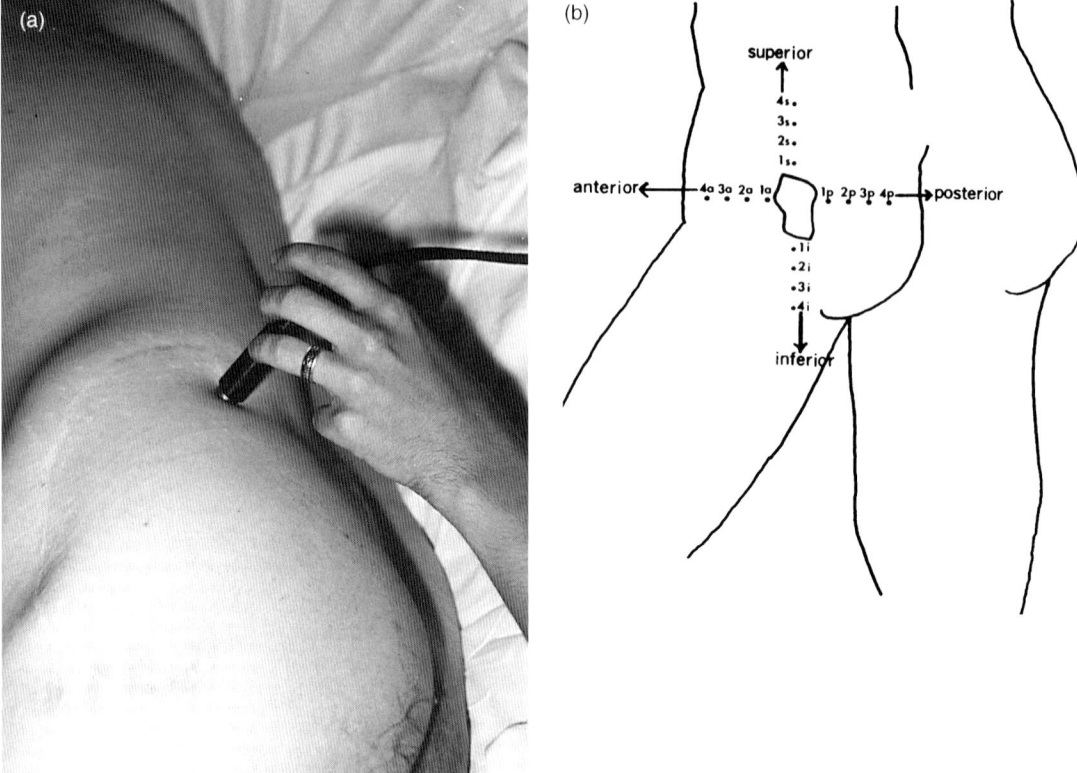

Figure 9-5.   (A) Position of probe placement; (B) Measurements taken around a right trochanteric pressure ulcer in a paraplegic patient.

Gradually the pressure is decreased until the wave-form reappears (Figure 9-6). The digital pressure at the point when the flow waveform reappears corresponds to the cutaneous pressure at that site, thus providing a systematic quantitative analysis of cutaneous pressure (Figures 9-7(A), (B)).

A review was conducted of surgical repairs of pressure ulcers including myocutaneous rotation flaps. The myocutaneous rotation flap is a single unit of skin and its underlying muscle, transferred to an area of defect such as a pressure ulcer, by means of a dominant vascular pedicle. The area to be covered may be adjacent to the flap or the flap may be floated to an area far removed from the donor site. The advantage of the myocutaneous rotation flap is that it brings new blood supply to an avascular area, while providing bulk in filling defects or covering bone grafts. The myocutaneous flap also supplies a mass of tissue to cushion a pressure-bearing area and functions in distributing the pressure and avoiding the recurrence of pressure ulcers.

As can be seen in Table 9-10, short-term success, defined as procedures not requiring additional surgery during the first month of follow-up, was comparable for all three techniques: myocutaneous rotation flap, conventional rotational flap, and primary closure. The long-term success, defined as those procedures not requiring additional surgery during follow-up, was greater for those patients with myocutaneous rotation flaps. The use of myocutaneous flaps offers the patient a distinct clinical advantage. The surgical management of a typical patient is presented in Figures 9-8 through 9-12.

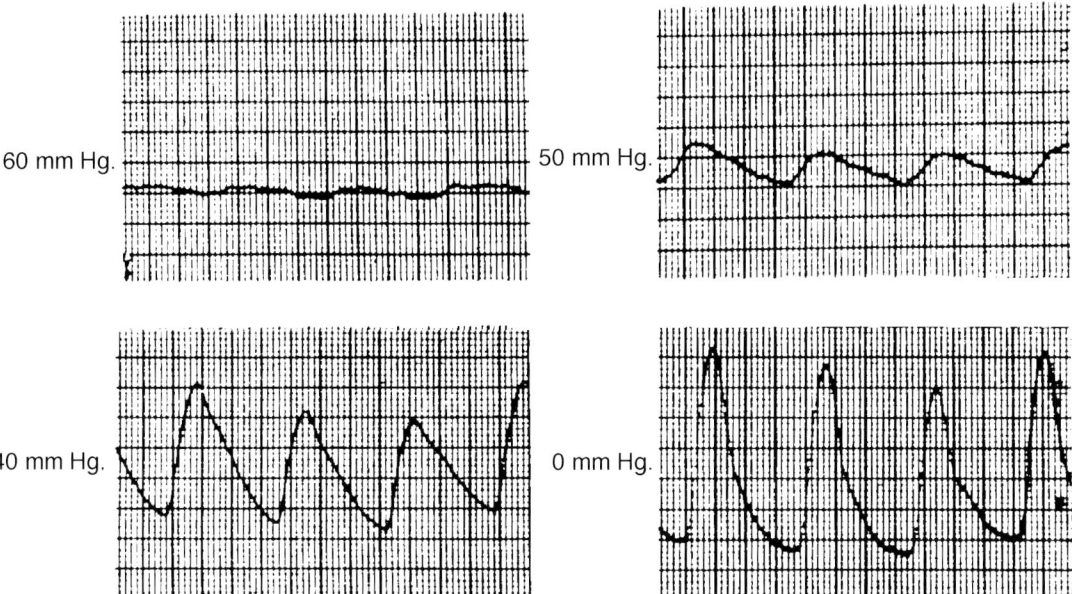

Figure 9-6. Effect of pressure on skin blood flow.

During surgery, viability of tissue may be evaluated. Skin blanching is a satisfactory method, although injection of an ampoule of fluorescein followed with examination after a 10-minute delay with a Wood's light is a superior method. Ostrander and Lee [133] evaluated prediction of flap survival using constant infusion fluorometry. They compared, in a dog model, wash-in slope and wash-out clearance, both measures of tissue perfusion, and compared sensitivity and specificity of the measurements in their ability to predict flap survival. The sensitivity of the two measurements was 100% and 95%, respectively. Specificity measurements were 97% and 86%, respectively. The authors concluded that both measurements have a high predictive potential for assessing tissue survival, with the wash-in method being preferable in providing results more rapidly and safely.

In paraplegics, control of minor bleeding with hemostats is counterproductive, because these will not vasoconstrict. Suction catheters should be placed in the wound under the skin flaps with continuous wall suction for at least five to seven days. This will reduce the risk of hematoma and increase the likelihood of tissue adherence [3, 81, 134].

Pressure ulcers on the occiput can be managed with split-thickness skin grafts if the ulcer is superficial. Ulcers extending through the periostium can be managed by decorticating the bone, waiting for granulation tissue to develop, and then applying a split-thickness skin graft. A second method is to decorticate the bone, create a skin flap including the galea, and transpose or rotate the flap onto the ulcer. The defect is filled with a split-thickness skin graft [3].

Sacral pressure ulcers are very common. They are usually centered over the sacral prominence and usually have large skin defects with overhanging edges. These pressure ulcers are completely excised removing all dead and necrotic tissue along with any concomitant bursae, leaving behind a rim of healthy tissue. The iliac spines may be removed, although total removal of bone is not necessary or recommended. The defect is generally converted into a triangle, which will allow flaps to fit in neatly. An inferiorly based large random cutaneous flap is the primary choice of closure for broad but shallow defects such as these. For defects that are larger than 10 cm in diameter or for recurrent ulcerations after previous random cutaneous flaps, gluteus maximus musculocutaneous V-Y flaps should be

(a) Inferior

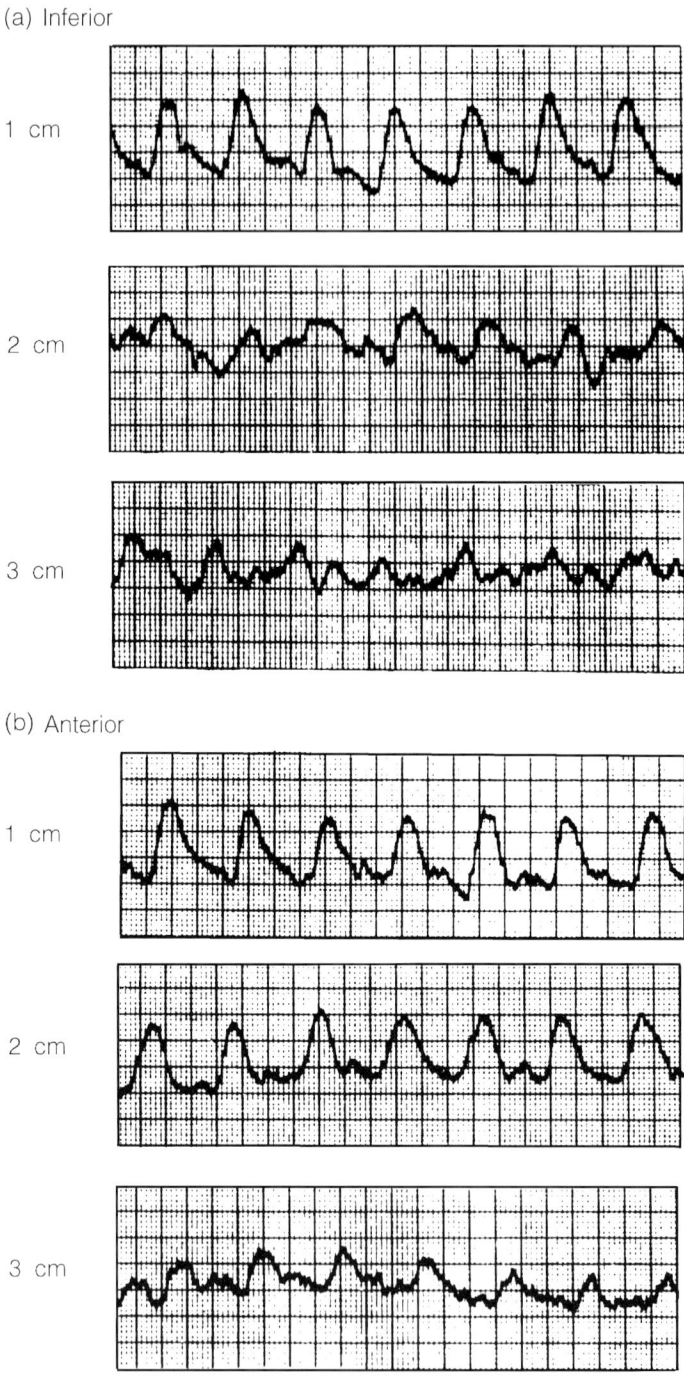

(b) Anterior

Figure 9-7(a),(b).   Systematic quantitative analysis at selected measurement sites. Photoplethysmographic waveforms around decubitus ulcer; D.A. Age 48 Male; Right Trochanter Pre-Op.

Table 9-9. Distribution of Pressure Ulcers by Body Area

Body area	Percent
Ischium	46.6
Sacrum	26.5
Trochanter	23.1
Os calcis	1.4
Hip	1.4
Ribs	0.7
Thorax	0.7
Thigh	0.7

Table 9-10 Outcome of Surgical Procedures

Procedures	Short-term[a] successes, (%)	Long-term[b] success, (%)
Myocutaneous rotational flap	90	87
Conventional rotational flap	86	72
Primary closure	89	62
Total	88	75

[a]Short-term success: No additional surgical procedures required during the first month of follow-up.

[b]Long-term success: No additional surgical procedures required during the entire duration of follow-up.

used [98]. Both the skin rotation flap and the muscle V-Y procedure can be reused if there are further ulcerations in this area. In patients with low-level spinal cord injury, reconstruction may be done using a sensate intercostal or tensor fascia lata flap [98].

Ischial pressure ulcers generally have smaller skin loss; however, the underlying cavity is frequently large with considerable undermining of the subcutaneous plane. Traditionally, this ulcer was treated with total ischiectomy [135]. This procedure, however, was frequently complicated by the occurrence of urethral strictures, for which reason partial ischiectomy became increasingly popular. Partial ischiectomy, on the other hand, resulted in the transfer of all weight-bearing function to the opposite ischium, thereby increasing the chances for pressure ulcers on the contralateral side. In the management of these conditions, the gluteus maximus transposition flap is the primary choice, or alternatively, an inferiorly based skin rotational flap may be used.

Greater trochanter defects generally show a modest amount of skin defect and have a similar size deeper defect with the trochanter at the base. A tensor fascia lata flap is the procedure of choice. This flap is based on the lateral femoral circumflex artery, allowing it to be used as an island transposition or as a free flap [136]. If

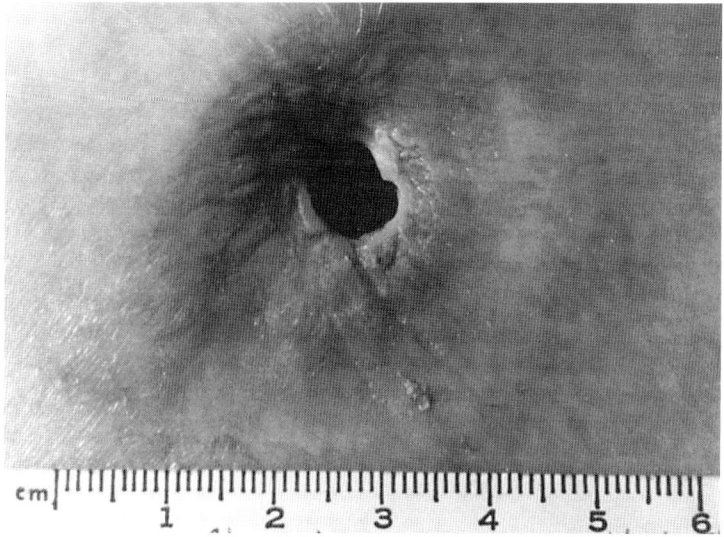

Figure 9-8. Preoperative right trochanteric ulcer in paraplegic patient.

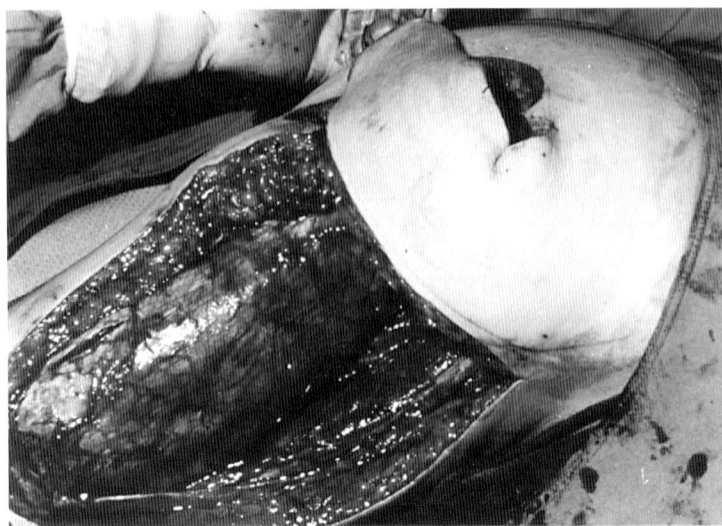

Figure 9-9.   Based on preoperative photoplethysmographic evaluation, the patient was scheduled for myocutaneous rotation flap. Myocutaneous flap was developed, and the vascularity was evaluated using blanching test.

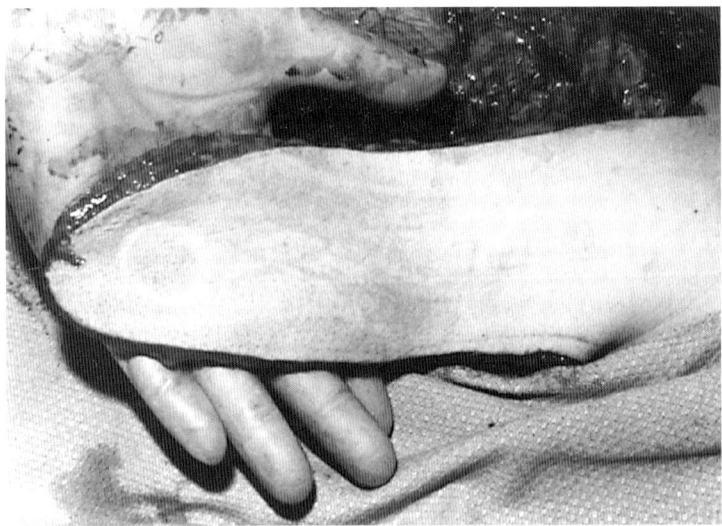

Figure 9-10.   The blanching test demonstrated good tissue perfusion of the flap. The flap was rotated into position.

this flap is not available, then the rectus femoris flap makes a good alternative. Other procedures available are vastus lateralis turnover flap, random skin rotation or transposition flaps, and the bipedicle fasciocutaneous flap.

Multiple ulcerations, as seen with ischial and trochanter ulcerations, represent a tremendous challenge to the plastic surgeon. The underlying bone

may have to be sacrificed, which will provide slack skin that can be used for reconstructive processes. For foot pressure ulcers, the utilization of a total contact cast is useful [137–140]. The other option is to use fasciocutaneous flaps based on the medial and lateral plantar arteries. In the lower limbs, the medial and lateral malleoli are the most common sites for ulcerations. These are closed most often

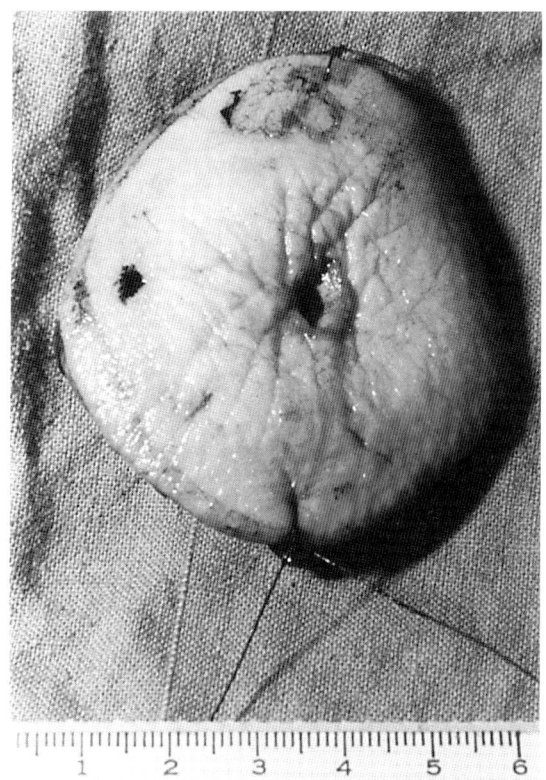

Figure 9-11. Excised area of pressure ulcer.

by unipedicle or bipedicle fasciocutaneous flaps. In the upper extremities, the olecranon is the most common site for ulceration and can be treated by excision and primary closure. Larger pressure ulcers, however, require flap coverage.

CONCLUSION

Pressure ulcers are a sign of acute illness caused most frequently by a failure of peripheral circulation and compounded by a patient's general physical status (comprising factors such as malnutrition, incontinence, immobility, and debilitating disease) as well as by attendant mental conditions such as dementia, depression, and other sensorium-altering cerebrovascular and neurological problems. Pressure ulcers have been identified as one of seven conditions affecting large numbers of patients, and requiring relatively expensive treatment and a correspondingly urgent necessity for strategies of prevention and cost containment. Although the incidence and prevalence of pressure ulcers within various institutions and countries may vary, overall, they are a serious concern in public health care policy.

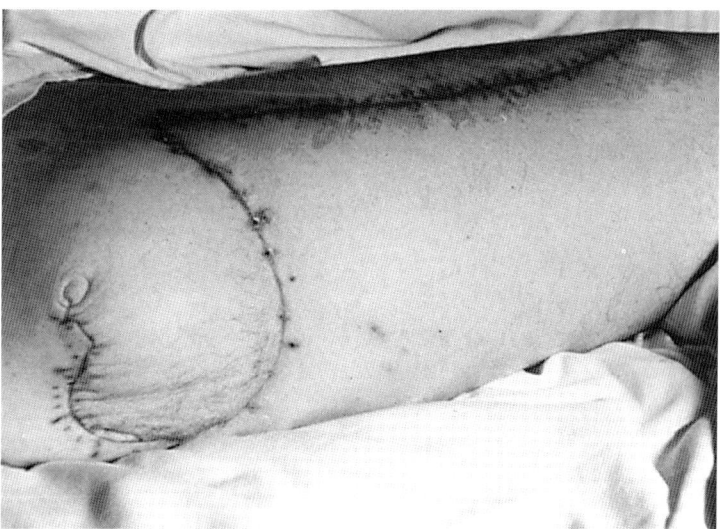

Figure 9-12. One month postoperative the myocutaneous rotation flap showed excellent healing.

Individual susceptibility for the development of pressure ulcers is as important as the various physical and environmental factors of causation. The goal is to identify individuals at risk for the development of pressure ulcers and to target these individuals for prevention. In the eventuality that pressure ulcers do develop, the goal shifts to optimizing management to achieve speedy recovery, improve the quality of life, and reduce mortality. Various risk assessment scales are available to help in such identification of at-risk individuals and to guide in the management of pressure ulcers. The Norton scale is the oldest of these and, despite its limitations, is in widest use. Classification systems proposed by the United Kingdom consensus and by the AHCPR have attempted, more recently, to meet the need for a standardized, widely adopted system to achieve uniformity in epidemiological studies, clinical trials, teaching, and outcome assessment. However, the usefulness of these scales will depend upon demonstrating continued reliability, reproducibility, and utility in varied settings.

Effective pressure ulcer management requires a coordinated effort by a multidisciplinary team and must include a major emphasis on education. Educational programs need to be structured, organized, comprehensive, and directed to all level of health care providers, the patients, and their families. They must be oriented to prevention, must describe each person's role in management, and be appropriate to the target audience in terms of the level of information presented and goals for expected participation. An educational program must be dynamically developed, implemented, evaluated, and updated on a regular basis so as to incorporate existing as well as newly innovating technology.

Pressure ulcers are no longer viewed as merely failures of nursing care, nor as inevitable complications that occur in anesthetic skin. They are now recognized as a highly preventable and treatable disorder, affecting about 10% of patients at risk, most of whom suffer silently and often die from the ulcers as a proximate cause. The time has come for physicians and providers to accept an increased responsibility for the management of this condition and to implement defined preventive strategies, as well as design and undertake educational and team-management plans to reduce morbidity and mortality from pressure ulcers and thus improve the overall quality of life in these patients.

REFERENCES

1. Fowler, E., Chronic wounds: An overview, in D. Krasner, ed., *Chronic Wound Care,* King of Prussia, PA: Health Management Publications, 1990:212–18.

2. Thompson, R. J., Pathological changes in mummies, *Proc Roy Soc Med* 1961; 54:409–415.

3. Vasconez, L. O.; Schneider, W. J.; and Lurkiewecz, M. J., Pressures sores, *Curr Probl Surg* 1977; 14:1–62.

4. Levine, J. M., Historical notes on pressure ulcers: The cure of Ambrose Pare, *Decubitus* 1992; 5:23–26.

5. *The Collective Works of Ambrose Pare* (1968) (Translated from the Latin by Thomis Johnson from the first English edition, London, 1634) Reprinted by Milford House, Poundridge, NY, p. 470.

6. Brown-Sequard, E., Experimental reseaches applied to physiology and pathology, New York: H. Bailliere, 1852.

7. Paget, J., Clinical lecture on bedsores, *Students J Hosp Gaz* 1873; 1:144–146.

8. Charcot, J. M., Lectures on the diseases of the nervous system, Delivered at Salpetriere (translated from 2nd ed.), Philadelphia: Henry C. Lea, 1879.

9. Snively, S. L., and Tebbetts, J. B., Pressure sores (overview), *Selected Readings in Plastic Surgery* 1986; 3:1.

10. Davis, J. S., Operative treatment of scars following bed sores, *Surgery* 1938; 3:1–7.

11. Brooks, B., and Duncan, G. W., Effects of pressure on tissues, *Arch Surg* 1940; 40:696–709.

12. Lamon, J. C., and Alexander, E., Secondary closure of decubitus ulcers with the aid of penicillin, *JAMA* 1945; 127:396.

13. White, J.; Hudson, A. H.; and Kenward, H., Treatment of bed sores by total excision with plastic closure, *Navy Med Bull* 1945; 45:454–463.

14. Conway, H., and Griffith, B. H., Plastic surgery for closure of decubitus ulcers in patients with paraplegia, *Am J Surg* 1956; 91:946–975.

15. Kostrubola, J. C., and Greeley, P. W., The problem of decubitus ulcers in paraplegics, *Plast Reconstr Surg* 1947; 2:403–412.

16. Furnas, D. W., Discussion of Sulibian, A. H.; Achauer, B. M.; Furnas, D. W.; The myocutaneous flap: A versatile approach to major reconstructive problems, *Am J Surg* 1980; 140:26–30.

17. Owens, N. A., A compound neck pedicle designed for the repair of massive facial defects: Formation, development and application, *Plast Reconstr Surg* 1955; 15:369–389.

18. Orticochea, M., The musculocutaneous flap method: An immediate and heroic substitute for the method of delay, *Brit J Plast Surg* 1972; 25:106–110.

19. McGraw, J. B.; Dibbel, D. G.; and Carroway, J. H., Clinical definition of independent myocutaneous vascular territories, *Plast Reconstr Surg* 1977; 60:341–352.

20. Bennett, G. C. J., Undergraduate teaching in chronic wound care, *Lancet* 1992; 339:249–250.

21. Rudman, D.; Slater, E. J.; Richardson, T. J.; and Mattson, D. E., The occurrence of pressure ulcers in three nursing homes, *J Gen Intern Med* 1993; 8:653–658.

22. Oot-Giromini, B. A., Pressure ulcer prevalence, incidence and associated risk factors in the community, *Decubitus* 1993; 6:24–32.

23. Brandeis, G. H.; Morris, J. N.; Nash, D. J.; and Lipsitz, L. A., The epidemiology and natural history of pressure ulcers in elderly nursing home residents, *JAMA* 1990; 264:2905–2909.

24. Allman, R. A., and Desforges, J. F., Pressure ulcers among the elderly, *N Engl J Med* 1989; 320:850–853.

25. Petersen, N. C., and Bittman, S., The epidemiology of pressure sores, *Scand J Plast Reconstr Surg Hand Surg* 1971; 5:62–66.

26. Barbend, J. C.; Jordan, M. M.; Nicol, S. M.; and Clark, M. O., Incidence of pressure ulcers in the greater Glasgow health board area, *Lancet* 1977; 2:548–550.

27. *Characteristic of Nursing Home Residents, Health Status, and Care Received: National Nursing Home Survey, United States, May–December 1977.* Hyattsville, MD: National Center for Health Statistics, 1981. U.S. Department of Health and Human Services publications PHS81-1712.

28. Barbanel, J. C.; Jordan, M. M.; Nichol, S. M.; and Clark, M. O., Incidence of pressure sores in the Greater Glasgow Health Board area, *Lancet* 1977; ii:548–550.

29. Guralnik, J. M.; Harris, T. B.; White, L. R.; and Cornoni-Huntley, J. C., Occurrence and predictors of pressure sores in the National Health and Nutrition Examination Survey follow-up, *J Am Geriatr Soc* 1988; 36:807–812.

30. Allman, R. M.; Lapraede, C. A.; Noel, L. B.; et al., Pressure sores among hospitalized patients, *Ann Intern Med* 1986; 105:337–342.

31. Allman, R. M., Epidemiology of pressure sores in different populations, *Decubitus* 1989; 2:30–33.

32. Berlowitz, D. R., and Wilking, S. V. B., Risk factors for pressure sores, *J Am Geriatr Soc* 1989; 37:1043–1050.

33. Michocki, R. J., and Lamy, P. P., The problem of pressure sores in a nursing home population: Statistical data, *J Am Geriatr Soc* 1976; 24:323–328.

34. Reed, J. W., Pressure ulcers in the elderly: Prevention and treatment utilizing the team approach, *Md Med J* 1981; 30:45–50.

35. Versluysen, M. J., Pressure sores in elderly patients: The epidemiology related to hip operations, *J Bone Joint Surg* 1985; 67:10–13.

36. Manley, M. T., Incidence, contributory factors and costs of pressure sores, *South Afr Med J* 1978; 53:217–222.

37. Lindan, O.; Greenway, R. M.; and Piazza, J. M., Pressure distribution on the surface of human body: Evaluation in lying and sitting position using a "bed of springs and nails," *Arch Phys Med Rehabil* 1965; 46:378–385.

38. Dansereau, J. G., and Conway, H., Closure of decubiti in paraplegics, *Plast Reconstr Surg* 1964; 33:474–480.

39. Lee, B. Y.; Shaw, W. W.; Madden, J. L.; Thoden, J. L.; and Lewis, J. M., Surgical management of pressure sores, *Contemporary Orthopaedics* 1982; 5:49–55.

40. Leigh, I. H., and Bennett, G., Pressure ulcers: Prevalence, etiology, and treatment modalities. A review. *Am J Surg* 1994; 167:25S–30S.

41. Reuler, J. B., and Cooney, T. G., The pressure sore: Pathophysiology and principles of management, *Ann Intern Med* 1981; 96:661–666.

42. Brandeis, G. H.; Ooi, W. L.; Hossain, M.; Morris, J. N.; and Lipsitz, L. A., A longitudinal study of risk factors associated with the formation of pres-

sure ulcers in nursing homes, *J Am Geriatr Soc* 1994; 42:388–393.

43. Spector, W. D., Correlates of pressure sores in nursing homes: Evidence from the National Medical Expenditure Survey, *J Invest Dermatol* 1994; 102:42S–45S.

44. Reichel, S. M., Shearing force as a factor in decubitus ulcers in paraplegics, *JAMA* 1958; 15:762–763.

45. Hofman, A.; Geelkerken, R. H.; Wille, J.; Hamming, J. J.; Hermans, J.; and Breslau, P. J., Pressure sores and pressure-decreasing mattresses: Controlled clinical trial, *Lancet* 1994; 343:568–571.

46. Henderson, J. L.; Price, S. H.; Brandstater, M. E.; and Mandac, B. R., Efficacy of three measures to relieve pressure in seated persons with spinal cord injury, *Arch Phys Med Rehabil* 1994; 75:535–539.

47. Meehan, M., Multisite pressure ulcer prevalence survey, *Decubitus* 1990; 3:14–17.

48. Bergstrom, N., and Branden, B., A prospective study of pressure sore risk among institutionalized elderly, *J Am Geriatr Soc* 1992; 40:747–758.

49. Meijer, J. H.; Germs, P. H.; Schneider, H.; and Ribbe, M. W., Susceptibility to decubitus ulcer formation, *Arch Phys Med Rehabil* 1994; 75:318–323.

50. Meijer, J. H.; Schut, G. L.; Ribbe, M. W.; Goovaerts, H. G.; Nieuwenhuys, R.; Reulen, J. P. H.; and Schneider, H., Method for the measurement of susceptibility to decubitus ulcer formation, *Med Biol Eng Comput* 1989; 27:502–550.

51. Dinsdale, S. M., Decubitus ulcers: Role of pressure and friction in causation, *Arch Phys Med Rehabil* 1974; 55:147–155.

52. Kosiak, M., Etiology of decubitus ulcers, *Arch Phys Med Rehabil* 1961; 42:19–29.

53. Kosiak, M., Etiology of pathology of ischemic ulcers, *Arch Phys Med Rehabil* 1959; 40:62–69.

54. Lindan, O., Etiology of decubitus ulcers, *Arch Phys Med Rehabil* 1961; 42:774–783.

55. Nola, G. T., and Vistnes, L. M., Differential response of skin and muscle in the experimental production of pressure sores, *Plast Reconstr Surg* 1980; 66:728.

56. Daniel, R. K.; Priest, D. L.; and Wheatly, D. C., Etiologic factors in pressures sores: An experimental model, *Arch Phys Med Rehabil* 1981; 62:429.

57. Reichel, S. M., Shearing forces as a factor in decubitus ulcers in paraplegics, *JAMA* 1958; 166:762–763.

58. Guttman, L., Problem of treatment of pressure sores in spinal paraplegics, *Brit J Plast Surg* 1958; 8:196–213.

59. Goossens, R. H.; Zegers, R.; Hoek van Dijke, D. A.; and Snijders, C. J., Influence of shear on skin oxygen tension, *Clin Physiol* 1994; 14:111–118.

60. Bennett, L.; Kavner, D.; Lee, B. Y.; and Trainor, F. S., Shear vs. pressure as causation factors in skin blood flow occlusion, *Arch Phys Med Rehabil* 1979; 60:309–314.

61. Bennett, L.; Kavner, D.; Lee, B. Y.; et al., Skin blood flow in seated geriatric patients, *Arch Phys Med Rehabil* 1981; 62:392–398.

62. Bennett, L.; Kavner, D.; Lee, B. Y.; et al., Skin stress and blood flow in sitting paraplegic patients, *Arch Phys Med Rehabil* 1984; 65:186–190.

63. Witkowski, J. A., and Parish, L. C., Histopathology of the decubitus ulcer, *J Am Acad Derm* 1982; 6:1014–1021.

64. Pinchafsky-Devin, G. D., and Kaminski, M. V., Correlation of pressure sore and nutritional status, *J Am Geriatr Soc* 1986; 34:435–440.

65. Husain, T., An experimental study of some pressure effects on tissue with reference to the bed sore problem, *J Pathol Bacteriol* 1953; 66:347–358.

66. Taylor, T. V.; Dymock, I. W.; and Tarrance, B., The role of vitamin C in the treatment of pressure sores in surgical patients, *Brit J Surg* 1974; 61:921.

67. Levine, J.; Simpson, M.; and McDonald, R., Pressure sores: A plan for primary care prevention, *Geriatrics* 1989; 44:75–90.

68. Shea, J. D., Pressure sores: Classification and management, *Clin Orthop* 1975; 112:89–100.

69. Johnson, A., A blueprint for the prevention and management of pressure sores, *CARE Science and Practice* 1985; 1:8–13.

70. Lowthian, P., The classification and grading of pressure sores, *CARE Science and Practice* 1987; 5:5–9.

71. Yarkony, G. M.; Kirk P. M.; Carlson, C.; et al., Classification of pressure ulcers, *Arch Derm* 1990; 126:1218–1219.

72. Reid, J., and Morison, M., Classification of pressure sore severity: Pressure-sore grading, *Nursing Times* 1994; 90:46–50.

73. *Pressure Ulcers in Adults: Prediction and Prevention,* in Clinical Practice Guideline Number 3, U.S. Department of Health and Human Services, Public Health Service, Agency for Health Care Policy and Research, Publication no. 92-0047, May 1992; 3:1–63.

74. Goldstone, L. A., and Goldstone, J., The Norton score: An early warning of pressure sores, *J Adv Nurs* 1982; 1:419–426.

75. Bergstrom, N.; Braden, B. J.; Laguzza, A.; and Holman, V., The Braden scale for predicting pressure sore risk, *Nurs Res* 1987; 36:205–210.

76. Williams, C., Comparing Norton and Medley, *Nursing Times* 1991; 87:66–68.

77. Waterlow, J., Risk assessment card, *Nursing Times* 1985; 81:49–55.

78. Editorials, Preventing pressure sores, *Lancet* 1990; 335:1311–1312.

79. Loader, S.; Delve, M.; and Hofman, D., A consultancy service that pays dividends; setting up a pressure sore resource group, *Professional Nurse* 1994; 9:259–266.

80. Taler, G.; Richardson, J. P.; Fredman, L.; and Lazur, A., The wound unit: A specialized unit for pressure sore management in long-term care facility, *Md Med J* 1994; 43:165–169.

81. Buntine, J. A., and Johnstone, B. R., The contribution of plastic surgery to care of the spinal cord injury patient, *Paraplegia* 1988; 26:87–93.

82. Gorse, G. J., and Messner, R. L., Improved pressure sore healing with hydrocolloid dressings, *Arch Derm* 1987;123:766–771.

83. Xakellis, G. C., and Chrischillis, E. A., Hydrocolloid versus saline-gauze dressings in treating pressure ulcers: A cost-effectiveness analysis, *Arch Phys Med Rehabil* 1992; 73:463–469.

84. Fowler, E., and Goupil, D. L., Comparison of wet-to-dry dressing and copolymer starch in the management of debrided pressure sores, *J Enterostomal Ther* 1984; 11:22–25.

85. Oleske, D. M.; Smith, X. P.; White, P.; Pottage, J.; and Donovan, M., A randomized clinical trial of two dressing methods for the treatment of low grade pressure ulcers, *J Enterostomal Ther* 1986; 13:90–98.

86. Kraft, M. R.; Lawson, L.; Pohlman, B.; Reid-Lokos, C.; and Barder, L., A comparison of Epi-Lock and saline dressings in the management of pressure ulcers, *Decubitus* 1993; 6:42–48.

87. Poteete, V., Case study: Eliminating odors from wounds, *Decubitus* 1993; 6:43–46.

88. Van Rijswijk, L., Full-thickness pressure ulcers: Patient and wound healing characteristics, *Decubitus* 1993; 6:16–21.

89. Pierce, G. F.; Mustoe, T. A.; Altrock, B. A.; Deuel, T. F.; and Thomason, A., The role of platelet derived growth factor in wound healing, *J Cell Biochem* 1991; 45:319–326.

90. Pierce, G. F.; Vande Berg, J.; Rudolph, R.; Tarpley, J.; and Mustoe, T. A., PDGF-BB and TGF-β1 selectively modulate glycosaminoglycans, collagen, and myofibroblasts in excisional wounds, *Am J Pathol* 1991; 138:629–646.

91. Pierce, G. F.; Tarpley, J. E.; Yanagihara, D.; Mustoe, T. A.; Fox, G. M.; and Thomason, A., PDGF-BB, TGF-β1 and basic FGF in dermal wound healing: Neovessel and matrix formation and cessation of repair, *Am J Pathol* 1992; 140:1375–1388.

92. Robson, M. C.; Phillips, L. G.; Thomason, A.; et al., Recombinant human platelet derived growth factor-BB for the treatment of chronic pressure ulcers, *Am Plast Surg* 1992; 29:193–201.

93. Grotendorst, G. R.; Martin, G. R.; Pencev, D.; Sodek, J.; and Harvey, A. K., Stimulation of granulation tissue formation by platelet derived growth factor in normal and diabetic rats, *J Clin Invest* 1985; 76:2323–2329.

94. Brown, G. L.; Nanney, L. B.; Griffen, J.; et al., Enhancement of wound healing by topical treatment with epidermal growth factor, *N Engl J Med* 1989; 321:76–79.

95. Robson, M. C.; Phillips, L. G.; Lawrence, W. T.; et al., The safety and effect of topically applied recombinant basic fibroblast growth factor on the healing of pressure ulcers, *Ann Surg* 1992; 216:401–408.

96. Mustoe, T. A.; Cutler, N. R.; Allman, R. M.; Goode, P. S.; Deuel, T. F.; Prause, J. A.; Bear, M.; Serdar, C. M.; and Pierce, G. F., A phase II study to evaluate recombinant platelet-derived growth factor-BB in the treatment of stage 3 and 4 pressure ulcers, *Arch Surg* 1994; 129:213–219.

97. Rudensky, B.; Lipschits, M.; Isaacsohn, M.; Sonnenblick, M., Infected pressure sores: Comparison of methods for bacterial infection, *Southern Med J* 1992; 85:901–903.

98. Linder, R. M., and Morris, D., The surgical man-

agement of pressure ulcers: A systematic approach based on staging, *Decubitus* 1990; 3:32–38.

99. Bryan, C. S.; Dew, C. E.; and Reynolds, K. L., Bacteremia associated with decubitus ulcers, *Arch Intern Med* 1983; 143:2093–2095.

100. Galpin, J. E.; Chow, A. W.; Bayer, A. S.; and Guze, L. B., Sepsis associated with decubitus ulcers, *Am J Med* 1976; 61:346–350.

101. Haley, R. W.; Hightower, A. W.; Khabbaz, R. F.; et al., The emergence of methicillin resistant *Staphylococcus aureus* infections in the United States hospitals; possible role of the house staff patient transfer circuit, *Ann Intern Med* 1982; 97:297–308.

102. Robertson, E. C., and Tisdall, F., Nutrition and resistance to disease, *Canad Med Assoc J* 1993; 40:282–284.

103. Joseph, B., Insulin in the treatment of non-diabetic bed sores, *Ann Surg* 1930; 92:318–319.

104. McCormick, W. J., The nutritional aspects of bed sores, *Med Rec* 1941; 154:389–391.

105. Mulholland, J. H.; Tui, C.; Wright, A. M.; Vinci, V.; and Shafiroff, B., Protein metabolism and bed sores, *Ann Surg* 1943; 118:1015–1023.

106. Claus-Walker, J.; Singh, J.; Leach, C. S.; Hatton, D. V.; Hubert, C. W.; and DiFerrante, N., The urinary excretion of collagen degradation products in quadriplegic patients and during weightlessness, *J Bone Joint Surg* 1977; 59A:209–212.

107. Claus-Walker, J., and Kretzer, F. L., Insensitive skin properties of spinal cord injury patients, *Arch Phys Med Rehabil* 1981; 62:521.

108. Daniel, R. K.; Priest, D. L.; and Wheatley, D. C., Etiologic factors in pressure sores: An experimental model, *Arch Phys Med Rehabil* 1981; 62:492–498.

109. Perkash, A., and Brown, M., Anemia in patients with traumatic spinal cord injury, *Paraplegia* 1982; 20:235–236.

110. Thompson, W. D.; Ravdin, I. S.; and Frank, I. L., Effect of hypoproteinemia on wound disruption, *Arch Surg* 1938; 36:500–508.

111. Thompson, W. D.; Ravdin, I. S.; Rhoads, J. E.; and Frank, I. L., Use of lyophile plasma in correction of hypoproteinemia and prevention of wound disruption, *Arch Surg* 1938; 36:509–518.

112. Chandra, R. K., Rosette forming T lymphocytes and cell mediated immunity in malnutrition, *Brit Med J* 1974; 3:608–609.

113. Geefhuysen, R. K.; Rosen, E. U.; Katz, J.; Ipp, T.; and Metz, J., Impaired cellular immunity in kwashiorkor with improvement after therapy, *Brit Med J* 1971; 41:527–529.

114. Chandra, R. K., Cell mediated immunity in nutritional imbalance, *Federation Proc* 1980; 39:3088–3092.

115. Stiehm, E. R., Humoral immunity in malnutrition, *Federation Proc* 1980; 39:3093–3097.

116. Dionigi, R.; Zonta, A.; Dominioni, L.; Gines, F.; and Ballabio, A., The effect of total parenteral nutrition on immunodepression due to malnutrition, *Ann Surg* 1977; 185:467–474.

117. Arora, N. S., and Rochester, D. F., Effects of general nutrition and muscular states on the human diaphragm, *Am Rev Resp Dis* 1977; 115:84.

118. Keys, A.; Brozek, J.; Henshel, A.; et al., *Biology of Human Starvation,* Minneapolis: University of Minnesota Press, 1950.

119. Winick, M., *Hunger Disease,* New York: Wiley, 1979.

120. Viart, P., Hemodynamic findings during protein-calorie malnutrition, *Am J Clin Nutr* 1978; 31:911–926.

121. Taylor, T. V.; Rimmer, S.; Day, B.; et al., Ascorbic acid supplementation in the treatment of pressure sores, *Lancet* 1974; 11:544–546.

122. Hallbook, T., and Lanner, E., Serum zinc and healing of venous leg ulcers, *Lancet* 1972; 11:780–782.

123. Pekarek, R. S.; Sandstead, H. H.; Jacob, R. A.; and Barcome, D. F., Abnormal cellular immune response during acquired zinc deficiency, *Am J Clin Nutr* 1979; 32:1466–1471.

124. Agarwal, N.; Del Guercio, L. R. M.; and Lee, B. Y., The role of nutrition in the management of pressure sores, Chapter 11 in *Chronic Ulcers of the Skin,* B. Y. Lee, ed., New York: McGraw Hill, 1985; 11:133–145.

125. Williamson, M. B.; McCarthy, T. H.; and Fromm, H. J., Relation of protein nutrition to the healing of experimental wounds, *Soc Exper Biol Med* 1951; 77:302–305.

126. Cannon, P. R.; Wissler, R. W.; Woolridge, R. L.; and Benditt, E. P., The relationship of protein deficiency to surgical infection, *Ann Surg* 1944; 120:514–525.

127. Meakins, J. L.; Pietsch, J. B.; Bubenick, O.; Kelly, R.; Rode, H.; Gordon, J.; and MacLean, L. D.,

Delayed hypersensitive: Indicator of acquired failure of host defenses in sepsis and trauma, *Ann Surg* 1977; 186:241–250.

128. Rhoads, J. E., and Alexander, C. E., Nutritional problems of surgical patients, *Ann NY Acad Sci* 1955; 63:268–275.

129. Christou, N. V.; Meakins, J. L.; and MacLean, L. D., The predictive role of delayed hypersensitive in preoperative patients, *Surg Gynecol Obstet* 1981; 152:297–301.

130. Harvey, K. B.; Ruggiero, J. H.; Regan, C. S.; Bistrian, B. R.; and Blackburn, G. L., Hospital morbidity-mortality risk factors using nutritional assessment, *Clin Res* 1978; 26:581.

131. Mullen, J. L.; Buzby, G. P.; Matthews, D. C.; Smale, B. F.; and Rosato, E. F., Reduction of operative morbidity and mortality by combined preoperative and postoperative nutritional support, *Ann Surg* 1980; 192:604–613.

132. Lee, B. Y.; Agarwal, N.; Corcoran, L.; Thoden, W. R.; and Del Guercio, L. R. M., Assessment of nutritional and metabolic status of paraplegics, *J Rehabil Res Dev* 1985; 22:11–21.

133. Ostrander, L. E.; Lee, B. Y.; Silverman, D. A.; and Groskopf, R. A., Constant infusion fluorometry to predict flap survival, *Decubitus* 1989; 2:40–46.

134. Tizian, C.; Brenner, P.; and Berger, A., The one stage treatment of multiloculated pressure sores using various myocutaneous island flaps, *Scand J Plast Reconstr Surg* 1988; 22:83–87.

135. Dansereau, J. G., and Conway, H., Closure of decubiti in paraplegics, *Plast Reconstr Surg* 1964; 33:474–480.

136. Nahai, F.; Silverton, J. S.; Hill, H. L.; and Vasconez, L. O., The tensor fascia lata musculocutaneous flap, *Ann Plast Surg* 1978; 1:372–389.

137. Helm, P. A.; Walker, S. C.; and Pullium, G., Total contact casts in diabetic patients with neuropathic feet ulcerations, *Arch Phys Med Rehabil* 1984; 65:691–693.

138. Barnett, O., Total contact cast, *Clin Podiatr Med Surg* 1987; 4:471–479.

139. Sinacore, D. R.; Mueller, M. J.; Diamond, J. E.; et al., Diabetic plantar ulcers treated by total contact casting. A clinical report, *Phys Ther* 1987; 67:1543–1549.

140. Mueller, M. J.; Diamond, J. E.; Sinacore, D. R.; et al., Total contact casting in treatment of diabetic plantar ulcers. Controlled clinical trial, *Diabet Care* 1989; 12:384–388.

141. Bergstrom, N.; Demuth, P. J.; and Braden, B. J., A clinical trial of the Braden Scale for predicting pressure sore risks, *Nurs Clin North Am* 1987; 22:417–428.

142. Richardson, R., and Meyer, P., Prevalence and incidence of pressure sores in acute spinal cord injuries, *Paraplegia* 1987; 19:235–247.

143. National Pressure Ulcer Advisory Panel, Pressure ulcers: Incidence, economics, risk assessment. Consensus development conference statement, *Decubitus* 1989; 2:24–28.

144. International Association of Enterostomal Therapy, Dermal wounds; pressure sores. Philosophy of the IAET, *J Enterostomal Ther* 1988; 15:4–17.

145. Hancock, K. A., and Leigh, I. M., Cultured keratinocytes and keratinocytes grafts, *Brit Med J* 1989; 299:1179–1180.

146. Hansborough, J. F.; Boyce, S. T.; Cooper, M. L.; and Foreman, T. J., Burn wound closure with cultured autologous keratinocytes and fibroblasts attached to a collagen-glycosaminoglycan substrate, *JAMA* 1989; 262:2125–2130.

147. Lee, B. Y., Plastic surgery for pressure sores, Chapter 18 in *The Spinal Cord Injured Patient Comprehensive Management,* B. Y. Lee, L. E. Ostrander, G. V. B. Cochran, and W. W. Shaw, ed., Philadephia: W. B. Saunders, 1991:223–230.

10

MECHANICAL LOADING AND PRESSURE ULCERS

David M. Brienza, Ph.D.
and Lee E. Ostrander, Ph.D.

MECHANICAL LOADING AND PRESSURE ULCERS

Unrelieved pressure upon weight-bearing tissues can produce lesions, identified by their etiology as pressure ulcers [1]. The purpose of this chapter is to discuss the role of pressure, and more generally the role of mechanics, in the formation of pressure ulcers (also referred to as decubitus ulcers or decubiti).

It is important to note that factors other than mechanics influence pressure ulcer formation. Many interrelated factors, intrinsic as well as extrinsic, have been shown to predispose load-bearing tissue to mechanical damage [2]. An extended accounting of pressure ulcer formation must include not only mechanics as a primary causative agent, but also contributing agents such as friction, heat, moisture, ischemia, and malnutrition [1, 3, 4]. The importance of these various factors also depends upon the particular patient population considered. For example, persons with spinal cord injury (SCI) are at greatest risk, subsequent to loss of sensory and motor functions, to loss of vasomotor control and tone, to changes and abnormalities in morphology of bone and soft tissue, and to altered neuromuscular activity (spastic or flaccid) [3, 5, 6].

The mechanics of pressure ulcer formation is characterized by key elements such as the magnitude of forces, the direction of forces, the distribution of forces over the surface, and the deformation of the tissues associated with the forces. Extrinsic pressure acting upon weight-bearing tissue is defined by the distribution of forces over a tissue area. The direction of the forces ranges from perpendicular to the tissue surface (referred to as "normal") to parallel or in line with the tissue surface (referred to as "shear"). The typical loading conditions will include a combination of normal and shear forces. The forces present at the surface of the tissue are transmitted into the tissue and cause deformation of the tissue. To complete this picture of mechanical loading, one can examine the tissue deformation that occurs with the loading [7–11].

TYPES OF MECHANICAL LOADING AND THEIR EFFECTS ON SOFT TISSUE

INTERFACE PRESSURE

Potentially harmful pressures are produced as the weight of the human body pushes down on its skeletal structure and becomes distributed through a relatively small volume of soft tissue located between bony prominences and supporting surfaces. For example, when a person is seated on a flat, hard surface (refer to Figure 10-1), a large percentage of the body weight is supported through the pelvis. The weight-bearing pelvis in this case acts in the same manner as a rigid indenter and presses down inside the body into the buttocks and into the associated tissues of muscle, fascia, fat, and skin. Reaction forces generated by the support surface oppose the weight-induced body forces, increasing the internal stress of the tissues and redistributing the soft tissue so that they become distorted by the applied forces [7, 8].

Although the idea of tissue compression is often present in the literature, soft tissue is a solid and fluid mixture that is essentially incompressible under the loading encountered with typical support surfaces. The external forces during normal sitting act predominantly in a direction perpendicular to the support surface. Soft tissue volume will reduce only a small amount with the applied force; that is, changes in tissue density and volume are negligibly small. Rather, the tissue is distorted and displaced to adjacent regions where the internal and external forces are lower. This physical response of the tissues continues as external forces are applied until a force equilibrium is reached. If the equilibrium condition causes an occlusion of capillary blood flow, the result can be ischemic injury [12]. The

impairment of lymphatic drainage or interstitial fluid flow under these same conditions has also been proposed as a primary cause of pressure ulcers [7, 8, 13, 14].

Coincident with tissue deformation is an increase in internal tissue pressure levels. The levels of internal pressure are dependent upon the heterogeneous mechanical properties throughout the soft tissues and also upon the directions in which these tissues are distended by the applied loading. If the tissues are confined so that no redistribution of tissue mass can occur, or if loading is applied hydrostatically through a fluid, the soft tissues can withstand relatively high pressures without significant risk of damage [9]. To illustrate this, consider the pressures externally applied to a scuba diver at depths of 50 or 100 feet. Although the pressure on the skin is far in excess of pressures considered harmful if applied nonuniformly, the diver is not at increased risk for pressure ulcers because the pressure is applied hydrostatically. Only when pressure is applied nonuniformly are tissues strained and consequently put at risk of tissue damage. While sitting, the soft tissue of the buttocks is not contained; therefore, support surface reaction forces can result in internal strain and ischemia. If excessive forces are not relieved, the result can soon be morbidity and ensuing tissue necrosis.

Variability of applied external forces (i.e., nonuniform external forces) over a body surface increases the potential for tissue damage as compared with equivalent forces applied uniformly. The variability in normal forces is sometimes described as vertical shear [15] or is quantified in terms of "gradients" of force or pressure [16]. As vertical shear increases, the likely effect is an increase in the deformation of the tissue with an increasing risk of tissue damage. Vertical shear should not be confused with the shear force acting parallel, or tangentially, to the surface, as described in the following section.

Muscle, fat, and connective tissues have different properties and distort differently in response to applied forces [7, 8]. Given the different tissues and their different mechanical properties, it is difficult to predict the internal conditions from external interface pressures. Although internal tissue forces

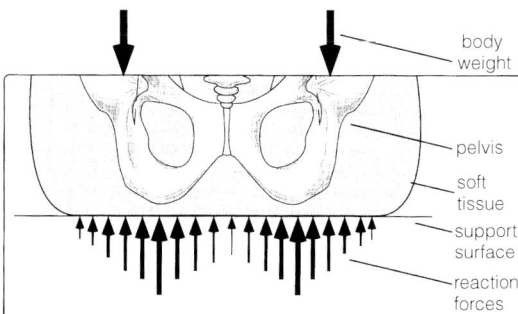

Figure 10-1.　Representation of body weight distribution through the cross section of pelvis and soft tissue of a subject seated on a flat non-compliant surface. Support surface reaction forces are concentrated in the region of the ischial tuberosities.

may result from and be related to external forces, it is important to note that the internal forces and pressures to be found in cutaneous, subcutaneous, and other tissues are generally not identical to the external pressures. The internal forces present in tissues can be substantial, even when the surface or interface pressures are low or moderate in value [17].

Reddy et al. used the wick catheter technique [18] to measure the interstitial fluid pressure in the forelimbs of ten Yorkshire pigs. External pressure was applied via a blood pressure cuff, and internal pressure was measured 2 to 5 mm below the skin. Reddy's results showed that interstitial fluid pressure reached approximately 72% of the externally applied pressure for external pressures to 150 mm Hg (Refer to Figure 10-2). When the experiments were repeated with a preinfusion of excess fluid in the tissue, internal pressure reached 100% of the externally applied pressure [7].

Le et al. measured internal and external pressures near the greater trochanter of Yorkshire pigs [17] and provided contrasting results to those of Reddy. In the second of the two in vivo experiments reported, the pig was laid horizontally on a clear plexiglass table. External pressure on the underside

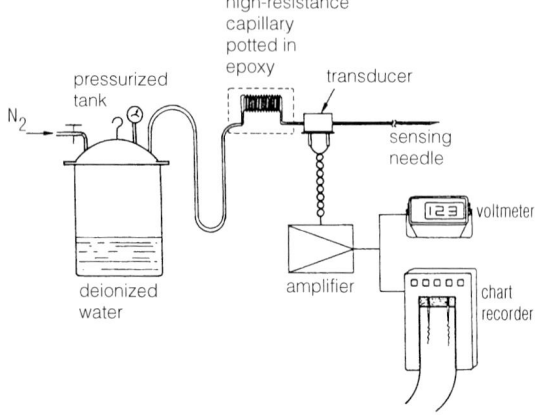

PRESSURE-SENSING SYSTEM

Figure 10-3.   Pressure-sensing system. The compressed nitrogen forces deionized water from the fluid reservoir into the flexible tubing and the high-resistance capillary network, past the sensor and the needle, and into the tissue. (From Le [17].)

of the pig was a result of the reaction forces of the table in response to the pig's body weight. Interface pressure between the table and the skin was measured using an air bladder device similar to the device used by Reddy in his experiments. Internal pressure was measured with a modified "needle method" [19] in which a miniature monolithic silicon pressure sensor measured fluid pressure, with fluid transmitted through a hypodermic needle. (Refer to Figure 10-3.) The needle was inserted perpendicular to the support surface from the underside through guide holes in the table. A sample of Le's results is shown in Figure 10-4 (Figure 10 from Le et al. [17]). The measured interstitial pressure was found to be maximum near the bony prominence and to decrease with position change vertically toward the surface and with position change horizontally away from the prominence. The peak internal pressures were found to be three to five times greater than externally measured pressures. Le concluded that these results supported clinical observations to the effect that pressure ulcers can "originate internally near bone and progress outward" toward the skin.

The apparent discrepancy between Le's and Reddy's results can be explained by analyzing the

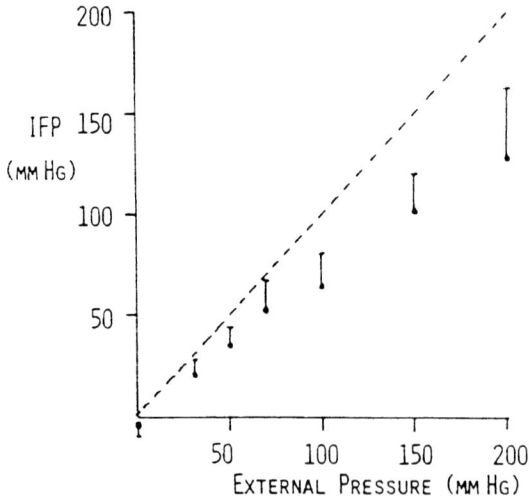

Figure 10-2.   Effects of external compression on interstitial fluid pressure (IFP). *Solid dots* are means of observations. *Bars* indicate standard deviation. (From Reddy [7], Figure 2.)

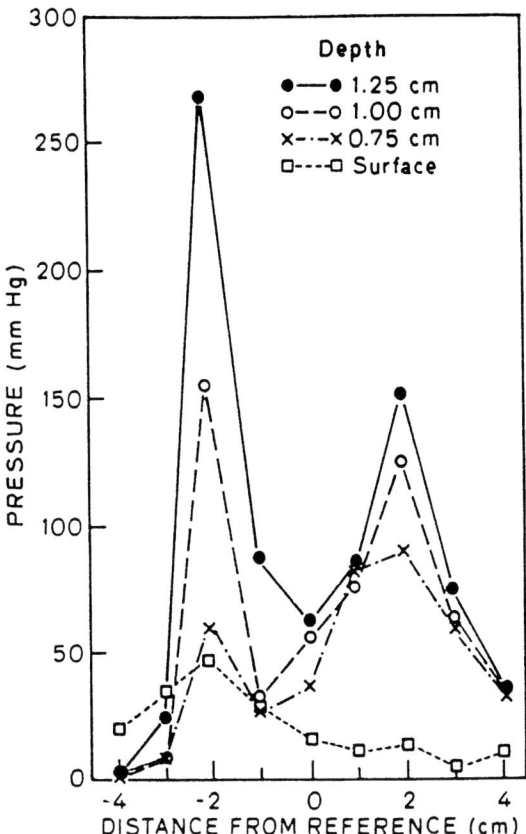

Figure 10-4. Pressure distribution sampled at different horizontal planes in the tissue underlying the left trochanter and the ischium and pressure distribution measured at the surface. The peak of the pressure distribution is also shifted from the reference. (From Le et al. [17], Figure 10.)

pressures more than five times higher than the internal pressures measured by Reddy.

In a separate study, Reddy et al. compared the surface pressures and subcutaneous interstitial fluid pressure in the posterior thighs of human subjects [20]. Subcutaneous pressures were measured using a wick catheter [18] and compared to interface pressures measured using an air bladder type interface pressure transducer (Scimedics Corp.). The wick was placed "close to the surface beneath the dermis." Pressures were measured at the interface and subcutaneously for three loading conditions on the thighs and for three thicknesses of soft foam pads. The interface pressure was varied both by adding weight to the free-hanging feet of the subjects and by using different thicknesses of padding as a support surface over the foam (Refer to Figure 10-5.)

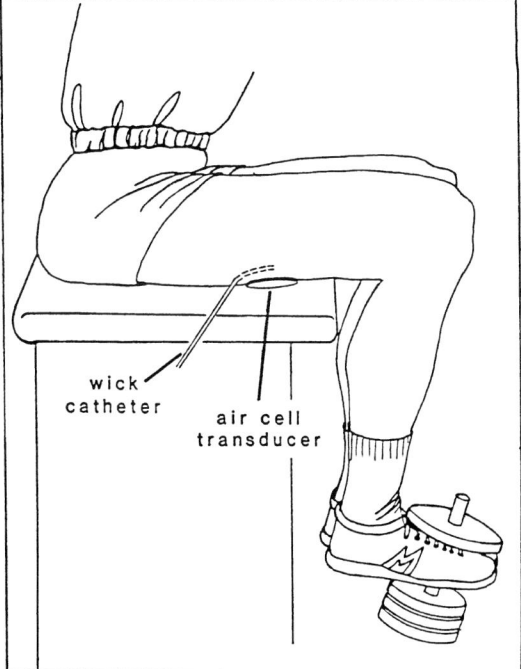

Figure 10-5. The experimental setup for comparison of interface and interstitial pressure measurements. Indentation of the soft tissue by the air cell transducer was minimal, but is exaggerated here to show the location. Muscles were relaxed during measurements so dead weight loading on legs compressed thigh against table surface covered by a 25-mm-thick soft foam pad. (From Reddy et al. [20].)

loading conditions for each of the experiments. In Reddy's experiments using Yorkshire pigs [7, 8], external pressure was applied with a wide pressure cuff on a relatively small limb. The ratio of cuff width to limb diameter was 1.3–1.4 to 1. Assuming that the forelimbs of the pigs were approximately round in cross section, the round cuff applied pressure in a uniform fashion. Although the deformation of the limb was not quantified, Reddy described the pattern qualitatively as a "uniform compression." In contrast, the mode of deformation seen by Le resulted from forces applied in a highly unidirectional fashion. For externally measured pressure in the range of 50 mm Hg, Le measured internal

The results showed that there were no significant differences between the interface and subcutaneous pressures. The measured external pressures ranged from 3.98 kPa (30 mm Hg) on 1/2-inch foam with no additional loading on the feet to 8.28 kPa (62 mm Hg) on 1/2-inch foam.

In this latter study by Reddy using human subjects, the external forces were applied approximately uniaxially through the foam support surface. (Refer to Figure 10-5.) Nonetheless, the results were consistent with his first experiments in that internally measured pressures were not significantly greater than the externally measured pressures. Although this is seemingly a contradiction of the conclusion postulated above concerning the relationship between the uniaxial nature of the applied forces and their adverse effect on internal pressure, an examination of the loading conditions can explain the contradiction. In Le's experiments, forces were applied to an area of the anatomy near a bony prominence, the trochanter of the Yorkshire pig. In contrast, Reddy examined the response of much thicker soft tissue, the posterior thigh of human subjects. The difference in the response of the soft tissues in terms of internal pressure may again be indicative of the difference in relative deformation of those tissues. The magnitudes of external pressures and the direction of force application were comparable; results are compared for external pressure in the range of 50 mm Hg, and the supporting surface transmitted force uniaxially. However, the thin tissues covering the bony prominences of the pigs investigated by Le were likely distorted by a much larger percentage of their original, unloaded thickness than the tissues investigated by Reddy in the posterior thigh of humans.

Sangeorzan et al. [21] used simultaneous measurement of tissue oxygenation via transcutaneous partial pressure of oxygen ($TcPO_2$) [22], as well as interface pressure, subcutaneous pressure, and skin deformation to investigate the relative effect of externally applied pressure on skin over bone versus skin over muscle. Responses to load were measured for the skin over the tibia and over the tibialis anterior muscle in 12 normal subjects. The applied normal force was used to estimate applied interface pressure. The $TcPO_2$ measurements showed that significantly less interface pressure was required to reduce $TcPO_2$ to zero for the skin over bone compared to skin over muscle. In contrast, at the points of zero $TcPO_2$, the subcutaneous pressures were not significantly different for skin over bone and skin over muscle. In other words, the subcutaneous pressure and $TcPO_2$ relationship was consistent for the skin over bone and skin over muscle sites, whereas the interface pressure and $TcPO_2$ relationship varied according to the site tested.

The implication of this result is that the relationship between interface pressure measurements and cutaneous perfusion, as measured by $TcPO_2$, is dependent on the mechanical properties of the underlying tissue. In this study, it was shown that skin above stiff underlying tissue, bone, was less tolerant to external loading than skin above more compliant underlying tissue, muscle. Other investigators have drawn attention to inconsistencies between $TcPO_2$ measurements and applied compressive forces. Xakellis [23] noted that one investigation found a linear relationship between $TcPO_2$ and increasing compressive force [24], whereas a second investigation found that $TcPO_2$ decreased parabolically with increasing compressive force [25].

TANGENTIAL SHEAR

Tangential shear forces act in a direction parallel to the supporting surface. For example, tangential shear forces appear when the body slides or has a tendency to slide across a support surface. For the patient in bed, elevating the head of a bed can increase tangential shear forces, particularly in the sacral area and on the heels, as the force of gravity pushes the individual toward the foot of the bed. Friction between the skin and the support surface may cause the skin to remain in place on the bed while the underlying deep fascia and skeletal structure slide toward the foot of the bed [1]. In the presence of tangential shear force, adjacent anatomical structures internal to the body slide across one another. This phenomenon, as illustrated by Jay [26], is shown in Figure 10-6.

Several theories have been proposed concerning the effect of shear on weight-bearing soft tissue. For example, Reichel hypothesized that blood vessels in the sacral area become twisted and distorted leading to ischemia and necrosis as a result of shear [27].

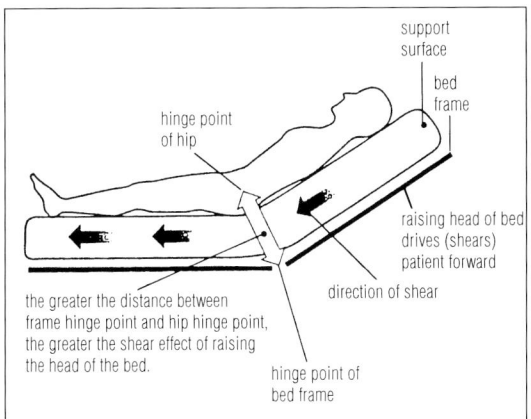

Figure 10-6. Shear effect of raising the head of the bed. (From Jay [26].)

Verification of alternative hypotheses has been problematic because there are inherent difficulties in investigating the effects of shear on the soft tissues between support surfaces and weight-bearing bony prominences. The problems include the heterogeneity of tissues and the dependence of shear force on normal force. Investigation is complicated further by the inability to directly measure the stress distribution within affected tissues.

Several researchers have investigated the skin's physiological responses to shear [28–31]. Bennett [28, 15] developed a noninvasive sensor for measuring pulsatile skin blood flow, normal pressure, and shear. Testing using four healthy subjects showed that occlusion of skin blood flow in the thenar eminence could be achieved with normal pressure alone for normal pressures in the range of 100 to 120 mm Hg. When shear of approximately 100 g/cm [2] was applied, approximately 60 to 80 mm Hg pressure was necessary to achieve occlusion. The conclusion was that normal pressure was roughly twice as effective as shear in reducing pulsatile blood flow. In these experiments, blood flow was measured using a blood flow photoplethysmograph. Pressure and shear were measured with cantilevered steel beams instrumented with strain gauges.

In further testing, Bennett et al. [29] used the sensor described above mounted flush in the flat rigid seat of a wheelchair to investigate the sitting-induced loading near the ischial tuberosity for normal ($n = 9$), paraplegic ($n = 16$), and ill elderly ($n = 16$) subject groups. Analysis of the results indicated that all three groups had median normal pressures approximately equal, in the range of 52 to 60 mm Hg. However, the shear was significantly higher and the blood flow rate was significantly lower for the paraplegic and elderly groups as compared to the normal group. Although this result does not identify a causal relationship between shear and skin blood flow [15], it has illustrated that factors other than load distribution may affect skin blood flow for paraplegic and elderly populations.

Bader et al. [30] studied the effect of shear force on the skin of the volar aspect of the forearm in 10 healthy subjects. A device was used to apply shear force to the skin—i.e., stretch the skin—between two pads placed in contact with the subject's forearm. Between the pads, tissue vasculature was monitored using vital capillary microscopy [32] while blood flow was measured using a laser doppler probe [33]. Strain was measured by monitoring the displacement of a grid stenciled onto the skin surface. This study revealed that more and more vertical and horizontal blood vessels in the skin collapsed as the tensile force applied to the skin increased. The mean force intensity required for occlusion of greater than 95% of the vessels was 1.99 N/mm. A reduction in the skin blood flow was also reported; however, quantitative results were not provided.

More recently, Schubert [31] studied the effects of pressure and shear on skin microcirculation over the sacrum in elderly stroke patients lying in supine and semirecumbent positions. The subjects were divided into high-risk ($n = 10$) and not-at-risk ($n = 20$) groups according to their Norton score [34]. The laser Doppler technique was used to quantify the circulation changes in the skin over a period of 30 minutes for each of two body positions, semirecumbent at a 45° angle and recumbent at 0°. Although pressure was not measured, it was assumed that the semirecumbent position provided more shear force than the recumbent position. The results showed that there were significant differences in skin blood flow between groups and between positions. Skin blood flow increased over time for the not-at-risk group for both positions, and it decreased over time for the high-risk group for both

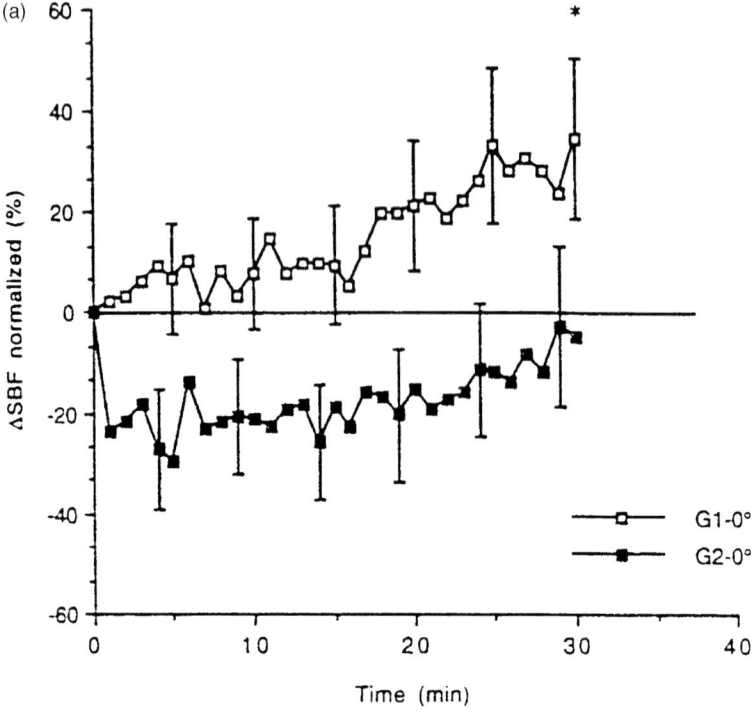

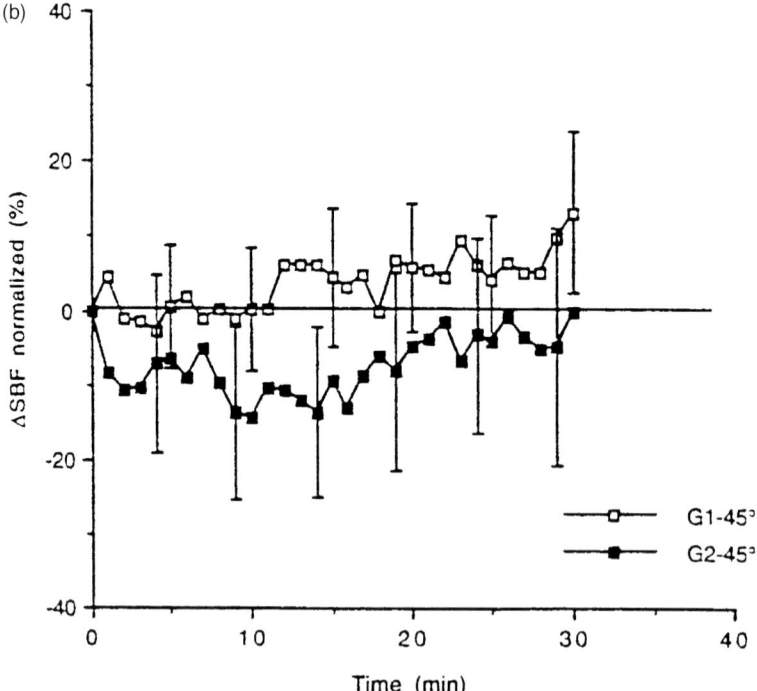

Figure 10-7.   Changes of normalized skin blood cell flux (ΔSBF_n, mean = SE) as a function of time measured in the sacral area of 20 patients (G1) not at risk or at low risk, and of 10 patients (G2) at high risk for developing pressure sores. The patients were lying in either (a) supine (0°) or (b) semirecumbent (45°) positions. (From Schubert and Herard [31], Figure 1.)

positions. The skin blood flow measurements are summarized in Figure 10-7. The surprising result from these experiments was that changes in skin blood flow for the high-risk group were lower in the recumbent position (high compressive force) as compared to the semi-recumbent (high shear) position. This led Schubert to the conclusion that the "findings favour the hypothesis of compressive force as the main external risk factor for developing tissue damage in the sacral area."

Although Bennett, Bader, and Schubert have provided valuable information regarding the skin's response to shear, there remain important unanswered questions concerning the effects of shear on deeper tissues and how deeper tissue effects factor into pressure ulcer risk.

FRICTION

Frictional forces are tangential shear forces that are limited to the skin and superficial fascia. They can be considered a subclassification of tangential shear forces. Friction between the skin and the support surface occurs when the skin moves against the support surface. Dinsdale [35] demonstrated that frictional forces caused pressure ulcers to form at lower normal pressures. In his experiments on normal and paraplegic swine, Dinsdale found that "friction increased the susceptibility to skin ulceration at constant pressures of less than 500 mm Hg. Friction and repetitive pressure of only 45 mm Hg resulted in skin ulceration."

TISSUE DEFORMATION AS A CHARACTERIZATION OF MECHANICAL LOADING

Interface pressure measurements are relatively easy to obtain. However, the apparent inadequacy of interface pressure measurements to predict harmful stresses, strains, and pressures in subcutaneous and deeper tissues has led investigators to seek alternate methods for predicting the loading conditions that increase the risk of pressure ulcer formation [23]. One such approach has been the estimation and prediction of the internal tissue stress and/or strain distributions based upon mathematical modeling of soft tissues with known geometries

and external loading. Using analytical techniques and in some cases using tissue-simulating test bodies, Chow et al. [36], Brunski et al. [37], Reddy et al. [38], and Todd et al. [39] have formulated models of stress and/or strain distributions in simulated human buttocks under various supportive loading conditions. The outcomes of these studies have generally supported the notion that higher stresses and strains exist near bony prominences in the deeper tissues. Caution must be used when interpreting the results from these studies because the geometric shape, tissue structure, Young's modulus, Poisson's ratio, and bulk modulus have been simplified to match the measurement techniques, the computational techniques, and the analytical techniques.

Levine et al. [9] has proposed that tissue shape and deformation measurements are superior to interface pressure measurements as a characterization of the loading condition between the buttocks and a seat support surface. Levine's rationale is twofold: (1) interface pressure measurements do not reliably predict adverse internal loading conditions; and (2) assuming that the optimum loading condition is the hydrostatic condition in which there is no tissue deformation, the degree of deformation is a measure of how close the loading is to the optimum condition. Several other investigators have drawn attention to the limitations of interface pressure in determining the efficacy of seating arrangements and have emphasized the importance of other factors. Using finite element analysis and in vivo soft tissue parameter measurements and verification, Todd reached the conclusion that "buttock-cushion interface pressure does not provide adequate information as to the performance of a particular cushion in decubiti prevention." [39]

Other investigators concur with Levine and have suggested that deformation of soft tissue is an important characterization tool. Levine sites Graebe [40], who advocates the use of "deformation patterns" to establish an individual's tolerance to external loading. Reddy, subsequent to investigating a model of interstitial fluid flow, concluded that "an adequate model should consider the responses of tissue matrix (deformation), and the responses of blood, lymphatic and interstitial fluid elements." [7]

A theoretical basis for the prediction of interface conditions between contacting bodies is provided by the "Contact Stress Theory" published by Heinrich Hertz in 1881 [41]. The Contact Stress Theory provides analytic equations for predicting peak interface pressure and body deformation based on the radii of curvature of the indenter and supporting surface, Poisson's ratios of the indenter and support body, and the applied force. Although the Contact Stress Theory requires assumptions that are not entirely met when human tissues and common seating materials are involved, the following may be implied from the characteristic equations: (1) matching a support to the unloaded shape of human body and optimizing the cushioning material would minimize the interface pressure, tissue deformation, and stress; (2) external loading (pressure or stress) of the tissue will approach a hydrostatic state as the cushion changes from a flat surface to a shape matching the unloaded body shape; and (3) peak pressures will decrease as Young's modulus of the cushion material decreases.

In 1974 Chow [42] described empirically the "envelopment" property of a cushioning support surface. Cushion surfaces were loaded with a gel model to simulate the human buttock. An x-ray method measured deformation of both gel and cushion and provided data from which to calculate interface pressure. Chow compared the effect of a flat cushion to a modified cushion with a surface profile matched to the buttock model shape. The matched cushion minimized distortion of the buttock model and cushion, provided a more uniform interface pressure, and significantly decreased distorting forces including normal and shear forces and tangential shear forces. Although Chow did not measure pressure within the buttock model, he concluded that, "in a highly enveloping cushion-surface, the hydrostatic pressure is predominant; in contrast, in a low enveloping surface the uniaxial pressure is predominant."

Sprigle [43] attempted to verify Chow's conclusion by measuring internal pressure at several locations in a gel-based buttock simulation model similar to Chow's. Sprigle found that the internal pressure was less hydrostatic for a flat foam support surface as compared to a support surface matched to the shape of the gel model or a support surface shaped to match the deflection obtained upon pressing the gel model into a flat foam contour gauge.

There was no difference in the degree of hydrostatic loading for the latter two conditions. Sprigle reasoned that because the support surfaces were made of compliant foam, an exact match was not necessary to approach hydrostatic loading.

The inherent problem with using tissue deformation measurements for mechanics characterization is that no practical clinical methods for direct measurement of deformations exist. In the laboratory, it is possible to use ultrasound transducers to quantify changes in tissue deformation for different loading conditions. Figure 10-8 shows an ultrasound image of the ischial tuberosity of a normal male subject seated on a contoured foam cushion. The ultrasound transducer was placed in contact with the subject through an access hole cut into the bottom of the cushion. As seen in the figure, there are obvious changes in deformation of the soft tissue located between the probe supplying external loading and the weight-bearing ischial tuberosity for the high and low loading conditions. Unfortunately, ultrasound imaging of soft tissue under load is not an economically feasible alternative. Magnetic resonance imaging was used by Protz et al. [44] to investigate the load-bearing buttocks tissue; however, this technology is also considered economically unfeasible.

As an alternative to direct measurement of tissue distortion, the use of soft tissue stiffness measurements as an indirect measure of deformation has been proposed [10, 11]. The load-deflection characteristic of soft tissue is nonlinear. A typical load-deflection characteristic for the soft tissue of the buttocks near the ischial tuberosity of a normal male subject is shown by plot T_2 of Figure 10-9. T_1 and T_3 are hypothetical curves that represent load deflection characteristics of thinner and thicker layers of tissue, respectively. For a given compressive load, the thinner tissue will exhibit a stiffer response to a change in load than the thicker tissue. As the relative deformation of the soft tissue increases, the load-deformation characteristic becomes stiffer. Sangeorzan [21] found that skin over the tibia bone in human subjects showed a significantly stiffer load-deformation relationship than skin over the tibialis muscle. For applied pressures of less than 20 mm Hg, the skin over bone was 2.5 times stiffer than skin over muscle. For applied

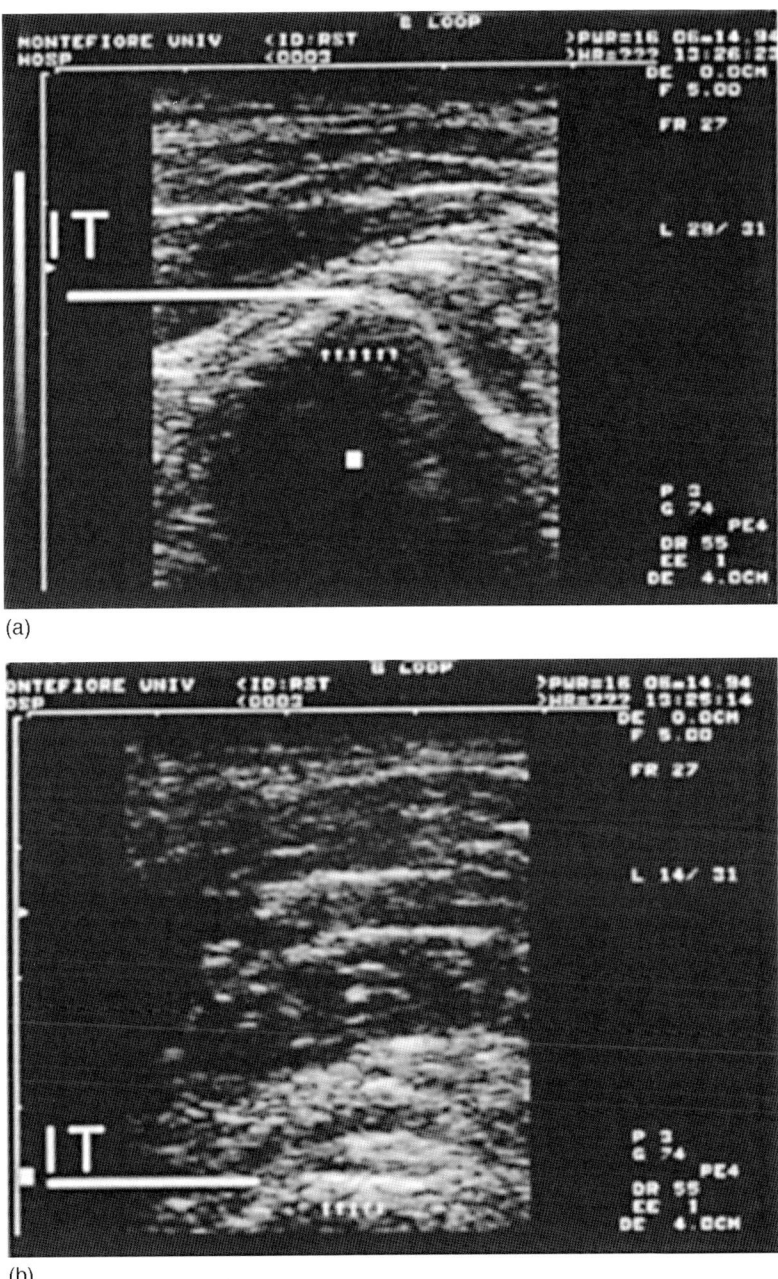

(a)

(b)

Figure 10-8. B-mode ultrasound images of the ischial tuberosity (IT) of an able-bodied male subject using a 5-MHz probe. The subject is seated on a custom-contoured foam with: (a) tissue under high compressive loading obtained by manually pushing the probe into soft tissue through an access hole cut into the cushion, and (b) tissue under minimal (low) compressive loading.

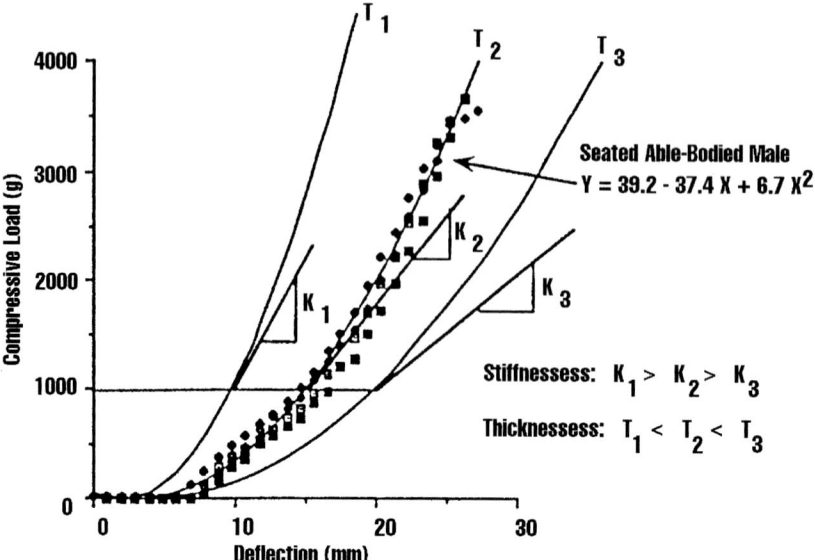

Figure 10-9. Typical force-displacement curve for tissue of the buttocks. (From Brienzo et al. [11], Figure 2.)

pressures greater than 40 mm Hg, the skin over bone was seven times stiffer than skin over muscle. Stiffness is therefore seen to be a measure of the relative deformation of the soft tissues.

SUMMARY

Strong evidence suggests that nonuniformly applied external loading is the prime factor by which soft tissues are damaged. Both shear and friction are also factors. The precise mechanisms for mechanical damage of tissue and pressure ulcer formation remain to be further delineated. The challenge for investigators studying the mechanics of soft tissue loading is to understand how externally applied loading affects internal tissues, placing them at risk of damage. The results from studies presented in this chapter suggest that interface pressure measurements, although common in clinical practice, do not always reflect high stresses or pressures in subcutaneous and deeper tissues. Tissue deformation, in combination with pressure measurements, appears to provide a more complete characterization of soft tissue loading; however, the practical application of deformation measurement is limited

at the present time by a lack of standards and proven methods.

REFERENCES

1. *Pressure Ulcers in Adults: Prediction and Prevention,* Clinical Practice Guideline no. 3, AHCPR Publication no. 92-0047, Rockville, MD: Agency for Health Care Policy and Research, Public Health Service, U.S. Department of Health and Human Services, 1992.

2. Crenshaw, R. P., and Vistnes, L. M., A decade of pressure sore research: 1977–1987 (review), *J Rehabil Res Dev* 1989; 26(1): 63–74.

3. Mawson, A. R.; Siddiqui, F. H.; and Biundo, J. J., Jr., Enhancing host resistance to pressure ulcers: A new approach to prevention (review), *Prevent Med* 1993; 22(3):433–50; ISSN:0091-7435.

4. Evans, J. M.; Andrews, K. L.; Chutka, D. S.; Fleming, K. C.; and Garness, S. L., Pressure ulcers: Prevention and management (review), *Mayo Clinic Proc* 1995; 70(8):789–99.

5. Rodriguez, G. P., and Garber, S. L., Prospective study of pressure ulcer risk in spinal cord injury patients, *Paraplegia* 1994; 32(3):150–8.

6. Ferguson-Pell, M. W., Seat cushion selection, *J Rehab Res Dev Clin Suppl* 1990; 2:49–74.

7. Reddy, N. P., and Cochran, G. V., Interstitial fluid flow as a factor in decubitus ulcer formation, *J Biomech* 1981; 14(12):879–81; ISSN:0021-9290.

8. Reddy, N. P.; Palmieri, V.; and Cochran, G. V., Subcutaneous interstitial fluid pressure during external loading, *Am J Phys* 1981; 240(5):R327-9; ISSN:0002-9513.

9. Levine, S. P.; Kett, R. L.; and Ferguson-Pell, M., Tissue shape and deformation versus pressure as a characterization of the seating interface, *Assist Tech* 1990; 2:93–99.

10. Brienza, D. M.; Chung, K.-C.; Brubaker, C. E.; and Kwaitkowski, R. J., Design of a computer-controlled seating device for research applications, *IEEE Trans Rehabil Eng* 1993; 1(1):63–67.

11. Brienza, D. M.; Inigo, R. M.; Chung, K. C.; and Brubaker, C. E., Seat support surface optimization using force feedback, *IEEE Trans Biomed Eng* 1993; 40(1):95–104.

12. Kosiak, M., Etiology of decubitus ulcers, 1961, pp. 19–29.

13. Krouskop, T. A.; Reddy, N. P.; Spencer, W. A.; and Secor, J. W., Mechanisms of decubitus ulcer formation—An hypothesis, Medical Hypotheses. 1978 Jan; 4(1): 37–9; ISSN: 0306-9877.

14. Krouskop, T. A. A synthesis of the factors that contribute to pressure sore formation, *Med Hypoth* 1983; 11(2):255–67.

15. Bennett, L.; Kavner, D.; Lee, B. Y.; Trainor, F. S.; Lewis, J. M. Skin stress and blood flow in sitting paraplegic patients. Archives of Physical Medicine & Rehabilitation. 1984 Apr; 65(4):186–90.

16. Garber, S. L., and Krouskop, T. A., Body build and its relationship to pressure distribution in the seated wheelchair patient, *Arch Phys Med Rehabil* 1982; 63(1):17–20.

17. Le, K. M.; Madsen, B. L.; Barth, P. W.; Ksander, G. A.; Angell, J. B.; and Vistnes, L. M., An in-depth look at pressure sores using monolithic silicon pressure sensors, *Plast Reconstr Surg* 1984; 74(6):745-56; ISSN:0032-1052.

18. Snashall, P. D.; Lucas, J.; Guz, A.; and Floyer, M. A., Measurement of interstitial "fluid" pressure by means of a cotton wick in man and animals: An analysis of the origin of the pressure, *Clin Sci* 1971; 41(1):35–53.

19. Brace, R. A., and Guyton, A. C., Transmission of applied pressure through tissues: Interstitial fluid pressure, solid tissue pressure and total pressure, *Proc Soc Exp Med* 1977; 154:164.

20. Reddy, N. P.; Palmieri, V.; and Cochran, G. V., Evaluation of transducer performance for buttock-cushion interface pressure measurements, *J Rehabil Res Dev* 1984; 21(1):43–50; ISSN:0748-7711.

21. Sangeorzan, B. J.; Harrington, R. M.; Wyss, C. R.; Czerniecki, J. M.; Matsen, FA 3d. Circulatory and mechanical response of skin to loading. Journal of Orthopaedic Research. 1989; 7(3): 425–31.

22. Tremper, K. K., Transcutaneous PO_2 measurement [review], *Canad Anaesth Soc J* 1984; 31(6):664–77.

23. Xakellis, G. C.; Frantz, R. A.; Arteaga, M.; and Meletiou, S., A comparison of changes in the transcutaneous oxygen tension and capillary blood flow in the skin with increasing compressive weights, *Am J Phys Med Rehabil* 1991; 70(4):172–7.

24. Seiler, W. O., and Stahelin, H. B., Skin oxygen tension as a function of imposed skin pressure: Implication for decubitus ulcer formation, *Geriatr Soc* 1979; 27(7):298–301.

25. Newson, T. P.; Pearcy, M. J.; and Rolfe, P., Skin surface PO_2 measurement and the effect of externally applied pressure, *Arch Phys Med Rehabil* 1981; 62(8):390–2.

26. Jay, R., Pressure and shear: Their effects on support surface choice (review), *Ost Wound Mgmt* 1995; 41(8):36–8, 40–2, 44–5.

27. Reichel, S. M., Shear force as a factor in decubitus ulcers in paraplegics, *JAMA* 1958; 166:762–3.

28. Bennett, L.; Kavner, D.; Lee, B. K.; and Trainor, F. A., Shear vs pressure as causative factors in skin blood flow occlusion, *Arch Phys Med Rehabil* 1979; 60(7):309–14.

29. Bennett, L.; Kavner, D.; Lee, B. Y.; Trainor, F. S.; and Lewis, J. M., Skin stress and blood flow in sitting paraplegic patients, *Arch Phys Med Rehabil* 1984; 65(4):186–90; ISSN:0003-9993.

30. Bader, D. L.; Barnhill, R. L.; and Ryan, T. J., Effect of externally applied skin surface forces on issue vasculature, *Arch Phys Med Rehabil* 1986; 67(11):807–11.

31. Schubert, V., and Heraud, J., The effects of pressure and shear on skin microcirculation in elderly stroke patients lying in supine or semi-recumbent positions, *Age & Ageing* 1994; 23(5):405–10.

32. Barnhill, R. L.; Bader, D. L.; and Ryan, T. J., A study of uniaxial tension on the superficial dermal

microvasculature, *J Invest Dermatol* 1984; 82(5):511–4.

33. Holloway, G. A. Jr., Watkins, D. W.; Laser Doppler measurement of cutaneous blood flow. J Invest Dermatol 69:306–309, 1977.

34. Norton, D.; McLaren, R.; and Exton-Smith, A. N., *An Investigation of Geriatric Nursing Problems in Hospital,* Edinburgh: Churchill-Livingstone, 1975.

35. Dinsdale, S. M., Decubitus ulcers: role of pressure and friction in causation, *Arch Phy Med Rehabil* 1974; 55(4):147–52; ISSN:0003-9993.

36. Chow, W. W., and Odell, E. I., Deformation and stresses in soft body tissues of a sitting person, *ASME J Biomech Eng* 1978; 100:79–87.

37. Brunski, J. B.; Roth, V.; Reddy, N. P.; and Cochran, G. V. B. Finite element stress analysis of a contact problem pertaining to formation of pressure ulcers, *Adv Bioeng* November, 1980: 3–59.

38. Reddy, N. P.; Patel, H.; Cochran, G. V.; and Brunski, J. B., Model experiments to study the stress distributions in a seated buttock, *J Biomech* 1982; 15(7):493–504; ISSN:0021-9290.

39. Todd, B. A., and Thacker, J. G., Three-dimensional computer model of the human buttocks, in vivo (see comments), *J Rehabil Res Dev* 1994; 31(2):111–9.

40. Graebe, R., Static forces-cushion, presented at 5th meeting of Wessex Tissue Viability Group, Odstock Hospital, Salisbury, England, 1980.

41. Thimosenko and Goodier, Theory of Elasticity, McGraw Hill Book Co., New York, 2nd ed., 1951.

42. Chow, W. W., Mechanical properties of gels and other materials with respect to their use in pads transmitting forces to the human body, Ph.D. dissertation, University of Michigan, Ann Arbor, MI, 1974.

43. Sprigle, S. H.; Haynes, H.; and Hale, J., Uniaxial and hydrostatic loading at the core of a gel buttock model, *Proceedings of the RESNA Annual Conference,* pp. 266–268, Nashville, Tennessee, June 17–22, 1944.

44. Protz, P. R., and Chung, K.-C. Implementing magnetic resonance imaging for the quantification of load-bearing buttocks tissues, *Proceedings of the RESNA 13th Annual Conference,* pp. 109–110, Washington, D.C., June 15–20, 1990.

11

ROLE OF ANTIMICROBIAL AGENTS IN INFECTED DECUBITUS ULCERS

Bok Y. Lee, M.D., V. J. Guerra, M.D., and Burton L. Herz, M.D.

HUMAN CUTANEOUS MICROFLORA

Infections encountered at the site of cutaneous pressure ulcers result from perturbation of the skin and surrounding tissues. Most of these infections are caused by microorganisms normally resident on the mucosa and skin. This resident microbial flora, usually referred to as the indigenous microflora or normal microbial flora, comprises a complex mixture of microbial species ranging from nonpathogenic saprophytes to pathogens. Local anatomic, physiologic, and environmental characteristics, which are different in different regions of the body surface, determine the density and composition of the normal flora. The number of aerobic and anaerobic bacterial species inhabiting the skin is relatively small. The simplicity of the cutaneous flora contrasts sharply with the complexity of the microflora of the alimentary and respiratory tracts. The composition of the normal cutaneous microflora changes with age. Normally, the fetus is sterile until shortly before birth, provided that the amniotic membrane remains intact. Colonization of the infant's skin proceeds rapidly during the first six hours of life. In adults, the normal cutaneous microflora consists of aerobic cocci of the family Micrococcaceae, aerobic diphteroids of the genera *Corynebacterium* and *Brevibacterium,* the anaerobic diphteroids *Propionibacterium acnes, P. granulosum, P. avidum,* and the yeasts *Pityrosporum orbiculare* and *P. ovale.* Other yeasts, such as *Candida albicans,* rarely inhabit intact glabrous skin. The distribution of these bacteria in the skin depends on the cutaneous microenvironment [1, 2].

Hospitalization, per se, alters the cutaneous microflora of seriously ill patients. Hospitalized patients manifest a number of significant changes. Gram-negative bacilli replace Gram-positive cocci as the predominant flora in the axilla, the anterior nares, the perineum, and the back. In patients with leukemia, these sites are frequently colonized with *Pseudomonas aeruginosa* and *Klebsiella pneumoniae.* In addition, the number of colonies in the axillae and perineum with *Candida* species are increased. It is unclear whether these changes in the microbial flora are related to the underlying illness or to the use of antibiotics. Patients may also acquire potential pathogens from medical personnel who are colonized or who transiently carry pathogens on their hands as a result of contact with other patients (i.e., MRSA, *C. difficile* and *E. faecalis*) [2].

GENERAL PRINCIPLES

When antimicrobial therapy is prescribed for surgery-related infections, four general principles apply [3]. First, the antimicrobial(s) should be selected on the basis of spectrum of activity, ability to achieve appropriate drug concentrations in specific tissues, results of culture and susceptibility testing (or most likely organisms if culture and susceptibility testing is unavailable), patient-specific factors (such as organ dysfunction or allergies), and cost. Second, antimicrobial therapy should be as specific as possible. Empiric broad-spectrum coverage is often used initially in surgery-related infections. However, as soon as culture and sensitivity information is available and if more than one drug was started empirically, it is reasonable to change to monotherapy. Changes in therapy should also be instituted if the patient's clinical condition is deteriorating and/or results of culture and susceptibility testing indicate inadequate or inappropriate coverage. It is important that surgical specimens (including anaerobic cultures when appropriate) be tested with Gram's stain early because cultures do not always grow out the important organism(s), especially after antibiotic therapy has been initiated. Third, unnecessary prolonged broad-spectrum antibiotic therapy should be avoided because it can promote development of bacterial antibiotic resistance and increase the likelihood for adverse events (such as pseudomembranous enterocolitis). Although inadequate treatment is occasionally encountered, prolonged treatment is more common. Fourth, antimicrobial agents should be prescribed at the correct dosage and frequencies. Factors such as age, weight, and renal and hepatic function (to estimate drug clearance) determine the optimal regimen for each patient [4]. Administering early repeated doses or using high doses of antibiotics may also be required in individuals with excessive blood or fluid losses. The pharmacodynamics of many antibiotics are still emerging and will ultimately have a significant impact on how antimicrobial regimens are designed [5]. Cost effectiveness is important when administering an antimicrobial agent. Monitoring peak and trough levels is an additional expenditure when aminoglycosides are used. Because of this, the administration of a single antimicrobial agent with high acquisition cost may in the long term be cheaper if it is either more effective or if the monitoring cost can be decreased.

MECHANISMS OF ACTION

Antimicrobials are either bactericidal (lethal) or bacteriostatic (inhibitory) at the standard clinical achievable concentrations. In patients with severe infections or neutropenia, bactericidal drugs are generally preferred. In general, it is more effective to combine antibiotics that act by different mechanisms than to combine drugs that compete for the same mechanism. However, bacteriostatic antibiotics may interact unfavorably with bactericidal drugs, such as β-lactam antibiotics, whose mechanisms of action require rapid microbial growth. One common exception is the bacteriostatic drug sulfamethoxazole, which acts synergistically in combination with the bactericidal drug trimethoprim.

Antibacterial agents can be divided into four general groups according to their mechanism of action; i.e., inhibition of cell wall, ribosomal proteins, folic acid, or DNA synthesis [6].

INHIBITORS OF CELL WALL SYNTHESIS

Most bacteria will die rapidly if they contain improperly formed cell walls that do not protect them from their environment. In order for the cell wall cross-linking in bacteria to occur, penicillin-binding protein must be present on the bacterial cytoplasmic membrane. β-lactam antibiotics, such as the penicillins, bind to this protein and thereby inhibit cell wall synthesis. Cephalosporins typically act by preventing septation, causing the bacteria to develop long filamentous form. Penicillin is effective against Gram-positive aerobic and anaerobic streptococci and some Gram-negative anaerobic organisms. The various congeners of penicillin include compounds with an increased Gram-negative spectrum (e.g., ampicillin), compounds that are β-lactamase resistant (e.g., nafcillin and methicillin), and compounds with greatly expanded Gram-negative coverage (e.g., ticarcillin/clavulanate, piperacillin and tazobactam).

Cephalosporin antibiotics inhibit cell wall synthesis in a manner similar to the penicillins and therefore are classified as bactericidal agents. The cephalosporins are classified as first, second, and third generation, depending on their spectrum of activity. First-generation cephalosporins are effective against most aerobic Gram-positive cocci, such as streptococci and staphylococci, and a limited number of Gram-negative organisms. They are not effective against enterococci or methicillin-resistant staphylococci. Second-generation cephalosporins are less effective than first-generation cephalosporins against Gram-positive organisms but are more effective against Gram-negative aerobes, such as *H. influenzae*. The cephamycins (cefoxitin, cefmetazole, and cefotetan) are also effective against anaerobes, such as *Bacteroides fragilis*. Third-generation cephalosporins are primarily effective against Gram-negative enteric organisms and some anaerobes. With the exception of cefoperazone and ceftazidime, third-generation cephalosporins have relatively little activity against *Pseudomonas*.

Imipenem/cilastatin is another cell wall inhibitor agent and has the broadest antimicrobial spectrum of any parenteral antibiotic. It is effective against most Gram-positive and Gram-negative organisms, including *Pseudomonas* and anaerobes, including *B. fragilis*. Because imipenem is rapidly metabolized by transpeptidase, a renal tubular enzyme, it is marketed in combination with cilastatin, an inhibitor of transpeptidase, to reduce urinary excretion and prolong the half-life.

Aztreonam also inhibits bacterial cell wall synthesis and has a broad spectrum of activity against Gram-negative bacilli, including *Pseudomonas*. It is ineffective against Gram-positive cocci or anaerobes, including *B. fragilis*. When used to treat mixed infections, aztreonam should be combined with clindamycin, which has some staphylococcal and streptococcal activity, as opposed to metronidazole, which is not effective against aerobes.

Vancomycin inhibits bacterial cell wall synthesis in earlier stages than the β-lactam antibiotics. It does this by blocking a pentapeptide from the cytoplasm to the cell membrane. It is effective against all staphylococci and streptococci, including enterococci and methicillin-resistant *S. aureus* (MRSA). However, vancomycin-resistant strains have been increasingly reported. Oral vancomycin, which is not absorbed, can be used to treat *C. difficile* colitis. However, new CDC (Centers for Disease Control) guidelines recommend oral metronidazole rather than vancomycin because of its induced enterococcus resistance. Metronidazole is also more cost effective than vancomycin.

INHIBITORS OF RIBOSOMAL PROTEIN SYNTHESIS

Aminoglycosides are bactericidal and function by inhibiting bacterial protein synthesis at the 30S ribosomal subunit. They require an oxygen-dependent transport mechanism to get inside the bacteria and are less effective in areas of necrosis or abscess where there is hypoxia and low pH. Aminoglycosides are primarily effective against most Gram-negative aerobic bacilli, including *Pseudomonas aeruginosa*. Combination antimicrobial therapy is recommended for synergy.

Tetracyclines are bacteriostatic agents that bind to the 30S ribosomal subunit. They are effective in the treatment of many Gram-negative aerobes, streptococci, and staphylococci, but many resistant strains have emerged.

Chloramphenicol, like the aminoglycosides, also inhibits bacterial protein synthesis, but at the 50S ribosomal subunit. It is bacteriostatic rather than bactericidal, but is highly effective against most Gram-negative bacilli and anaerobes, including *B. fragilis*.

Clindamycin also inhibits protein synthesis at the 50S ribosomal subunit and is effective against nearly all anaerobic bacteria, except *C. difficile*. It is also effective against streptococci and staphylococci, but not methicillin-resistant staphylococci.

Erythromycin binds to the 50S ribosomal subunit in a position similar to clindamycin and is bacteriostatic. It is primarily active against Gram-positive organisms.

INHIBITORS OF FOLIC ACID SYNTHESIS

All sulfonamides inhibit the enzyme tetrahydrofolic acid synthetase in the folic acid pathway to purine synthesis. Sensitive organisms are unable to use host folic acid and therefore must synthesize their own supply. Sulfonamides are broadly active against Gram-positive and Gram-negative organisms, including enteric Gram-negative organisms, but have no activity against staphylococci, enterococci, *Serratia*, or *Pseudomonas*.

Trimethoprim is a folic acid antagonist that inhibits dihydrogenase reductase and purine synthesis. It is commonly used in combination with the sulfonamides for synergy, resulting in action at two different sites in the same metabolic pathway. It is effective against most aerobic Gram-negative bacilli except *Pseudomonas aeruginosa*. The combined agent trimethoprim/sulfamethoxazole has a broad-spectrum activity against staphylococci, streptococci, Enterobacteriaceae, *Shigella, Salmonella,* and *Xanthomonas,* but it is ineffective against *P. aeruginosa*.

INHIBITORS OF DNA SYNTHESIS

Metronidazole is thought to act by disrupting DNA transcription and microbial replication. It has a limited-activity spectrum to anaerobes, including all *Bacteroides* species.

Quinolone antibiotics inhibit the DNA gyrase enzyme needed to package DNA into dividing bacteria. Quinolones have a broad antimicrobial spectrum effect against Gram-positive aerobes including enterococci, *Staphylococcus aureus* and *S. epidermidis,* and most Gram-negative aerobes, including all *Bacteroides* species. Quinolones are ineffective against anaerobes. The newer quinolones, such as ciprofloxacin and ofloxacin are currently the only oral antibiotics effective against *P. aeruginosa*.

Rifampin blocks DNA synthesis by inhibiting DNA-dependent RNA-polymerase. It has a broad spectrum of activity, but resistant bacteria emerge rapidly as if a single agent were used. Therefore, rifampin is often given with penicillinase-resistant penicillins or vancomycin.

ANTIFUNGAL AGENTS

Amphotericin B is a polyene macrolide that combines with surface sterols to increase cell membrane porosity, which leads to the death of the fungus. It is currently the most effective antifungal agent available and is effective against virtually all fungal pathogens. Amphotericin B has generally been considered to be quite toxic, but, when given properly, it is actually relatively safe.

Nystatin is an oral antifungal agent related to amphotericin B, but it is not systemically absorbed. It can be used in a swish-and-swallow technique to help prevent fungal overgrowth in the gastrointestinal tracts of critically ill patients receiving broad-spectrum antibiotics.

Ketoconazole interferes with the formation of membrane sterols. It has excellent activity against *Candida* and is effective for the treatment of mucocutaneous and mucosal candidal infections.

Fluconazole is a recently marketed, relatively nontoxic, fungistatic agent that can be used instead of amphotericin B in many fungal infections involving *Candida*. It is highly effective for the treatment of localized infections and may be effective for many systemic infections. However, resistance has been reported, and close observation is warranted.

An even newer agent, oral itraconazole, has been used to treat a variety of superficial and systemic infections. However, well-controlled, comparative studies are needed to assess its place in therapy [7].

ANTIMICROBIAL RESISTANCE

Antimicrobial resistance has become an increasingly important problem. Some of the mechanisms through which resistance can develop include changes in the antimicrobial target, production of detoxifying enzymes, and decreased uptake [6].

Changes in the antimicrobial target occur when alterations in ribosomal proteins, enzymes of folic acid metabolism, penicillin-binding proteins, or DNA gyrase modify the sites where antibiotics act to such an extent that binding cannot occur, thus rendering the antibiotic ineffective. Enterococci have become resistant to many penicillins because they possess a low-affinity penicillin-binding protein that reduces the activity of these drugs on the cytoplasmic membrane enzymes needed for cell wall synthesis. Vancomycin blocks cell wall synthesis by binding to peptidoglycan. Resistance has developed to vancomycin in a few bacteria that can synthesize a protein to selectively inhibit such binding. In addition, resistance to ciprofloxacin has occurred through mutations of bacterial DNA gyrase subunits to reduce inhibition by that antibiotic.

Some bacteria produce detoxifying enzymes such as β-lactamases and aminoglycoside-modifying enzymes that break down penicillins and aminoglycosides, rendering them ineffective. Nearly all Gram-negative bacteria possess a chromosomal gene for production of different types of β-lactamases. Up to 90% of *S. aureus* have β-lactamases and, therefore, are resistant to penicillin. Penicillinase-resistant penicillins (e.g., cloxacillin, methicillin, nafcillin) are effective against β-lactamase producing staphylococci. In addition, β-lactam inhibitors such as clavulanate, sulbactam, and tazobactam inhibit β-lactamases produced by bacteria, thereby allowing antibiotics that are usually susceptible to hydrolysis by β-lactamases to reach their target and be effective. Methicillin-resistant staphylococci are able to produce another enzyme that maintains cell wall integrity during growth and division. The native enzymes needed for cell wall synthesis are inactivated by a β-lactam inhibitor antibiotic.

Many aminoglycoside-resistant bacterias are able to synthesize aminoglycoside-modifying enzymes that are transmissible through plasmids. These enzymes can cause phosphorylation, adenylation, or acetylation of the antibiotic, preventing its binding to ribosomes. Some Gram-negative bacteria have modified their 30S ribosomes so that they fail to effectively bind to aminoglycosides.

To be effective, an antimicrobial agent needs to be incorporated into the microbe. Decreased uptake will prevent antimicrobial action. The outer membrane porosity of some bacteria, such as *Pseudomonas,* can decrease, which reduces accumulation of ciprofloxacin or other agents in the bacteria. In addition, some *Pseudomonas* exhibit diminished aminoglycoside uptake as a resistant organism.

INFECTION IN PRESSURE ULCERS

Pressure ulcers are a common clinical problem, especially in patients with spinal cord injury (SCI) and in the ever-growing geriatric population. Although they represent mainly local wound problems and often respond to local wound care, infected decubitus ulcers are a source of bacteremia associated with significant mortality. Surgical debridement is the definitive treatment of septic decubiti in addition to antibiotics [8, 9].

The bacteriology of chronic ulcers, such as decubitus and diabetic ulcers, is notoriously difficult to define because of contamination by colonizing surface flora. A reliable identification of true infecting organisms could guide the clinician in prescribing a more definitive antibiotic treatment. Sapico et al. [10] showed a poor correlation between the results obtained by deep tissue culture versus swab or needle aspiration. Lee et al. [11] found a fine needle aspiration technique to be reliable and clinically applicable. Their study, however, involved only a small number of chronic soft tissue infections and conclusions cannot be drawn. Rudensky et al. evaluated three methods of specimen collection from 72 pressure sores. Specimens taken by swab or by needle aspiration were compared with deep biopsy specimens for diagnostic reliability. They found that swab specimens reflected surface colonization and that needle aspiration seemed to underestimate bacterial isolates as compared to deep tissue biopsy specimens. Their final conclusion, for septic patients, was to select the antibiotic therapy based on deep biopsy specimens [9].

Pressure ulcers (decubitus ulcers) develop because of tissue death due to ischemia and are one of the most common problems encountered following traumatic spinal myelopathy. There are usually multiple ulcers, and they can vary in severity from mild erythema of the skin to large necrotic excavations with extensive destruction of underlying connective tissue and bone. Pressure sores impede rehabilitation and have major socioeconomic consequences. They are recurrent and often serve as foci for local and systemic sepsis. The devitalized, ischemic tissue adjoining pressure sores is conducive to the growth of microorganisms. Gram-negative infections frequently complicate these wounds and are often caused by organisms susceptible to aminoglycoside antibiotics. Bacteremia can be anticipated to occur following debridement of pressure sores, and septicemia or cellulitis associated with pressure ulcers is a significant cause of morbidity and mortality in patients with spinal cord injuries [12, 13].

Most bacterial infections are localized in the soft tissues. The interstitial fluid in tissue contiguous with a pressure ulcer serves as a medium for propagation of infection. Interstitial fluid is a primary path by which antibiotics are transported to a site of infection and is a major determinant of antimicrobial therapy efficacy. The concentration of a drug in the interstitial fluid that is free, unbound to proteins, and generally considered to be biologically active is of greater therapeutic significance than the corresponding total concentration [14].

Although not all patients with pressure sores have bacteremia, pressure ulcers can be a source of severe septicemia with a subsequent poor prognosis. As many as 50% of the cases of bacteremia due to pressure ulcers will be polymicrobial. In the Rudensky report [9], polymicrobial infections were diagnosed by swabs in 68% of the ulcers, by needle aspirations in 50%, and by deep tissue biopsies in 41%.

Because it is difficult to reliably identify the exact organisms causing infection, patients with sepsis related to decubitus ulcers are usually treated empirically with broad-spectrum, potentially toxic, and expensive antibiotic regimens. The choice of antibiotic depends on the anatomic site of the lesion, the duration of the illness, the findings on Gram's stains obtained by drainage or tissue aspiration with subsequent cultures, the odor of the pus, and the prior condition of the patient. Deep tissue sampling of decubiti should be considered for specific identification of the infective agent, but it is an invasive procedure. A relatively noninvasive procedure that could rival in reliability with deep tissue sampling would be a most important contribution to the clinician, because isolation and identification of the true causative organisms would permit the use of the most active and least toxic antibiotics.

Although surface swabs are unreliable indicators of deep tissue infection, they may be useful in monitoring the presence and spread of dangerous multiresistant pathogens, such as methicillin-resistant *Staphylococcus aureus* [15]. Awareness of these particular organisms, especially among patients transferred between institutions, can allow prompt initiation of required isolation and infection control procedures. Patients with decubitus ulcers transferred from other institutions should be isolated when arriving, and cultures should be immediately obtained in order to rule out the presence of MRSA. These patients should be suspected of having more severe infection as opposed to those coming from their homes.

The tissue penetration of various antibiotics in patients with pressure ulcers is rather poor [14]. It has been found that the percentage of positive cultures obtained by any method has been high even when the patient is receiving antibiotics. Few organisms growing in biopsy specimens or aspirates have been shown to be sensitive to the antibiotic that the patient had been receiving. It appeared that the decubiti became infected with resistant bacterial strains. Antibiotic therapy does not seem to lower the incidence of colonization in pressure ulcers but simply affects the ecology of the infecting flora.

Although penetration of antibiotics into living tissue has been extensively studied, the measurement of antibiotic concentration in viable tissue surrounding pressure ulcers in SCI patients had not been described until Segal et al. [12] conducted a study with amikacin on patients with pressure ulcers. Strategies for the use of antimicrobial agents have come about in the absence of information concerning the concentrations in tissue and pharmacokinetic behavior at the precise location where infection originates and is propagated. Segal et al. found that in SCI patients the optimal use of amikacin in the treatment of infected pressure ulcers is contingent upon accurate characterization of the pharmacokinetic behavior of the aminoglycoside in serum and in the interstitial fluid in contact with these lesions [12]. Only methods that quantitate amikacin concentration and protein binding in the interstitial fluid and incorporate a model that can simultaneously simulate nonlinear and linear disposition processes should be relied upon to influence therapeutic decision making.

The key to successful treatment of decubitus ulcer infections is early recognition of those infections requiring prompt surgical drainage and debridement. It is appropriate to classify lesions into those that are focal, such as cutaneous abscesses and pyoderma gangrenosum, and those that are diffuse and often require emergency treatment, such as cellulitis and necrotizing cellulitic infections. The clinician should initially decide if there is an infection and/or the presence of any important systemic disease. If infection is indeed present, appropriate antibiotics should be administered followed by the required surgical procedure [12].

There is no consensus about the relationship of infection to the etiology of pressure ulcers. Some studies suggest that infections can cause ulcers, whereas others state that bacteria are opportunistic colonizers of the wound but do not promote skin breakdown [16, 17]. Nevertheless, it is generally agreed that microbial infections have a profound effect on healing, as well as serving as potential sources for bacteremia and sepsis. Infection may be the sole cause of nonhealing of pressure ulcers. It usually provides an environment for wound enlargement, along with some of the noninfectious causes of ischemia such as anemia, malnutrition, continued pressure, vascular disease, heterotopic bone, and spasticity. It has been shown that infections can delay the wound healing process by depriving cells of the oxygen required by phagocytes to function properly and by generating anaerobic waste [18].

Epidemiological, clinical, and experimental information indicate that malnutrition is associated with depression of cellular immunity. The degree of this impairment has been shown to be related directly to the degree of erosion of body cell mass. Protein deprivation results in impaired synthesis of deoxyribonucleic acid and interferon, and atrophy of thymus and lymphoid tissue with a reduction of serum thymic hormone activity. Consequently, a reduction of thymus-dependent T lymphocytes occurs, specifically T cells with a marker for Fc-IgM (T lymphocytes), with no change in the number of antibody-producing B lymphocytes. Nutritional replenishment breaks the vicious cycle of malnutrition and immune deficiency [19]. Copeland et al. have shown that malnourished patients exhibited improved immunocompetence after 11 to 18 days of total parenteral nutritional support. Meakins et al. have shown that restoration of delayed hypersensitivity responses by nutritional support was associated with a 14-fold decrease in mortality and a 3-fold decrease in infections. The constituents of nutritional therapy have an equally important role. Jose et al. suggested that protein is the key dietary substrate for maintenance of adequate cell immu-

nity. Daly et al. showed that amino acids alone are not efficient, but a balanced nutritional regime, providing adequate amounts of both protein and nonprotein calories, is most effective for restoration of immunocompetence [19].

Bacterial counts greater than 100,000 per gram of tissue markedly affect wound healing. This is demonstrated by the fact that 95% of skin grafts will be successful in patients with bacterial counts of less than 100,000, compared to a success rate of 20% with counts greater than 100,000 per gram of tissue [20]. Persistent bacteremia originating from pressure ulcers has an estimated mortality rate of between 50–75% [21]. Galpin et al. [22] reported that in 21 patients with sepsis and pressure ulcers, 50% involved obligate anaerobes and 50% were polymicrobial. The predominant anaerobe was *Bacteroides fragilis* [22]. These results have been validated by other studies of bacteremia and sepsis from infected pressure ulcers (Peromet et al. [23] in 1973 and Rissing et al. [24] in 1974) and have led to the recommendations of initiating therapy with clindamycin or chloramphenicol with an aminoglycoside to cover coliform organisms in septic patients with pressure ulcers. Both aerobic and anaerobic organisms are found in large numbers in pressure ulcers that present with an extensive amount of tissue necrosis. In wounds that are free of necrotic tissue, anaerobic organisms are not found at all; the predominant organisms are *Pseudomonas aeruginosa* and *Staphylococcus aureus* [25].

PERIOPERATIVE PERIOD

Given the results of past studies, it becomes evident that an effective antimicrobial regimen needs to be evaluated in the perioperative period for the surgical treatment of pressure ulcers. The treatment of the pressure ulcer begins with surgical debridement and local dressing changes. These are designed to rid the ulcer of any necrotic, nonviable tissue and to minimize the bacterial contamination of the wound to less than the critical level of 10^5 per gram of tissue. The debridement may be surgical, chemical, or mechanical; surgical debridement is the most expeditious. Abramowicz [26] demonstrated that antimicrobial agents are most effective when present in therapeutic levels in the tissues during or soon after the surgical intervention. He pointed out that it is during this period that bacterial shedding reaches its maximum activity. Stahl and colleagues [27] stated that, "Short term prophylaxis is recommended in relatively clean cases. Postoperative antibiotics chosen on the basis of either preoperative or intraoperative cultures are, therefore, therapeutic rather than prophylactic in design." The duration and dosage of the postoperative systemic antimicrobial therapy is then tailored to the extent of wound destruction and involvement of underlying tissue.

In a survey by Salzberg et al. [17] done at 85 centers, several consistent findings were obtained. Fifty-eight percent (*n*=29) of the respondents stated that they routinely use preoperative antibiotics for flap surgery, whereas 48% (*n*=24) do not. Fifty-nine percent (*n*=30) believe that their use of antibiotics was prophylactic, whereas 40.7% (*n*=20) thought their use of antibiotics was essentially therapeutic.

The preoperative use of antibiotics involved an "on call" regimen in 60% (*n*=31) of the centers surveyed, whereas 8% (*n*=4) initiated the antibiotics 48 hours preoperatively, 24% (*n*=12) initiated the preoperative antibiotics 24 hours prior to the surgical procedure, and 8% (*n*=4) employed some other preoperative regimen. Only 6% (*n*=3) reported an antibiotic prep prior to flap surgery.

The coverage with antibiotics after surgery varied from 48 hours to one week. Cephalosporins were the overwhelming choice for antibiotic coverage, being utilized by 69% of surgeons in flap surgery. A small percentage of the respondents said antibiotic coverage was based on culture specificity. Seven percent used no antibiotics at all. Cultures were taken by 80 percent. Suction drains were left in place by all the surgeons questioned.

CLINICAL ENTITIES

CONFINED CUTANEOUS ABSCESS (FIRST PRESENTATION)

A cutaneous abscess is a walled-off collection of pus that presents as a painful fluctuant mass, surrounding erythema, and firm granulation tissue. The standard treatment is incision and drainage.

Gram's stains and culture of the pus are not routinely performed, because antibiotics are not administered unless the patient is toxic or there is a cellulitic component present. However, antibiotics may be helpful in immunocompromised patients. The findings on Gram's stains can suggest an appropriate antibiotic. Gram-positive cocci in clusters indicate *Staphylococcus aureus,* which may be treated with an oral semisynthetic penicillin such as cloxacillin. Mixed Gram-positive and Gram-negative bacilli on the smear represent an infection by aerobic, and facultative and nonfacultative anaerobic organisms, which can be treated with an oral cephalosporin such as cephalexin [8].

CLASSIC PYODERMA GANGRENOSUM

This entity is characterized by a painful raised postular lesion that progresses to a spreading ulceration with a typical necrotic center, bluish undermined edges, and surrounding erythema. Investigations should include Gram's stain and culture of the biopsy specimen. An underlying disease with immunosuppression is present in 60–80% of the cases. Treatment should include pressure-relieving devices, such as egg crates or air beds. Useful antimicrobials include sulfasalazine, minocycline and rifampin, sulfasalazine and clofazimine. Massive intravenous doses of methlyprednisolone or high-dose oral prednizone will bring about rapid improvement. Local wound care may be successful when used alone [28, 29].

POSTOPERATIVE PROGRESSIVE BACTERIAL GANGRENE OF MELENY

This entity is usually caused by a Gram-positive and a Gram-negative bacteria. The original description by Meleny stated this entity to be caused by a Gram-positive aerobe and a Gram-positive anaerobe. It is considered to be a variant of classic pyoderma gangrenosum. It has been reported to occur in pressure ulcers. The lesion appears two weeks or more after accidental trauma or after operative management of purulent peritoneal or pleural infections. It is characterized by wound edema, redness, and tenderness that progresses to the three characteristic zones of pyoderma gangrenosum: a necrotic center, bluish undermined edges, and surrounding erythema. Fever, muscle wasting, and toxicity are often present. A swab taken from the central necrotic area shows the usual growth to be hemolytic *S. aureus* on culture. Later in the course of the illness, a culture may show Gram-negative bacilli. Needle aspirate from the outer zone may grow microaerophilic nonhemolytic streptococci. Penicillin (or cloxacillin) and tobramycin are the antimicrobials of choice. Antibiotic therapy is followed by wide excision of the necrotic portion of the skin lesion, and the tissue is left to granulate. Primary closure, if possible, can be attempted later. Supportive therapy may be of benefit in those patients having marked systemic manifestations and significant muscle wasting [27, 30, 31].

SUPERFICIAL ATYPICAL MYCOBACTERIAL LESIONS

In cases of nonhealing ulcers unresponsive to conventional surgical and antibiotic treatment, the possibility of an atypical mycobacterial infection should be considered. *Mycobacterium smegmatis, M. kansasii,* and *M. chelonei* have been isolated. These bacterias have been present in chronic ulcerations with violaceous edges, rolled margins, and nongranulating base. Treatment should include debridement and intravenous antibiotic therapy followed by oral antibiotics. Effective antibiotics against these three species are cefoxitin and ciprofloxacin [27, 32].

DIFFUSE NECROTIZING INFECTIONS

In the clostridial type of infections two entities are recognized: (1) necrotizing cellulitis—early local signs, moderate pain, and involvement of superficial tissue (skin and subcutaneous tissue) and (2) myonecrosis—early systemic signs, severe pain, and involvement of deeper layers of tissue (primarily muscle). Surgery must be performed early to limit tissue damage. The extent of surgical debridement depends on operative findings and cannot be predicted before surgery.

NONCLOSTRIDIAL DIFFUSE NECROTIZING INFECTIONS

Three subgroups have been identified: (1) monomicrobial necrotizing cellulitis—caused in streptococcus (gangrene) and vibrio necrotizing infections. It has a rapid onset (one to three days), there is a single causative organism, and there is involvement of superficial tissue (skin and subcutaneous tissue); (2) necrotizing fasciitis—there two types, one caused by classic bacteria and the other by a phycomycotic type. It has a slower onset (four to seven days), bacterial synergy, some anaerobic activity, and involvement of deeper layers of tissue); (3) synergistic necrotizing cellulitis—caused by Gram-negative bacteria. It has the slowest onset (five to ten days), bacterial synergy, with greatest anaerobic activity, and involvement of deepest layers of tissue (deep fascia and possibly muscle).

In the treatment of necrotizing diffuse tissue infections, the first step is to recognize the clinical presentation, the anatomic site of primary tissue involvement, and the microbiology of the causative organisms. Antibiotics plus surgical intervention will be the main treatment of soft tissue infection. The main goal is to limit tissue damage. The extent of surgical debridement depends on operative findings and cannot be predicted before surgery. It is very difficult to assess the depth of involvement without incising the skin [27, 33].

SELECTION OF ANTIBIOTIC THERAPY

Several important advances in antimicrobial therapy were made in the early 1980s. Among the most significant of these advances are: (1) the improved understanding of the microbiological spectrum of so-called optimal therapy, (2) better application of pharmacokinetic principles to drug administration, (3) the development of several new classes of antibiotics, and (4) greater insight into the interplay of host resistance factors, microorganisms, and chemotherapy.

To make a rational decision regarding empirical therapy, the surgeon must be familiar with organisms that are likely to be encountered when a particular infection is suspected. Selection of the agent or agents is based on the patient history, physical examination, where the infection was likely to have been acquired, host defense status, overall clinical severity of the infection, and the response of the host. Definitive therapy is initiated after the host response to the infection and to the empirical treatment has been monitored and the results from the microbiology laboratory—specifically, identification of the isolated organisms and the minimal inhibitory concentrations (MIC) of various antimicrobial agents—have been assessed [13].

The primary development in the area of antibiotic treatment in surgical infections in the last five years has been the expanded clinical importance of β-lactamases that protect Gram-negative organisms against previously active drugs. To counter this problem, a series of new antibiotic agents has been developed, including new cephalosporins, carbapenems, quinolones, and β-lactamase inhibitors.

Antibiotic treatment for the established infections encountered by surgeons is an important element of therapy and has considerable impact on outcome. Of all the adjunctive treatment measures provided, appropriate antibiotic therapy is the only measure clearly shown to affect treatment success or failure [34].

β-lactamases are ubiquitous, and therapeutic use of β-lactam antibiotics has selected strains with increased amounts of enzymes and/or enzymes with an extended spectrum of activity. The most important chromosomal enzymes are the class I enzymes, which occur in Enterobacteriaceae and *Pseudomonas* species. These enzymes have a high affinity for β-lactams but exhibit a slower hydrolysis of the drugs. Some bacteria are able to synthesize large amounts of β-lactamases if challenged with a β-lactam. This induced expression is important for *Pseudomonas aeruginosa, Enterobacter, Citrobacter, Serratia, Morganella, Proteus vulgaris,* and *Providencia* species and in bacteria in which enzyme activity is constantly derepressed. Some investigators claim that some antibiotics are able to induce enzyme expression [36]. The claim is made that such antibiotics tend to cause treatment failure, as was true with cefamandole. This is true only if the inducing agent is susceptible to the β-lactamase. Once selected, derepressed mutants remain sensitive to carbapenems, cafepime, cefpirome, quinolones, and aminoglycosides. The side chain MTT present in some cephalosporins has caused bleeding disorders in patients receiving these antibiotics. Vitamin K has been administered to patients receiving cephalosporins such as cefotetan [35–38].

ANTIBIOTIC PRESCRIBING PRIVILEGES

Antibiotics continue to be used in an appropriate and excessive fashion in many areas of surgery today. Systemic antimicrobial agents have been proven to be of value for prophylaxis in many operative procedures, but no benefit has been shown for extended postoperative prophylactic administration. Although cultures are routinely produced, the results are often disregarded. This results in the frequently seen empirical, polypharmaceutical choices being continued for extended periods of time without appropriate changes. Anaerobic bacteria are important pathogens that require specific therapy. The consequences of wholesale overuse of antimicrobial agents has led to excessive expense, microbial resistance, and compromise of host defenses. Despite endless programs that have championed strategies for appropriate utilization of antibiotics in surgery, a certain tedium and cynicism with respect to the utilization of antibiotics, has resulted, as observed in trends during the last two decades. Compliance audits and continual education efforts result in little long-term change in behavior. In conclusion, the only strategy that will ensure compliance with accepted standards of antibiotic utilization is a rational prescription of prophylactic and therapeutic antimicrobial agents. An alternative would be to have guidelines for antibiotic use in each surgical specialty. Consultation with an infectious disease specialist should be made in cases of severe infection. Bacteriologic cultures and sensitivity should be obtained in every case with follow-up every three days. Algorithms, when properly used, are useful in the treatment of infected pressure sores. Clinical signs of improvement are more important than the laboratory information. The attending physician, resident, and nurse in charge of the patient should communicate regarding ulcer appearance, time of antibiotic administration, presence or absence of systemic infection, need for isolation, nutritional status, need of surgical debridement, and results of bacteriologic cultures and sensitivity. The holistic approach to patients with infected decubitus ulcers is as important as the selection of the proper antibiotic [39, 40].

REFERENCES

1. Larson, E. L.; McGinley, K. J.; Foglia, A. R.; et al., Composition and antimicrobic resistance of skin flora in hospitalized and healthy adults, *J Clin Microbiol* 1986; 23:604.

2. Bjornson, H. S., Microbiology of surgical infection, in J. L. Meakins, *Surgical Infections. Diagnosis and Treatment,* New York: Scientific American, 1994:1–2.

3. Sabath, L. D.; Simmons, R. L.; and Howard, R. J., Antimicrobial agents, in R. J. Howard, R. L. Simmons, eds., *Surgical Infectious Diseases,* 2nd ed., Norwalk, CT: Appleton and Lange, 1988; 259–306.

4. Ericsson, C. D.; Fischer, R. P.; Rowlands, B. J.; Hunt, C.; Miller-Crotchett, P.; and Reed, L., Prophylactic antibiotics in trauma: The hazards of underdosing, *J Trauma* 1989; 29:1356–1361.

5. Carbón, C., Single-dose antibiotic therapy: What has the past taught us? *J Clin Pharmacol* 1992; 32:686–691.

6. Simmons, R. L., and Kispert, P. H., Infection and host defenses, in R. L. Simmons, D. L. Sneed, eds., *Basic Science Review for Surgeons,* Philadelphia: W. B. Saunders, 1992:56–83.

7. Wilson, R. F., Antimicrobial therapy, in R. F. Wilson, ed., *Handbook of Antibiotic Therapy for Surgery Related Infections,* Springfield, N.J. Scientific Therapeutics Information, 1994:79–100.

8. Allman, R. M., Pressure ulcers among the elderly, *N Engl J Med* 1989; 320:850–853.

9. Rudensky, B.; Lipschits, M.; Isaacsohn, M.; and Sonnenblick, M., Infected pressure sores: Comparison of methods for bacterial identification, *Southern Med J* 1992; 85:901–903.

10. Sapico, F. L.; Witte, J. L.; Canawati, H. N.; et al., The infected foot of the diabetic patient: Quantitative microbiology and analysis of clinical features, *Rev Infect Dis* 1984; 6:S171–176.

11. Lee, P. C.; Turnidge, J.; and McDonald, P. J., Fine needle aspiration biopsy in diagnosis of soft tissue infection, *J Clin Microbiol* 1985; 22:80–83.

12. Segal, J. L.; Brunnemann, S. R.; and Eltorai, I. M., Pharmacokinetics of amikacin in serum in tissue contiguous with pressure sores in humans with spinal cord injuries, *Antimicrob Agents Chemother* 1990; 34:1422–1428.

13. Glenchur, S.; Patel, B. S.; and Pathmarajh, C., Transient bacteremia associated with debridement of decubitus ulcers, *Mil Med* 1981; 146:482–533.

14. Bagley, D. H.; MacLowry, J.; Beazley, R. M.; Gorschboth, C.; and A. S. Ketcham, Antibiotic concentration in human wound fluid after intravenous administration, *Ann Surg* 1978; 188:202–208.

15. Rhinehart, E.; Shlaes, D. M.; Keys, T. F.; et al., Nosocomial clonal dissemination of methicillin-resistant *Staphylococcus aureus:* Elucidation by plasmid analysis, *Arch Intern Med* 1987; 147:521–524.

16. Bendy, R. H., Jr., *Relationship of Quantitative Wound Bacterial Counts of Healing Decubiti: Effects of Topical Gentamicin, Antimicrobial Agents, and Chemotherapy,* Ann Arbor, MI: American Society of Microbiology, 1964.

17. Salzberg, C. A.; Gray, B. C.; Petro, J. A.; and Salisbury, R. E., The perioperative antimicrobial management of pressure ulcers, *Decubitus* 1990; 3:24–6.

18. Babior, B. M., Oxygen dependent microbial killing by phagocytes, *N Engl J Med* 1978; Vol 298 659.

19. Agarwal, N.; Del Guercio, L. R. M.; and Lee, B. Y., The role of nutrition in the management of pressure sores, in B. Y. Lee, ed., *Chronic Ulcers of the Skin,* New York: McGraw-Hill, 1985:133–146.

20. Schneider, M., and Vildozola, C. W., Quantitative assessment of bacterial invasion of chronic ulcers, *Am J Surg* 1983; 145:26.

21. Longe, R., Current concepts in clinical therapeutics: Pressure sores, *Clin Pharm* 1986; 5:669.

22. Galpin, J. E.; Chow, A. W.; Bayer, A. S.; and Guze, L. B., Sepsis associated with decubitus ulcers, *Am J Med* 1976; 61:346.

23. Peromet, M.; Labbe, M.; Youssaowsky, E.; et al., Anaerobic bacteria isolated from decubitus ulcers, *Infection* 1973; 1:205.

24. Rissing, J. P.; Crowder, J. G.; Dunfee, T.; et al., Bacteroides bacteremia from decubitus ulcers, *Southern Med J* 1974; 67:1179.

25. Sapico, F.; Ginunas, V. J.; et al., Quantitative microbiology of pressure sores in different stages of healing, *Diag Microbial Infect Dis* 1986; 5:31.

26. Abramowicz, M., Antimicrobial prophylaxis for surgery, *Med Lett Drugs Ther* 1981; 23:17.

27. Stahl, S.; Serum, S.; Donovan, W.; and Spira, M., The perioperative management of the patient with pressure sores, *Ann Plast Surg* 1983; 11:347.

28. Lewis, R. T., Soft tissue infection, in J. L. Meakins, *Surgical Infections. Diagnosis and Treatment,* New York: Scientific American, 1994:269–290.

29. Holt, P. J. A.; Davies, M. G.; Saunders, K. C.; et al., Pyoderma gangrenosum, *Medicine* (Baltimore) 1980; 59:114.

30. Grainger, R. W.; Mackenzie, D. A.; and McLachlin, A. D., Progressive bacterial synergistic gangrene: Chronic undermining ulcer of Meleney, *Canad J Surg* 1967; 10:439.

31. Ledingham, I. M. A., and Tehrani, M. A., Diagnosis, clinical course and treatment of acute dermal gangrene, *Brit J Surg* 1975; 62:364.

32. Plaus, W. J., and Hermann, G., The surgical management of superficial infection caused by atypical mycobacteria, *Surgery* 1991; 110:99.

33. Bongard, F. S.; Elings, V. B.; and Markison, R. E., New uses of fluorescence in the surgical management of necrotizing tissue infection, *Am J Surg* 1985; 150:281.

34. Christou, N. V., Antibiotics, in J. L. Meakins, *Surgical Infections. Diagnosis and Treatment,* New York: Scientific American, 1994:441–474.

35. Bush, K., Characterization of beta-lactamases, *Antimicrob Agents Chemother* 1989; 33:259–263.

36. Livermore, D. M., Clinical significance of beta-lactamase and stable depression in gramnegative rods, *Eur J Clin Microbiol* 1987; 6:439–445.

37. Livermore, D. M., Interplay of impermeability and chromosomal beta-lactamase activity in imipenem-resistant *Pseudomonas aeruginosa, Antimicrob Agents Chemother* 1992; 36:2046–2048.

38. Sanders, W. E., Jr., and Sanders, C. C., Inducible beta lactamases: Clinical and epidemiologic implications for use of newer cephalosporins, *Rev Infect Dis* 1988; 10:830–838.

39. Fry, D. E.; Harbretch, P. J.; and Polk, H. C., Jr., Systemic prophylactic antibiotics: Need the costs be so high? *Arch Surg* 1981; 116:466–469.

40. Fry, D. E., PRO: Antibiotic prescribing privileges should be restricted by hospital committees, Postgraduate course, American College of Surgeons meeting, Chicago, IL, 1994.

12

THE CARBON DIOXIDE LASER: DECUBITUS DEBRIDEMENT AND STERILIZATION

Gordon D. Lutchman, M.D., David A. Staffenberg, M.D., and Burton L. Herz, M.D.

INTRODUCTION

The first step in the treatment of any decubitus with a significant amount of necrotic tissue is the *debridement* of that wound to a healthy base. Methods of debridement can be classified as (1) chemical (2) mechanical, and (3) surgical.

The tedium and frustration suffered by the medical personnel associated with repetitive bedside debridement is well known. In addition, because it is a relatively less efficient way of removing necrotic tissue, there is a significant time lag, usually weeks, between the initiation of debridement and the arrival at the final product of a clean, granulating wound.

The carbon dioxide (CO_2) laser is an efficacious, precision tool, offering controllable vaporization of tissues, that greatly expedites the debriding process. The more rapid attainment of a clean, granulating, odor-free wound facilitates care by nurses and family members and has obvious advantages to the patient.

HISTORY

The first CO_2 laser was developed in 1964 by Patel working at AT&T Bell Laboratories [1]. Lasers have been in clinical use only since the 1960s, and since then sporadic reports have appeared in the literature extolling their virtues for wound sterilization and debridement.

Hinshaw and Lanzafame et al. from Rochester demonstrated the ability to debride, sterilize, and close infected necrotic wounds primarily, using the CO_2 laser [2].

It was Stellar et al. in 1972 [3], who showed that decubiti can also be debrided, sterilized, and closed primarily. Kori and Glantz in 1985 [4] and, more recently, Lutchman et al. in 1991 [5] presented larger series of patients with decubiti resulting in consistently good results. Lutchman has also demonstrated that the procedure can be done effectively under local anesthesia, as well as on an ambulatory surgery basis.

Juri and Palma of Argentina [6] published a prospective, randomized study in which a number of parameters were rigidly controlled, and statistically significant results were obtained when laser debridement was compared to conventional surgical debridement. The study demonstrates greater efficacy, decreased blood loss, and shorter hospital stay in the laser-treated group.

CO_2 LASER PHYSICS

White light, when broken down into its components by diffraction through a prism, is revealed to consist

Radiation	The Electromagnetic Spectrum		Wavelength
Cosmic			0.00001 nm
X-rays			0.1 nm
Ultraviolet			10 nm
VISIBLE	Violet		400 nm
	Blue		500 nm
	Green		
	Yellow		
	Orange		600 nm
	Red		700 nm
Infrared			10,000 nm
Microwave			1 cm
TV and FM radio			100 cm
AM radio			10,000 cm

Figure 12-1. Overview—Electromagnetic spectrum.

of many different wavelengths, scattered. In contrast, laser light [1] consists of one wavelength, the beam is parallel, and all waves are synchronized in time and space. The net effect of these features is that the energy of the laser can be efficiently harnessed and controlled to perform precise functions in a predictable fashion (see Figure 12-1).

The wavelengths of the commonly used lasers are found in that part of the electromagnetic spectrum corresponding to ultraviolet through visible

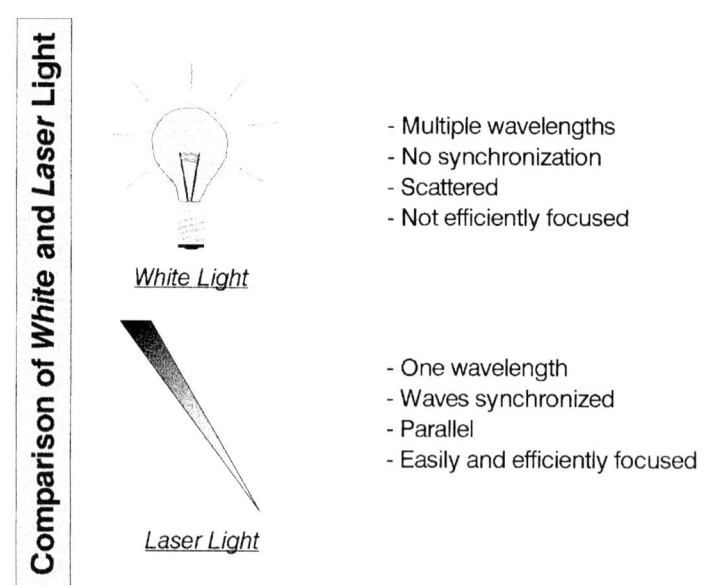

Figure 12-2. Comparison of laser light and white light.

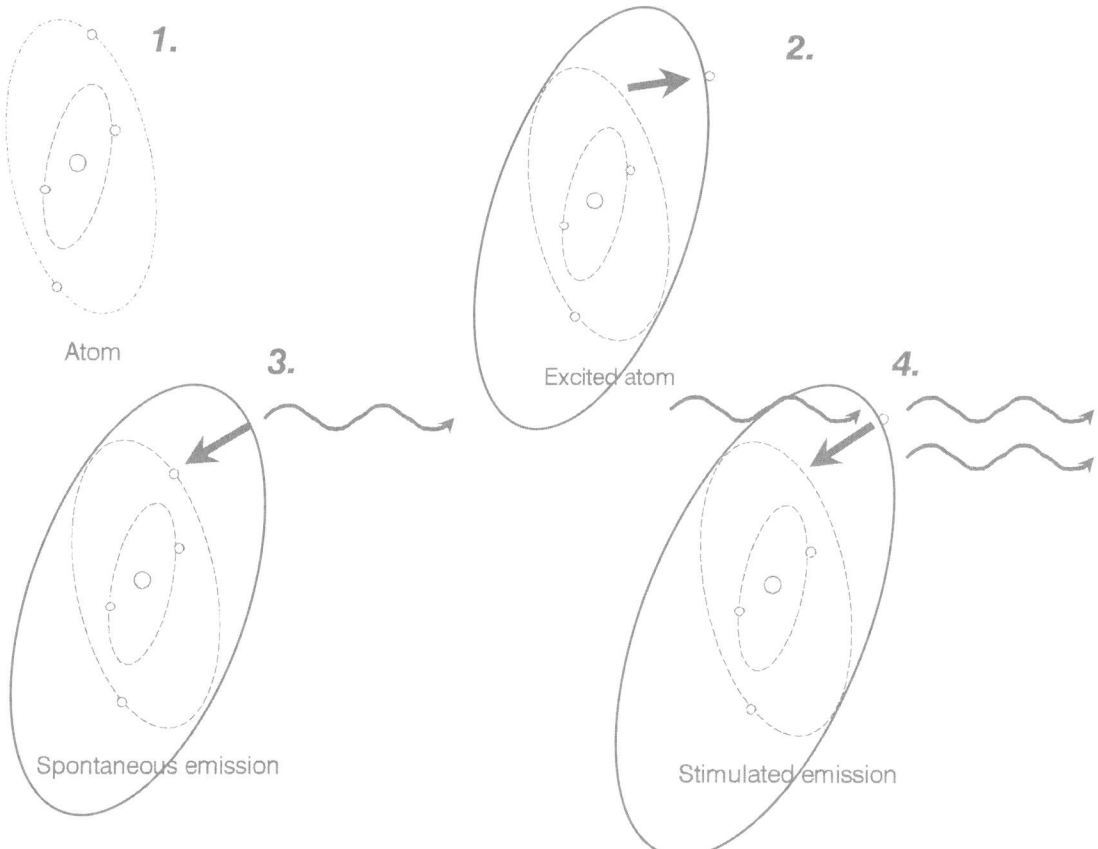

Figure 12-3. Basics of stimulated emission of radiation.

light into the infrared range (Figure 12-2). The individual wavelength of each laser is dependent upon the active medium used to produce that laser, the medium being solid, liquid, or gas. Each element or molecule used produces its own specific wavelength. The first laser ever made consisted of a solid ruby rod. The CO_2 laser uses pumped CO_2 gas as its medium and produces a beam of wavelength 10,600 nm, which lies in the far infrared.

The basic process at the atomic/molecular level that produces laser light is *stimulated emission of radiation,* hence the acronym LASER (*L*ight *A*mplification by *S*timulated *E*mission of *R*adiation) described by Einstein in 1917. The principle is that the normal release of energy that occurs when an excited orbiting electron returns to baseline (spontaneous emission of radiation) can be magnified to produce more quanta of energy of exactly the same wavelength, by applying external energy to the system (Figure 12-3). This process is further magnified by allowing it to occur in an optical resonant chamber (Figure 12-4).

The active medium is CO_2 gas pumped into the optical chamber, and the energy source is electrical. Because the CO_2 beam is invisible, a further inflow of a gas combination of helium and neon (HeNe), which produces a visible red laser, is delivered coaxially with the CO_2 beam, permitting visualization of the beam. This beam is delivered by an articulating arm with a system of mirrors arranged in a periscope fashion. This parallel beam of light is focused by a 125-mm convex lens in the handpiece of the laser delivery system.

The ability to focus the beam creates spot sizes

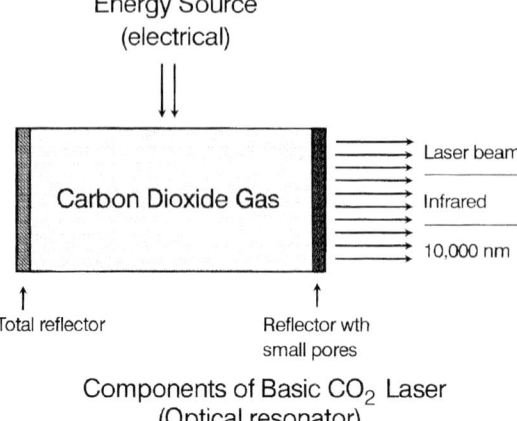

Figure 12-4.   Basic principles of structure of CO_2 laser.

of different diameters and surface areas. The spot size at the focal point of the lens is the smallest possible area into which the greatest concentration of energy or energy density occurs (Figure 12-5).

The interaction of lasers of different wavelengths on different types of tissues is unique and is a function of the particular wavelength. The CO_2 laser beam, at 10,600 nm, is selectively absorbed by water as opposed to, for example, the argon laser beam (532 nm) which is selectively absorbed by pigmented tissues (e.g., blood, retina). It is this high coefficient of absorption in water that makes the CO_2 laser the perfect debridement tool. By ren-

dering it as a surface-acting laser, the depth of penetration can be controlled.

TISSUE EFFECTS OF CO_2 LASER

VAPORIZATION

Cells are 70% water. The water of the surface cells absorbs the energy of the CO_2 beam, the water is converted to steam by flash boiling, and the resulting expansion that occurs exceeds the limits of the cell membrane. The cell explodes, resulting in vaporization of the tissue. The resultant steam, smoke, and intracellular particles is called a *plume*. A secondary effect is that some heat is generated, and a thin film of carbonaceous ash may be left on the surface. See Figures 12-6(a), (b).

The understanding of the concept of vaporization is the key to the appreciation of the CO_2 laser as a debridement tool, especially in precision *vaporization* and *surface sterilization*. Confusion arises because of a tendency to assume that there is a strong electrocautery-like effect. However, the electrocautery does not cause vaporization but only causes coagulation necrosis and desiccation with some smoke as a byproduct. The laser works primarily by exploding cells and creating an exuberant smoke or plume, heat generation being secondary.

SURFACE STERILIZATION

Bacterial cells on the surface of the wound or in the superficial levels are subject to vaporization in the same manner as tissue cells. Manipulation of the beam to allow this effect to occur over the entire surface of a wound has been shown to sterilize the surface [2, 8–10].

TISSUE WELDING

Laser tissue welding is the topic of much research in vascular surgery and in surgery on the fallopian tubes, the gastrointestinal tract, and the ureters.

The mechanism of tissue welding is not completely understood but is thought to involve the creation of covalent bonds in the collagen of the tissues being welded. The tissues just below the layer of ablation are subject to less intense laser

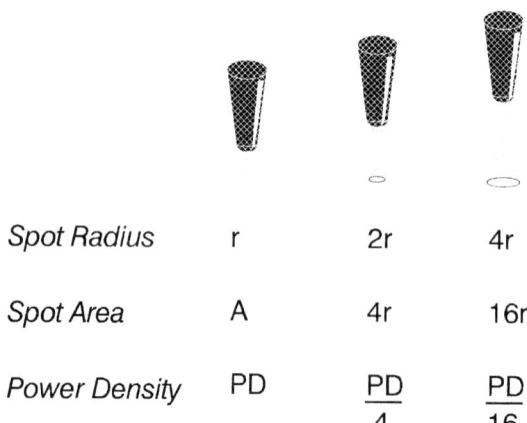

Spot Radius	r	2r	4r
Spot Area	A	4r	16r
Power Density	PD	$\dfrac{PD}{4}$	$\dfrac{PD}{16}$

Figure 12-5.   Relationship between spot radius, spot area, and power density with distance of laser to tissue.

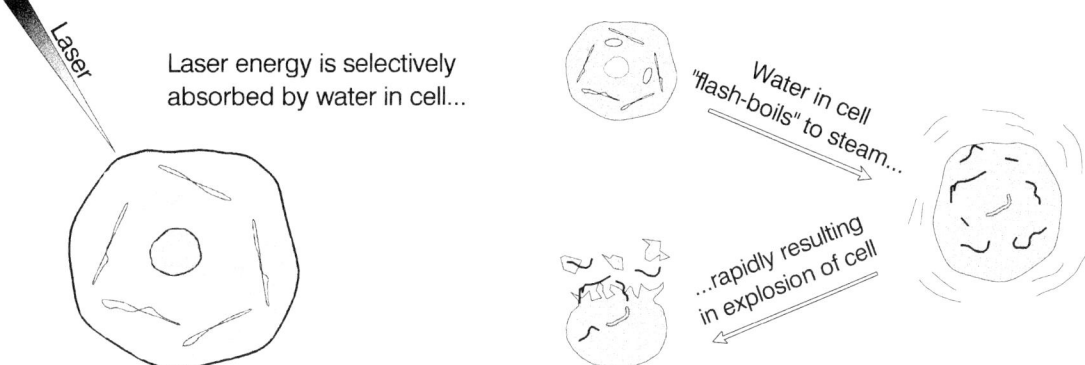

Figure 12-6. Mechanism of cellular vaporization by CO_2 laser.

energy, resulting in a degree of welding that causes the capillaries smaller than 1.5 mm in diameter to be welded shut. This mechanism may be responsible for the decreased amount of bleeding observed with laser debridement. In fact, there is so little bleeding that patients with coagulopathy or who are on anticoagulants can still be debrided [11, 12].

TECHNIQUE OF LASER DEBRIDEMENT

BASIC PRINCIPLES

Ninety-eight percent of laser debridement procedures [6, 8, 9] have been performed under local anesthesia, combined with intravenous sedation when necessary. This is ideal for the population of elderly, often acutely ill, patients requiring decubitus debridement. It also makes it ideal for home-bound and nursing home patients who can be treated on an *ambulatory surgery* basis. A clear understanding of the variables under the control of the operator have to be well understood in order to achieve optimal benefit from the technique.

The technique utilizes a hand-held laser. The varying effects on the various parts of a necrotic wound result from different, dynamic combinations of power, degree of focus of the beam, and hand speed.

Power

The power (watts) delivered by most CO_2 lasers ranges from a fraction of a watt to 60 or 100 watts.

Most debridement can be done at 40–55 watts. Smaller and more delicate tissues require lower power, and a higher power generally expedites the debridement of larger decubiti.

Beam Focus

At the focal point of the beam (0.1 cm) the thinnest, most efficacious vaporization occurs, and this is tantamount to excision using a knife or electrocautery. As the beam is defocused, the spot size gets bigger, and so a less intense effect is achieved in a wider area. This allows vaporization of thin sheets of necrotic tissue in a layer-by-layer manner. Further defocusing of the beam results in no depth of penetration, but an effect only on the surface of the wound, resulting in vaporization of surface cells and *bacteria*. This allows surface sterilization.

Hand Speed

This is the final "fine-tuning" that also determines the *depth of debridement*. A *static* beam will drill a hole into the tissue proportional to the energy and size of the beam. The same beam that is kept moving in a circular side-to-side manner now enables the operator to "sculpt" the tissue to an appropriate contour and depth.

DETAILS OF OPERATIVE TECHNIQUES

The actual manner of debridement is performed in three distinct stages: excision, vaporization, and surface sterilization.

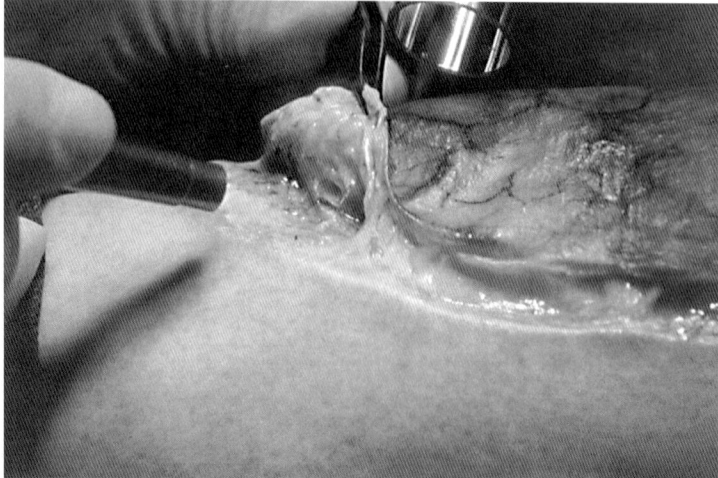

Figure 12-7.   Excision with laser in focus.

Excision

Large areas of necrotic tissue are more easily excised than fully vaporized. The beam is used at the focal point (0.1 cm) for vaporization in a thin line, which is tantamount to an incision. See Figure 12-7.

Vaporization

This is the function of the CO_2 laser that renders it superior to other debridement tools. The thin, irregular layer of remaining necrotic tissue, especially when friable and difficult to grasp with forceps, is very *precisely and easily* debrided to the exact interface of viable and nonviable tissue. This is effected by a defocused beam (~1.0 cm), and the necrotic tissue is vaporized layer by layer until the interface zone is reached. There is no need to attempt to grasp the tissue, and accessibility to necrotic tissue in the depths of wounds and under flaps is easily attained with a beam of light (Figures 12-8 through 12-10). The transformation of the wound from one with layers of liquefaction necrosis to a clean base with minimal capillary oozing is accomplished very precisely with the laser.

Surface Sterilization

The beam is now further defocused (1.5 cm or greater), and the hand speed and power are adjusted to allow the wound to be "airbrushed." This results in a sterilized wound that can now undergo primary closure.

ENDPOINT OF DEBRIDEMENT

The presence of cellulitis, edema, incomplete demarcation, or poor tissue perfusion can make the identification of viable tissue difficult. The following primary guidelines have been adopted based on experience of over 1000 debridements [12].

Fat. Small punctate bleeding has proven to be a reliable sign of viability even when the pallor of the fat may wrongly suggest tissue death. The operator should leave such potentially viable fatty tissue intact.

Fascia. Punctate bleeding is less readily seen in fasciae, but the maintenance of defined striations has proven reliable as an indicator of viability, and fasciae retaining this characteristic should be left intact.

Tendon. The loss of paratenon and even some necrosis of superficial layers of tendon do *not* mean death to the whole tendon if deeper layers have retained morphology and punctate bleeding.

Muscle. Very edematous, pale muscle may appear dead, but any evidence of punctate bleeding warrants ending the debridement at that point, often with preservation of large areas of muscle.

Bone. Debrided areas of exposed bone, including cortical bone, can be salvaged and obtain coverage by "drilling" holes with the laser to the marrow. These "islands" allow granulating tissue to cover the de-

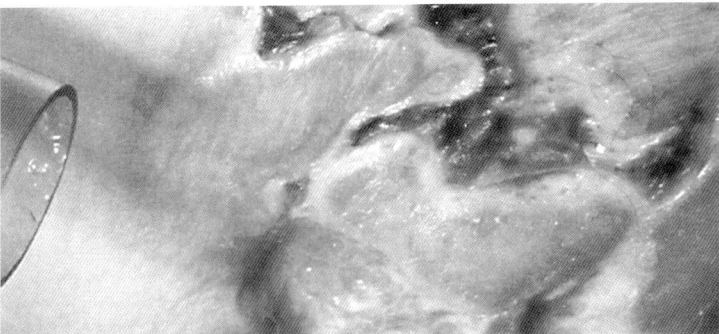

Figure 12-8. Vaporization with laser defocused.

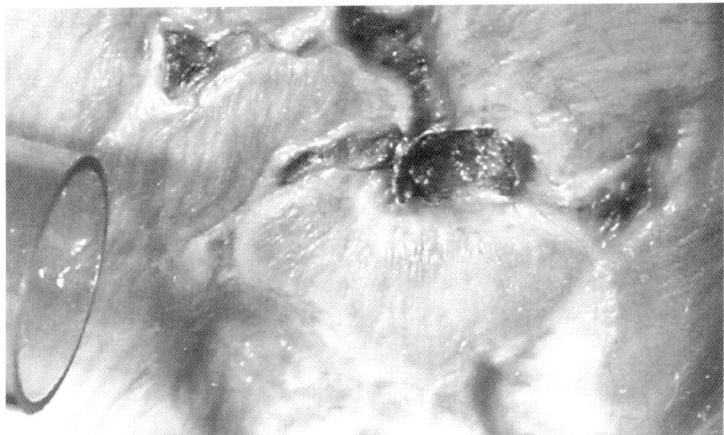

Figure 12-9. End of vaporization—Small amount of char on wound.

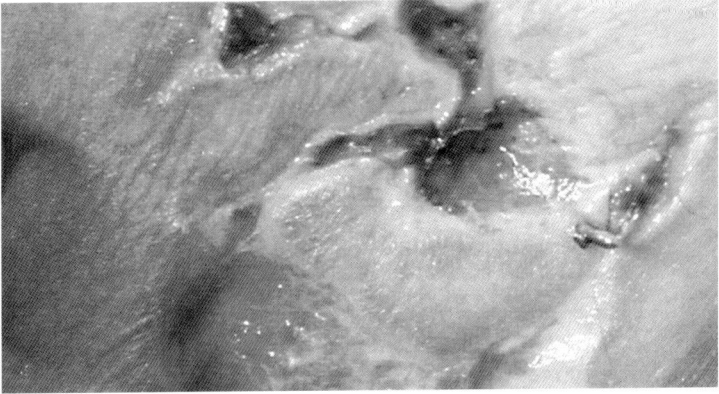

Figure 12-10. After irrigation of char—Precisely debrided to viable tissue interface.

nuded bone. Obvious dead bone can be excised or vaporized [13].

AFTER CARE

The general care of the patient must include adequate turning and all other decubiti-preventive methods, including the use of specialty beds, attention to nutrition with appropriate vitamin and mineral supplementation, and attention to keeping the patient clean and dry.

Wound care

In general, there is no need for wound packing. In cases where continued oozing is encountered, temporary (24–48 hours) packing is used for hemostasis. In larger undetermined areas, a thin tongue of Vaseline gauze is placed to facilitate drainage. Chemical debriding agents are used; e.g., Collagenase with or without Polysporin powder (both from Knoll Pharmaceutical Company, New Jersey).

Vaseline gauze is ubiquitous and inexpensive. Used in a single layer, it allows egress of excess fluid to the overlying dry dressings, thus allowing the wound to remain *moist,* without becoming macerated.

Excellent patient tolerance is noted because such dressings do not stick to the wound and allow easy, pain-free removal. The mechanical effect of dressing changes is not needed after a complete laser debridement, and, because the Vaseline gauze keeps the wound moist, the dressing need only be changed once daily.

Further operative care

The decision as to whether the wound or decubitus requires further laser debridement, maintenance of open wound care, or progression to flap closure (if delayed closure was elected) is made every five to seven days.

The beneficial effects of laser debridement are not limited to pressure ulcers. Similar results can be obtained when laser debridement is used in the treatment of ischemic ulcers, necrotic wounds, necrotizing fasciitis, abscesses, and infected muscle. It is especially useful in deep wounds with undermining, as the beam can be directed into deep crevices

that would not be easily accessed with fingers or surgical instruments. The versatility is further extended when working near vital structures, as the beam can be defocused and intact necrotic tissue can be debrided in a layer-by-layer manner, precisely to the interface of viable tissue.

DISCUSSION

In the senior author's first 200 cases, the success rate was 97% with laser debridements, 90% with only two laser treatments. Success was defined by the establishment of a clean granulating wound or one that was successfully closed primarily. This rate of success has continued to be the experience with an additional 600 cases including over 1000 decubiti. Figures 12-11 through 12-13 show laser debridement with primary closure. Figures 12-14 through 12-16 show a granulating wound following repeat debridement with healing by secondary intention.

As long as a moist dressing is provided for the wound, the consistent, and often striking, finding is the early appearance of odor-free, pink granulation tissue. This raises the question of an additional induction of wound healing resulting from the laser. The issue is raised here not to substantiate it, but to acknowledge the research being done to clarify the effects of low- and middle-energy-level lasers on cellular physiology (biostimulation).

A number of patients with partially necrotic Achilles tendons—a notoriously difficult area to heal—have been successfully treated with the laser, including one patient with peripheral vascular disease and chronic renal failure.

Wounds with significant areas of denuded bone have also been successfully treated by the drilling techniques mentioned previously. One of the most striking patients was an elderly woman with a revascularized lower extremity, who suffered ischemia to the muscles of the anterior compartment. The deep necrotic ulcers had been treated conventionally for weeks without significant improvement, and she was referred for laser debridement. After one laser treatment, a bed of viable tissue was obtained over 5 to 6 cm of exposed tibia. This area continued to heal without further debridements or

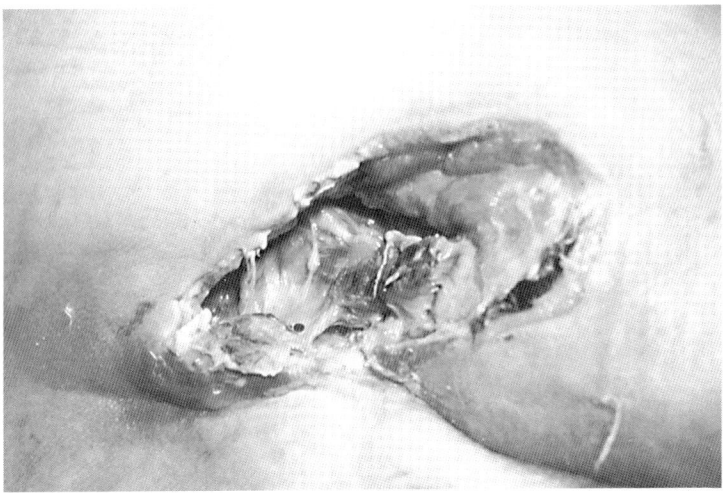

Figure 12-11. Stage IV sacral decubitus with deep necrosis.

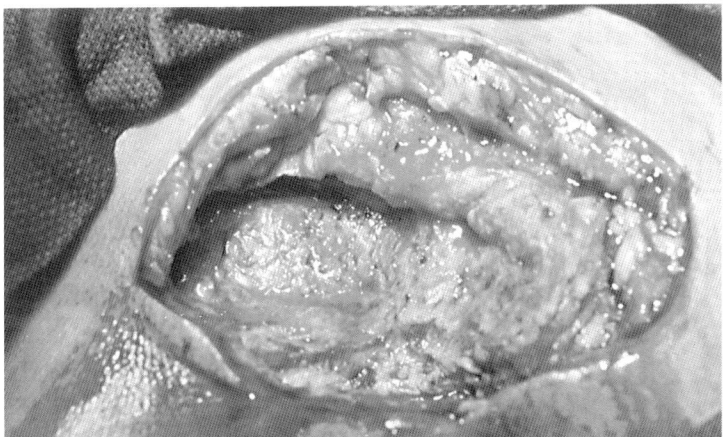

Figure 12-12. Stage IV sacral decubitus post debridement and surface sterilization.

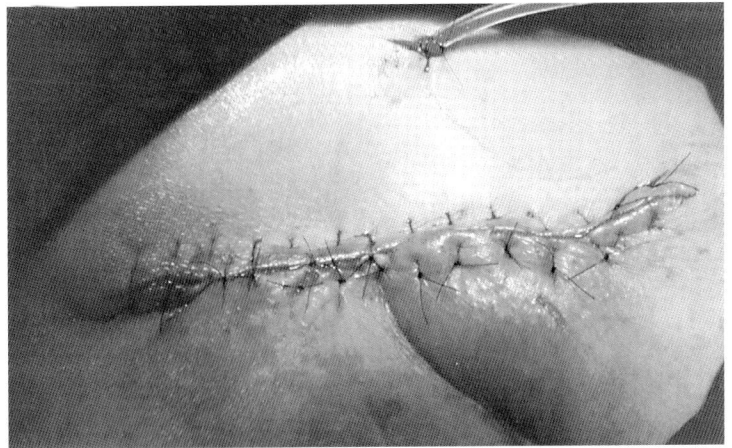

Figure 12-13. Primary closure post laser debridement and flap advancement.

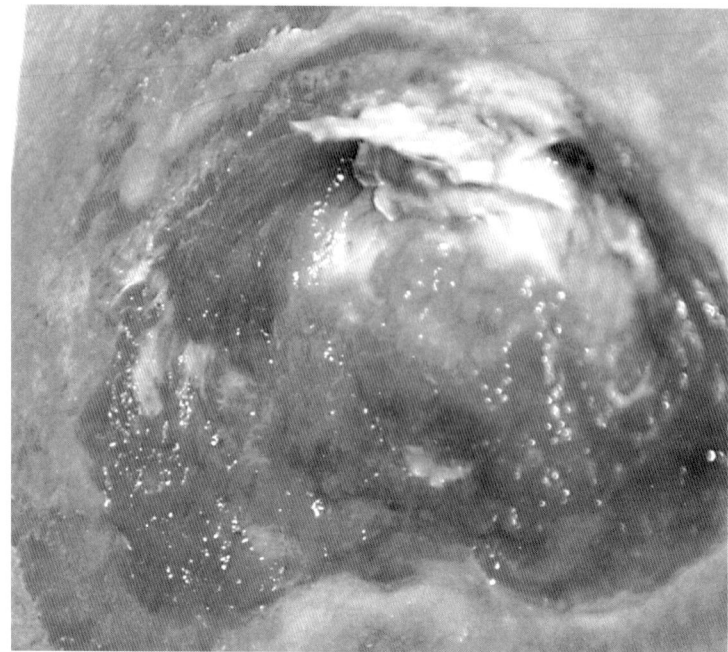

Figure 12-14.   Previously debrided ulcer with small residual necrosis, four weeks—half size.

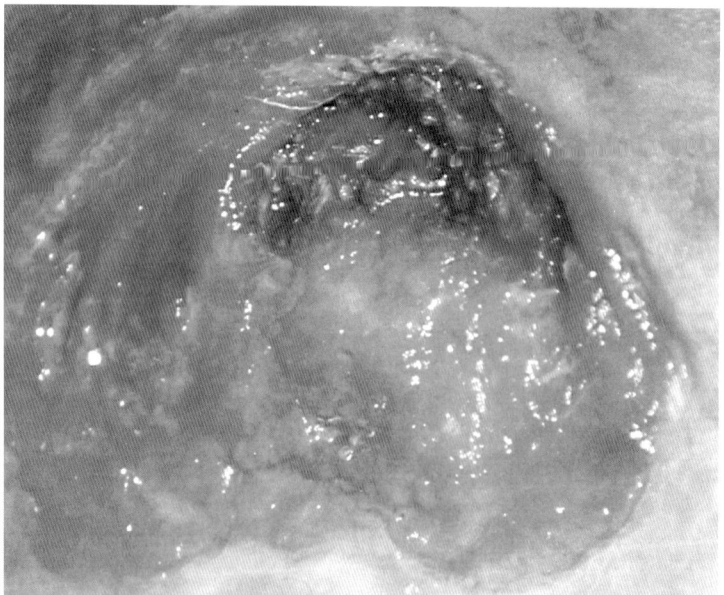

Figure 12-15.   Immediately after follow-up debridement.

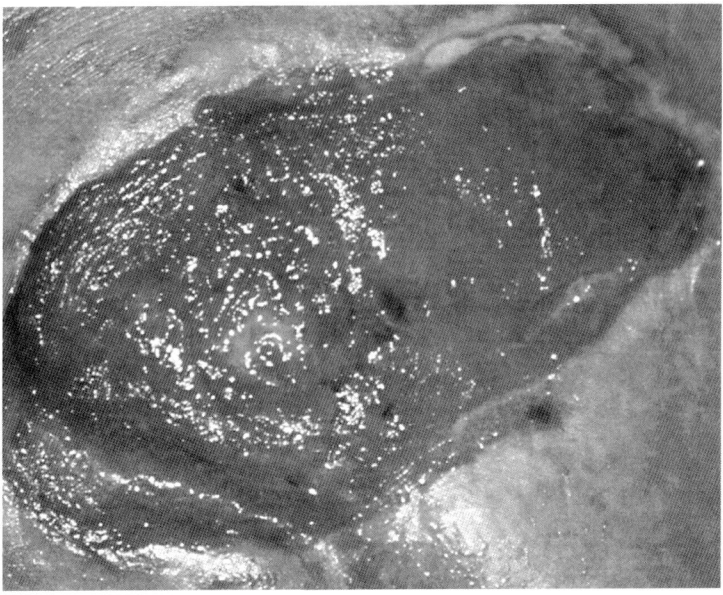

Figure 12-16. Clean, granulating, shallow smaller ulcer after two weeks.

skin grafting. The success with long bones as well as cancellous bone is noted, including metatarsals.

The erosion of ulcers into joint spaces is easily treated by vaporizing the articular cartilage, allowing granulation tissue to fill the bed.

The potential for cost savings is evident and occurs at many levels: Decreased hospital stay, decreased need for materials, elimination of sources of generalized sepsis, and the inherent cost factor of the laser. A dramatic case that serves to underscore this potential is that of an elderly nursing home patient admitted with sepsis from a deep sacral collection under an eschar. The ulcer was debrided, surface sterilized, and covered with an advancement flap. The drain was removed after seven days, and the patient was discharged on postoperative day 10. It can be readily appreciated that this patient could easily have spent weeks in the hospital with repeated debridements, as well as the continuing need for daily, or twice daily, dressing changes as an outpatient. A second case that further attests to the utility of the laser in debridement and steril-

ization concerns an elderly gentleman who presented to the emergency department in septic shock from a subcutaneous abscess tracking from the scrotum to the sixth rib on the right side. Initial treatment included broad-spectrum antibiotics and incision and drainage of the abscess. The patient improved, and on the fourth hospital day, he returned to the operating room for laser debridement. In this procedure the CO_2 laser was used to excise necrotic debris and then to surface sterilize the cavity. At this time the skin was closed primarily over two closed suction catheters. On the seventh postoperative day the drains were removed, and the patient was changed to appropriate oral antibiotics. He was discharged home on the eighth day. The patient recovered without wound sequelae and required no home care whatsoever See Figures 12-17 through 12-20.

Finally, patient comfort is improved with laser debridement. It is readily evident that patients and their families appreciate the many features already discussed. Whether the patient is in the hospital, at

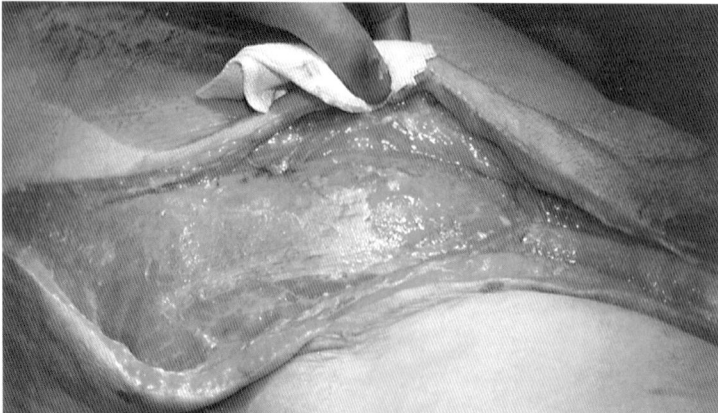

Figure 12-17. Partially debrided, extensive abscess cavity.

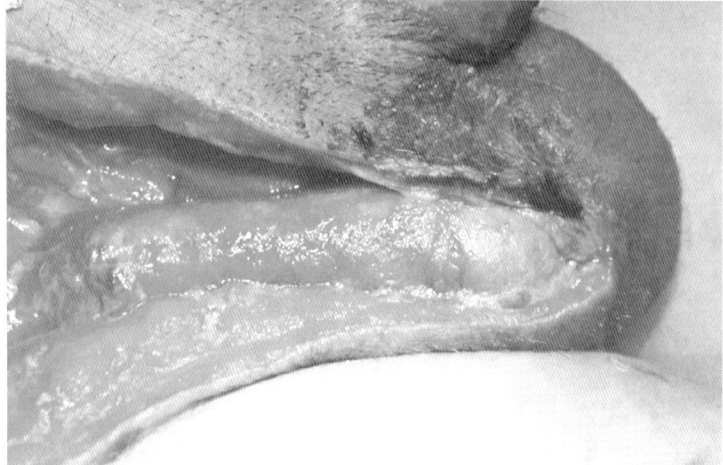

Figure 12-18. Necrotic scrotal skin, pus in scrotum and around testicle; testicle mobilized, sterilized, and replaced into scrotum.

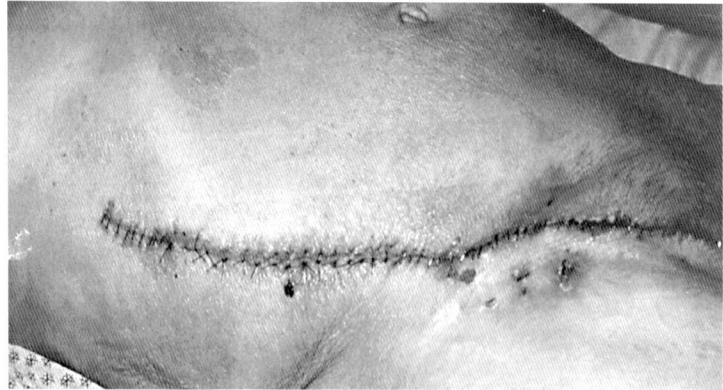

Figure 12-19. Postoperative day 7. Jackson-Pratt drains removed; suture line intact.

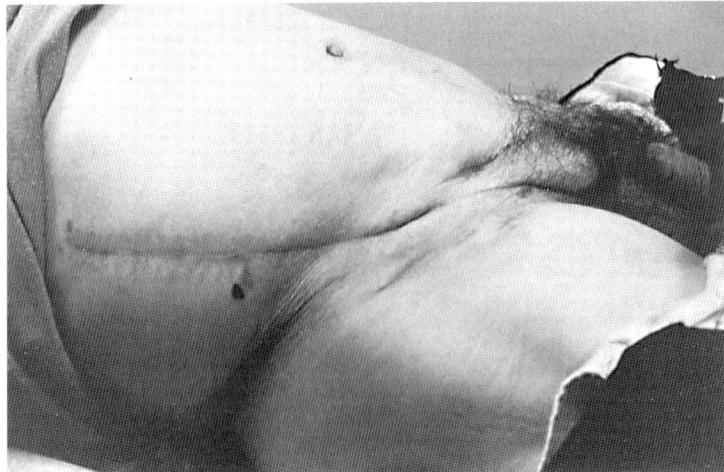

Figure 12-20. Office visit at three months. Fully healed. No infection.

home, or in a nursing home, the presence of a malodorous wound is very distressing to the patient and family. As simple as it appears, providing a clean, *non*odorous wound makes a tremendous difference.

LIMITATIONS

The main contributing factor to the inability to debride a wound successfully is the presence of severe ischemia of the tissues. Under normal circumstances, there is a very small zone of thermal injury beyond the zone of vaporization. In ischemic tissues this zone is increased and is manifested by a new line of necrotic tissue 24 hours after surgery.

Modifications of conventional technique make use of higher energy for shorter duration, or the use of intermittent or pulsed beams instead of a continuous beam.

Further work is needed in this area to treat the patient with ischemia who cannot be revascularized.

COMPLICATIONS

Complications of this procedure have proven to be exceedingly few. Patients require monitoring for the following:

1. **Bleeding.** Capillary ooze and small vessel bleeding are actually *decreased* as compared with conventional surgery, so much so that patients with coagulopathy or on anticoagulants can still be debrided. The larger bleeders still have to be cauterized or suture ligated.

2. **Further necrosis.** This may be caused by nonadherence to all standard decubitus care protocol in the postoperative period, inappropriate wound care, or injudicious laser use, causing an increased zone of thermal injury and resulting in new necrosis.

Complications related to the laser itself are (a) the beam: The main danger of using a monochromatic beam of light is the potential to cause damage *remote* from the operative site –this includes potential damage to the patient, as well as to the medical personnel; (b) the plume: The plume produced by laser vaporization is thick and profuse and can be very readily evident in the operating room if not properly evacuated. In addition, it has been shown in other arenas that live viral particles have been present in the plume. This raises concern over the possible transmission of viral infections via this route.

It is obvious that all laser safety precautions have to be strictly observed to avoid potential mishaps, specifically the use of appropriate suction devices at the immediate operative site and the use of specially designed masks that filter to 0.3 µm as well as specially designed goggles.

SUMMARY/FUTURE

The CO_2 laser continues to be an extremely efficacious precision instrument for the debridement and sterilization of decubiti. The advantages are more rapid debridement, earlier control of infection, greater patient comfort, decreased manpower and material requirement for wound care, decreased hospital stay, and the potential for tremendous cost savings.

The anticipated technological advancements in an instrument that is only thirty years old hold a promise of a smaller, more mobile unit.

The hope, by workers who have seen the clear supremacy of the CO_2 laser over conventional surgery, is that use of this very precise instrument will become the standard for treating stage III and IV decubiti and indeed any wound that requires debridement.

REFERENCES

1. Dixon, J. A., *Surgical Applications of Lasers,* 2nd ed., Chicago: Year Book Medical Publishers, 1987.
2. Hinshaw, J. R.; Herrera, H. R.; Lanzafame, R. J.; and Pennino, R. P., The use of the carbon dioxide laser permits primary closure of contaminated and purulent lesions and wounds, *Lasers Surg Med* 1987; 6(6):581–3.
3. Stellar et al. 1972.
4. Kori, A., and Glantz, G. J., The use of CO_2 laser in general surgery, *Proceedings of the Trans 6th International Congress, Society of Lasers in Medicine and Surgery,* Jerusalem, 1985, p. 7.
5. Lutchman, G. D., et al., The use of the CO_2 laser as a debriding tool. *Proceedings of the 17th International Congress of the Society for Laser Medicine and Surgery,* San Diego, 1991.
6. Juri, H., and Palma, J. A., CO_2 laser in decubitus ulcers: A comparative study. *Lasers Surg Med* 1987; 7(4):296–9.
7. Lanzafame, R. J., and Hirshaw, J. R., ed., *Atlas of Laser Surgical Techniques,* St. Louis, MO: Ishiyaku EuroAmerica Publishing, 1989.
8. Eltorai, I.; Glantz, G.; and Montroy, R., The use of the carbon dioxide laser beam in the surgery of pressure sores, *Internat Surg* 1988; 73(1):54–6.
9. Chegin, V. M., et al., Laser surgery for soft tissue purulent diseases, *Lasers Surg Med* 1984; 4(3):279–82.
10. Takiguchi, S., et al., Carbon dioxide laser surgery and hemorrhagic tendencies, in K. Atsumi, N. Minsakui, eds., *Laser Tokyo '81,* Tokyo: Inter-Group, 1981:9–11.
11. Herrera, R. H.; Mackay, R.; and Hinshaw, J. R., Use of the CO_2 laser in surgery of the hemophiliac patient, *Proceedings of the 6th Congress of the International Society for Lasers in Medicine and Surgery,* 1985, p. 48.
12. Lutchman, G. D., Unpublished personal series of over 1800 cases, 1988–1997.
13. Bailin, P. L., and Wheeland, R. G., Carbon dioxide laser perforation of exposed cranial bone to stimulate granulation tissue, *Plast Reconstr Surg* 1985; 75:898–902.

13

NURSING CARE OF PATIENTS WITH PRESSURE ULCERS

Mary Lou Shannon, Ed.D., R.N.

INTRODUCTION

The role of the nurse in the management of pressure ulcers has changed radically in the past decade because of: (1) a better understanding of wound healing, (2) the realization that effective wound healing cannot take place unless both systemic and local factors that affect the individual and the wound are controlled to the greatest extent possible, (3) an understanding of the importance of nonionic cleansers and their role in safe wound cleansing, (4) an understanding of the appropriate use of topical and/or systemic antibiotics and antiseptics, (5) the addition of new dressing materials/substances that interact with the wound to enhance healing, (6) an understanding of the indications for use of surgical, mechanical, chemical, or autolytic debridement, and (7) the continuing research directed toward modifying the wound environment and/or accelerating wound healing through the use of such technological developments as growth factors, electrostimulation, hyperbaric oxygen therapy, and lasers. These changes have created both a new knowledge base on wound healing and a new therapy base for wound management.

In addition to the changes affecting the wound and its management, the practice of professional nursing is also undergoing major alteration. This is due in part to the major health care changes aimed at cost containment in the United States. These changes impact where patient care will be given—hospital, nursing home, or home setting; when or if hospitalization is indicated for patient care; the length of hospitalization if determined to be necessary for treatment; which health professional groups may legally provide different aspects of patient care; what care will be reimbursed; federal and/or state policies and guidelines affecting professional practice and patient care; and the nurse's employing agency's policies.

In addition to the changes wrought by alterations in the health care system, changes are occurring within the nursing profession that will impact the expanded role that nurses with advanced preparation are prepared to assume. A cadre of acute care nurse practitioners will be prepared to assess and manage patients with certain types of health care problems in conjunction with physicians. These practitioners are envisioned to represent a melding of the current nurse practitioner and clinical nurse specialist roles. The patient with a chronic wound is a good prototype of the type of health problems that these professional nurses are well equipped to manage. Such management assumes that the patient's general health condition is stable, and that the wound is not complicated to the degree that

155

sepsis or surgical treatment, beyond minor debridement, is necessary.

THE NURSE'S ROLE IN THE PROMOTION OF PRESSURE ULCER HEALING

Professional nurses are acutely aware of the pressure ulcer problem because they deal with it so frequently. Nursing is often blamed for allowing pressure ulcers to develop because of poor care. Although this can never be totally refuted, it is much more likely that pressure ulcers occur for a variety of reasons, such as the following:

(1) Preventive measures were not started in time to prevent skin damage.

(2) Preventive measures chosen for use were ineffective for the specific patient situation.

(3) Changes in patient acuity levels on nursing units require more nursing contact time, but there are fewer staff to provide it.

(4) There is a deterioration in the patient's condition of a preterminal nature.

(5) Surgery or other diagnostic procedures have been performed that require long periods of immobilization on inadequately padded surfaces.

(6) Agency cost containment policies affect nurse-patient staffing ratios, equipment, and other supplies necessary for the prevention and/or management of pressure ulcers.

(7) Iatrogenic causes are responsible for tissue damage, such as placing a patient in restraints for safety or having to move a patient up in bed without sufficient help to lift his/her body.

(8) Unusual causes may be to blame, such as occult soft tissue injury occurring prior to hospitalization (e.g., a fall in the home), factitious injury (e.g., SCI persons have been reported to develop pressure ulcers to facilitate admission to the hospital), internal orthopedic devices such as plates and screws that can cause abrasion of the overlying muscle, congenital or acquired bony anomalies, casts that create undue pressure, depression, etc.

In order to plan effective pressure ulcer management, the professional nurse must perform a thorough patient assessment on admission. This carefully documented assessment must include physical, mental, and emotional baselines. It is axiomatic that no wound can heal if major systemic pathologies such as uncontrolled diabetes interfere.

Physical assessment by the nurse begins with a comprehensive history. Questions should be both objective and open ended in order to elicit the greatest amount of useful information. The patient who is asked to "tell me about your wound" may volunteer significant information that objective questioning would not elicit. It is also important to recognize that the elderly patient gives a better history when he/she is not rushed. Physical assessment of the patient should cover all body systems. Of special importance to wound healing considerations are the circulatory, respiratory, and neurological system assessments, as well as the patient's nutritional, metabolic, and immunologic status. There should be careful examination of his/her ability to perform the activities of daily living (ADL) such as feeding himself and moving about without assistance, the nature of any sensory impairments that might create safety concerns such as visual defects, elimination patterns/difficulties, and ability to communicate. If there are limitations involving any aspect of ADLs, these should be described and plans made for dealing effectively with them. It is essential that the nurse perform *and record* a head-to-toe skin examination in order to ensure that no occult skin problems exist at the time of admission.

Mental assessment should include the patient's degree of orientation. Assessment of this dimension is accomplished by asking not only questions that require factual answers, such as, "Who is the President of the United States?", but also questions that require limited explanation that any patient could be expected to know. An example of such a question is: "Tell me the difference in the shape of an orange and the shape of a banana." Asking questions such as "What is the date?" or "What day of the week is this?" are not useful because patients lose track of this information when ill. It is necessary that the patient's mental status be sampled sufficiently to ensure that an accurate assessment of orientation is made. If family or friends are present, their input can be helpful in making such a determination.

Psychological assessment is important because it has an impact on both the patient's general health status and the pressure ulcer. Of particular importance is the presence of anxiety, depression, or disregard of the wound. Anxiety increases metabolic demand, which adds to the perfusion problems that helped create the pressure ulcer. Depression may be a causative factor in pressure ulcer development or the patient's reaction to a hard-to-heal chronic wound. As an etiologic agent in pressure ulcer development, the depressed patient may not move himself at intervals that are sufficiently frequent to prevent skin damage. Fuhrer et al. [1], found that spinal cord injury (SCI) patients, a population known to be at increased risk for pressure ulcers, had high mean depression scores. Shannon and Skorga [2] found that 98% of the 40 SCI patients who were admitted to a large Veterans Administration spinal cord service were admitted with pressure ulcers. According to spinal cord personnel, many of these patients developed their skin lesion(s) purposely in order to be admitted to the hospital where they could be with other veterans who had SCI. The physician in charge of the SCI service felt that depression and inability to adjust to life outside the hospital was a major factor in their development of pressure ulcers. In the same study, the authors found that 33% of patients who developed pressure ulcers in a private general hospital were found to be alert and oriented *and able to move without assistance*. It is possible that depression played a part in the etiology of their skin breakdown.

Disregard of a wound by the patient raises several possibilities. The first is that the wound is anxiety producing and represents a threat to the patient's well-being. A second possibility is that patient depression interferes with concern about the wound. A third possibility is that medications may alter patient perception of discomfort/pain, and the individual does not perceive the need to move. A fourth possibility is seldom appreciated: the wound is factitious; e.g., the patient purposely developed the wound. Yet this is strongly suspected in certain populations such as the one reported in the Shannon and Skorga study [2].

PRESSURE ULCER ASSESSMENT

Every nurse who cares for pressure ulcers must be readily conversant with the staging system that is used to determine wound depth. The system that is recommended by the Panel for the Prediction and Prevention of Pressure Ulcers in *Pressure Ulcers in Adults: Prediction and Prevention and Treatment of Pressure Ulcers* published by the Agency for Health Care Policy and Research; the National Pressure Ulcer Advisory Panel; and the Wound, Ostomy and Continence Nursing Society is as follows:

Stage I. Nonblanchable erythema of intact skin; the heralding lesion of skin ulceration. In individuals with darker skin, discoloration of the skin, warmth, edema, induration, or hardness may also be indicators. Note: Reactive hyperemia can normally be expected to be present for one-half to three-fourths as long as the pressure occluded blood flow to the area (Lewis and Grant, [3]). This should not be confused with a stage I pressure ulcer.

Stage II. Partial-thickness skin loss involving epidermis and/or dermis. The ulcer is superficial and presents clinically as an abrasion, blister, or shallow crater.

Stage III. Full-thickness skin loss involving damage or necrosis of subcutaneous tissue that may extend down to, but not through, underlying fascia. The ulcer presents clinically as a deep crater with or without undermining of adjacent tissue.

Stage IV. Full-thickness skin loss with extensive destruction, tissue necrosis, or damage to muscle, bone, or supporting structures (for example, tendon or joint capsule). Note: Undermining and sinus tracts may also be associated with stage IV pressure ulcers.

Staging definitions recognize these assessment limitations:

1. Identification of stage I pressure ulcers may be difficult in patients with darkly pigmented skin.

2. When eschar is present, accurate staging of the pressure ulcer is not possible until the eschar has sloughed or the wound has been debrided ([4], pp. 8, 145).

Although it is recognized that staging is not the only assessment measure needed, it is the one that is in common use by health care professionals who manage pressure ulcers. Barr [5] has pointed out that staging is designed to identify the anatomical depth of the wound. In order to be able to use staging accurately, the clinician must be able to identify the types of tissue involved. Those nurses who have had preparation as clinical nurse specialists, acute care nurse practitioners, and enterostomal therapists should be proficient at determining whether the tissue involved is subcutaneous tissue, muscle, etc. However, it is not clear whether the generalist in nursing is skilled to the same degree in tissue identification.

Other concerns about staging exist. The main one is its use to indicate the progression of healing. Pressure ulcers heal by different processes. Stages I and II pressure ulcers are partial-thickness wounds. They heal by epithelization; e.g., the wound heals with the same cell type as was damaged and normal function is restored. Stages III and IV are full-thickness pressure ulcers. The cells that eventually cover the wound defect are not the same as those originally lost. This means that the wound heals by scarring. Scar tissue never restores normal tissue strength or normal tissue continuity. It is avascular and lacks elasticity. This makes it more prone to subsequent damage. These examples point out the fallacy of using staging to describe healing. Pressure ulcers do not heal from stage IV to III to II to I. Deep lesions cannot do this because they do not epithelialize; stages III and IV ulcers can never progress to become stage II or I ulcers. There are also other concerns about staging, but at present, it is a commonly accepted tool for communication among wound care professionals.

In addition to staging, there are a number of methods/instruments available for wound assessment in the clinical setting. The AHCPR Treatment of Pressure Ulcers Guideline Panel [6] feels that there is no assessment and monitoring instrument that can be recommended at present. However, Bates-Jensen's pressure sore status tool [7, 8] with its thirteen areas of assessment (wound size, depth, edges, undermining, necrotic tissue type and amount, exudate type and amount, surrounding skin color, edema, induration, granulation tissue, and epithelization) furnished much of the basis for the AHCPRs Assessment Guide, shown in Figure 13-1.

Other instruments/methods to assess wounds are discussed by Cooper [9]. She describes the wound assessment inventory; the wound characteristics instrument; the red, yellow, black method; the wound severity score; the Wells incisional category; staging; measurement methods—linear, photography, wound tracings, planimetry, Kundin wound gauge, molds, foam, and water instillation. The instruments/equipment are designed for varied purposes. It is an area of continuing research and development.

Lazarus et al., [10] discuss the guidelines for assessment of wounds and evaluation of their healing in an excellent article that points out that complete wound assessment "must include the extent of the wound, associated attributes of the wound, host factors that influence wound status, and environmental factors that impact on optimum wound management."

Until a valid and reliable wound assessment instrument is available, the nurse might find a mnemonic developed by Ayello [11] useful in assessing pressure ulcers:

A = anatomical location, age of wound
S = size, stage
S = sepsis
E = exudate type and amount, erythema
S = surrounding skin color, swelling, saturation of
      dressing
S = sinus tract, undermining
M = maceration
E = edges, epithelialization
N = nose (odor), necrotic tissue type and amount,
      neovascularization
T = tenderness to touch, tension (induration),
      tautness, tissue bed (granulation)

The nurse performing the physical examination of the pressure ulcer wound should pay particular attention to see if there is undermining, where the wound extends under the surface wound margins, if there are sinus tracts that extend from the bottom or sides of the wound to involve other structures, and if there is dead space; e.g., a cavity remaining in the wound. Any of these conditions will require careful assessment so that appropriate measures can be used to manage them.

Attachment A. Sample Pressure Ulcer Assessment Guide

Patient Name: _____ Date: _____ Time: _____

Ulcer 1:		Ulcer 2:

Ulcer 1:
Site _____
Stage[a] _____
Size (cm)
 Length _____
 Width _____
 Depth _____

	No	Yes
Sinus Tract	☐	☐
Tunneling	☐	☐
Undermining	☐	☐
Necrotic Tissue	☐	☐
Slough	☐	☐
Eschar	☐	☐
Exudate	☐	☐
Serous	☐	☐
Serosanguineous	☐	☐
Purulent	☐	☐
Granulation	☐	☐
Epithelialization	☐	☐
Pain	☐	☐

Surrounding Skin:

	No	Yes
Erythema	☐	☐
Maceration	☐	☐
Induration	☐	☐

Description of Ulcer(s):

Ulcer 2:
Site _____
Stage[a] _____
Size (cm)
 Length _____
 Width _____
 Depth _____

	No	Yes
Sinus Tract	☐	☐
Tunneling	☐	☐
Undermining	☐	☐
Necrotic Tissue	☐	☐
Slough	☐	☐
Eschar	☐	☐
Exudate	☐	☐
Serous	☐	☐
Serosanguineous	☐	☐
Purulent	☐	☐
Granulation	☐	☐
Epithelialization	☐	☐
Pain	☐	☐

	No	Yes
Erythema	☐	☐
Maceration	☐	☐
Induration	☐	☐

_____

_____

Indicate Ulcer Sites:

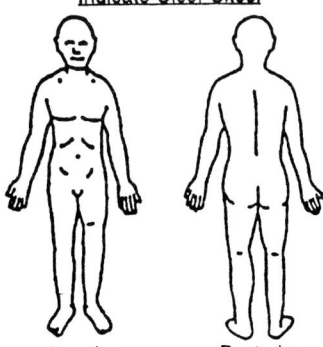

Anterior   Posterior

(Attach a color photo of the pressure ulcer[s] [Optional])

[a]Classification of pressure ulcers:
Stage I: Nonblanchable erythema of intact skin, the heralding lesion of skin ulceration. In individuals with darker skin, discoloration of the skin, warmth, edema, induration, or hardness may also be indicators.
Stage II: Partial thickness skin loss involving epidermis, dermis or both.
Stage III: Full thickness skin loss involving damage to or necrosis of subcutaneous tissue that may extend down to, but not through, underlying fascia. The ulcer presents clinically as a deep crater with or without undermining adjacent tissue.
Stage IV: Full thickness skin loss with extensive destruction, tissue necrosis, or damage to muscle, bone, or supporting structures (e.g., tendon or joint capsule).

Figure 13-1. AHCPR Sample Pressure Ulcer Assessment Guide. (From [4].)

It is essential that regular wound evaluations be made in order to determine if the wound is progressing toward a healing state or if wound deterioration is taking place. During the healing phase of a full-thickness wound, the nurse should expect to see a well-vascularized wound that is pink and has a good granulation tissue bed, no purulent exudate, no erythema around the wound margins, no signs of infection. A fully healed partial-thickness wound is one that achieves restoration of normal structure, function, and appearance; whereas a full-thickness wound is a minimally healed wound. It achieves a restoration of cover by scar tissue and does not possess the preinjury functional result. This type of wound is at risk to recur. The presence of infection, poor granulation tissue, necrotic tissue, purulent exudate, and enlargement of the wound are signs associated with wound deterioration.

The healing of a pressure ulcer is facilitated by removing the products of soft tissue breakdown: slough, exudates, and metabolic byproducts. Removal of these products along with surface wound contaminants decreases the likelihood of subsequent infection.

The first step in cleansing is to select a cleansing solution that is not harmful to tissue. Research on the effects of various agents routinely used to cleanse wounds started to appear in the 1970s. However, it was not until Rodeheaver [12] explained the dangers of using most commercially available wound cleansers at the Symposium on Advanced Wound Care that the dangers of ionically charged agents was appreciated by many wound care nurses.

All ionically charged agents interact with cell membranes, causing the membrane to lose normal permeability and inhibiting the cell's ability to withstand external invasion by bacteria. Hexachlorophene, chlorhexidine, and povidone-iodine all cause damage to normal cells in the wound, especially fibroblasts. Povidone-iodine, for example, kills all of the white blood cells in the wound and allows bacteria to proliferate. Rather than being protective to the wound, it is detrimental [12].

If the pressure ulcer is a clean wound with evidence of granulation tissue, it requires *only* gentle cleansing using isotonic saline (0.9%), a nonionic cleanser that will not damage normal cells. If the

wound is infected or contains much necrotic material, additional cleansing measures may be indicated. These include irrigating the wound with normal saline under a pressure of not less than 4 psi (pounds per square inch) or more than 15 psi. A 35-ml syringe with a 19-gauge blunt-tipped needle or an angiocath delivers cleansing solutions at 8 psi, a level that effectively removes bacteria. To be most effective, the needle tip should be 1 to 2 inches from the wound surface. The AHCPR guideline [6] states that, "Wounds with adherent materials may benefit from the use of those commercial wound cleansers that do not contain harmful chemicals."

The toxicity indices for some wound and skin cleansers are listed in Table 13-1.

Whirlpool treatment should be reserved for cleaning pressure ulcers that have thick exudate, slough, or necrotic tissue. Effective disinfection of the whirlpool tub between patients is *absolutely essential*. Otherwise, there can be sharing of organisms from one patient to another. See the Association for Practitioners in Infection Control (APIC) guidelines (Rutala [13]) for the correct methods to achieve disinfection. It should also be remembered that placing the patient's pressure ulcer close to a

Table 13-1.   Toxicity Index for Wound and Skin Cleansers

Test agent	Toxicity index[a]
Shur Clens	1:10
Biolex	1:100
Saf Clens	1:100
Cara Klenz	1:100
Ultra Klenz	1:1,000
Clinical Care	1:1,000
Uni Wash	1:1,000
Ivory Soap (0.5 percent)	1:1,000
Constant Clens	1:10,000
Dermal Wound Cleanser	1:10,000
Puri-Clens	1:10,000
Hibiclens	1:10,000
Betadine Surgical Scrub	1:10,000
Techni-Care Scrub	1:100,000
Bard Skin Cleanser	1:100,000
Hollister	1:100,000

Source: AHCPR [6].

[a]The dilution required to maintain white blood cell viability and phagocytic efficiency.

whirlpool jet could result in very high pressures being exerted against the wound bed, thus causing damage. It has been found that a clean pressurized rinse used after the whirlpool treatment is more effective in removing bacteria from the wound than using the whirlpool alone (Neiderhuber et al. [14], Bohannon [15]).

The AHCPR [6] makes the following recommendations for wound cleansing:

- Cleanse wounds initially and at each dressing change.

- Use minimal mechanical force when cleansing the ulcer with gauze, cloth, or sponges.

- Do not clean ulcer wounds with skin cleansers or antiseptic agents (e.g., povidone iodine, iodophor, sodium hypochlorite solution [Dakin's solution], hydrogen peroxide, acetic acid).

- Use enough irrigation pressure to enhance wound cleansing without causing trauma to the wound bed. Safe and effective ulcer irrigation pressures range from 4 to 15 psi.

- Consider whirlpool treatment for cleansing pressure ulcers that contain thick exudate, slough, or necrotic tissue. Discontinue whirlpool when the ulcer is clean.

Wound cleansing not only aids healing but also helps to reduce wound odor. Some chronic wounds such as pressure ulcers and fungating tumors can be particularly odoriferous. The odor is distressing to patients, their families, visitors, and personnel and contributes both physical and psychological isolation of the patient.

Although there are a number of wound deodorizers on the market such as charcoal-impregnated dressings, oral deodorizer tablets, and sprays, they vary greatly in effectiveness. One of the most promising treatments for the control of wound odor is the use of metronidazole. This antimicrobial agent has been shown to be effective against odors in several studies. Metronidazole is effective against many of the Gram-negative and Gram-positive anaerobic bacteria that cause odor such as *Bacteroides, Fusobacterium, Clostridium* and some strains of *Eubacterium*, peptococcus, and peptostreptococcus. Ashford et al. [16] performed a randomized, double-blind crossover study comparing

metronidazole 200 mg p.o. t.i.d. with a placebo for fourteen days in nine patients with malodorous fungating tumors. The odor was significantly less in the treated patients ($p < 0.01$). Witkowski and Parish [17] applied a topical preparation of Metro-Gel to pressure ulcers in ten patients who had sacral ulcers with clinical signs of infection. The drug was then covered with fluffed gauze and an abdominal dressing pad. Treatment was repeated every 12 hours. Odor was eliminated from the wound in all cases, frequently within the first 36 hours of use. Similar findings were reported by Poteete [18] in a case study of thirteen patients.

The use of topical forms of metronidazole has several advantages over the systemic administration of the drug. First, it necessitates cleaning and inspecting the wound each time it is used; this means that any wound changes will be noted quickly. Second, direct application to the wound surface places the drug where the odor-causing bacteria are concentrated, and third, systemic levels of the drug are much lower with topical drug use, so the risk of side effects from the drug is decreased.

Providing treatment and protection for the pressure ulcer wound may include the use of topical agents (including growth factors), wound dressings, and pressure reduction/relief support surfaces. Currently, the only topical medications that are advocated for use on pressure ulcers are antibiotics that are effective against a wide variety of bacteria. The AHCPR [6] recommends that the physician do the following:

> Consider initiating a 2-week trial of topical antibiotics for clean pressure ulcers that are not healing or are continuing to produce exudate after 2 to 4 weeks of optimal patient care. The antibiotic should be effective against gram-negative, gram-positive, and anaerobic organisms (e.g., silver sulfadiazine, triple antibiotic).
>
> Do not use topical antiseptics (e.g., povidone-iodine, iodorphor, sodium hypochlorite [Dakin's solution], hydrogen peroxide, acetic acid) to reduce bacteria in wound tissue.

The only other topical preparations thought to hold promise in wound healing are growth factors and skin equivalents. Growth factors are not yet available outside controlled clinical trial settings. Both platelet-derived growth factor and fibroblast growth factor are being evaluated for use in wound healing. More than 36 growth factors have been identified to date. It is possible that others will be found to have a role in wound healing as well.

Wound care products represent an $8 billion dollar industry in the United States [19]. The number and type of products are difficult to track. Hess [20] states that there are more than 2000 wound care products. The *1995 Wound Care Products Resource* [19] lists 980. To discuss them in detail is beyond the scope of this chapter. However, it is possible to describe the classifications of the wound dressings currently available as well as some of the factors to keep in mind when choosing a dressing.

There are two major classifications of wound dressings: nonocclusive and occlusive/semiocclusive. Nonocclusive dressings allow free exchange of gases between the wound surface and the atmosphere. Occlusive dressings do not allow the exchange of gases between the wound and the atmosphere. Semiocclusive dressings allow gases from the wound surface to diffuse through the dressing to the atmosphere.

Nonocclusive dressings include silk and gauze. Silk is commonly used over newly sutured wounds and donor sites because its small mesh weave causes it to not adhere to the wound surface to the same extent as gauze. Gauze is used primarily to cover surgical wounds. Its use as a acute wound covering is widespread. Surgical incisions are essentially closed wounds, biologically speaking, so within the first 24 hours there is little likelihood of an external dressing serving as anything more than a protection from mechanical trauma. Gauze is also used for mechanical wound debridement in a wet-to-dry form. The use of mechanical debridement is acceptable when other forms of debridement are not readily available. It is a nonselective method that removes both necrotic and nonnecrotic tissue from a wound. If wet-to-dry debridement is ordered, the nurse should be sure that it is performed properly, because frequently it is not. The correct way to perform wet-to-dry debridement is to saturate unfilled 4×4 cotton dressings with sterile isotonic saline and wring them out so that they are moist but not dripping. They are then lightly packed into the wound and allowed to remain until they dry

out. When dry they are pulled off the wound surface to which they had adhered. When the gauze is removed, it debrides the necrotic tissue in the wound, but it also pulls off normal tissue. Other methods of debridement—surgical, conservative sharp, enzymatic, and autolytic—do not share this shortcoming.

Surgical debridement is the method of choice for removing *adherent* necrotic tissue from the pressure ulcer wound bed. It is also the method of choice for management of the patient with risks that directly affect the wound, such as blood clotting problems or infections. Surgical debridement is usually performed by a surgeon in the operating room. Its disadvantages include the necessity for anesthesia, the cost of the procedure, and the fact that it is not available to patients in nursing home and home care settings.

Laser debridement is a more recent technique used by surgeons to removed adherent necrotic tissue. Its use allows for immediate hemostasis, which cuts blood loss and allows minimal dissection of viable tissue. In the hands of a surgeon trained in its use, it is a very safe and effective technique. Its disadvantages are the same as those for surgical debridement.

Conservative sharp debridement is used to remove *loosely adherent* necrotic tissue. Such debridement usually takes place without causing pain and bleeding. Conservative sharp debridement can be performed by professional nurses if the provisions of the Nurse Practice Act in their state allow it. Only nurses who have had instruction in sharp debridement through an approved continuing education course, or who have received this training in accredited ET programs or wound management specialty courses, are legally able to perform the technique. Nurses wishing to perform conservative sharp debridement should be certain that their Nurse Practice Act, their employing agency, and the patient's physician allow it, and that they are adequately prepared to perform it (WOCN News [21]). The disadvantages of conservative sharp debridement are few. It takes longer than surgical debridement to create a clean wound, and it may be uncomfortable for the patient.

Enzymatic debridement is a chemical method of ridding the wound of necrotic, devitalized tissue.

When applied to the wound surface, enzymatic agents proteolytically debride the wound. These agents have varying properties. Some products are supposed to be able to moisturize the wound surface and help to revascularize it. They may be used in both infected and noninfected wounds. They may also be used in pressure ulcers from stage I to stage IV, depending on the product. The nurse should always follow the product insert directions carefully. For activation of the enzyme, a moist wound environment is needed. If there is dry eschar, it must be crosshatched with a scalpel prior to applying the enzyme. These agents may be used in hospital, nursing home, and home settings; however, their use requires a physician's order. Their disadvantage is that they can cause burning, and they take longer than sharp debridement to achieve a satisfactory result. They are also expensive.

Autolytic debridement is a natural process of debridement that the body is able to mount if there is necrotic tissue present. It is literally the self-digestion that occurs in tissues or cells by enzymes in the cells themselves, even after death and in the absence of putrefactive bacteria. Occlusive dressings provide an environment conducive to this type of debridement. The disadvantage is that the process is slow. If there is a large amount of necrotic tissue in the wound, autolysis is not satisfactory. Infection may occur before the process is completed.

Occlusive dressings have various properties and different indications for use. The chief property of these dressings as opposed to nonocclusive dressings is that they can control the wound's tissue hydration and oxygen tension. Examples of occlusive and semiocclusive dressings are nonadherent dressings, polyurethane film dressings, polyurethane foams, hydrocolloids, hydrogels, absorptive products (calcium alginates, hypertonic saline dressings, absorptive powders, pastes, beads, and granules), and impregnated dressings.

The advantages of occlusive dressings include protection from bacterial invasion; promotion of more rapid healing by keeping the wound surface moist and allowing more rapid epithelization, debridement of necrotic material, reduction of pain by reducing drying and by insulating and protecting sensitive nerve endings in the wound that may be

exposed, waterproof protection to the wound surface. They also require fewer dressing changes than nonocclusive dressings, and offer ease of use for nursing and medical personnel.

There are some disadvantages to the use of occlusive dressings. They should not be used on infected wounds because anaerobic organisms proliferate well in occlusive environments. Some occlusive dressings are opaque or semiopaque and make the wound surface difficult or impossible to monitor. This means that infection can develop without the nurse's knowledge. Such a "silent infection" does not become evident initially and may manifest first with systemic symptoms such as fever. Infection should be strongly suspected, however, in the elderly patient who becomes lethargic, loses his/her appetite, and manifests confusion for no other apparent reason. Many occlusive dressings cannot handle large amounts of wound drainage and will leak. Special occlusive dressings such as pouches or absorptive products must be used for this purpose. Some occlusive dressings may stick to new tissue that forms on the wound surface and will disrupt it when they are removed. Folliculitis (inflammation around the hair shafts) can occur with some adhesive-type occlusive dressings.

Types of occlusive/semiocclusive dressings include:

1. **Nonadherent dressings.** Do not stick to the wound surface under ordinary circumstances. They are semipermeable. Useful for treating skin tears, donor sites, skin grafts, and wounds where the skin around the wound is friable. They have very little absorptive ability. They are applied to the wound surface and held in place by conforming roller gauze or by tubular bandage. Examples are Telfa pads and nonadhesive film dressings.

2. **Polyurethane film dressings (transparent films).** Adhesive, semipermeable, and transparent. They allow passage of oxygen from the atmosphere and water vapor from the wound surface to vent to the atmosphere. The pores of the dressing are small enough to prevent bacteria or atmospheric particles from penetrating to the wound from the environment. They may be used to protect superficial wounds, I.V. sites, donor sites, abrasions, and certain other wounds. These films maintain a moist wound environment that pro-

motes granulation tissue formation and the body's autolysis of necrotic tissue. The film dressings do not have absorptive properties, and normal wound fluid builds up under them quickly. They are prone to leak if wound fluids are allowed to collect. Examples are OpSite, Tegaderm, and Bi-occlusive.

3. **Polyurethane foams.** Semipermeable dressings that are both nonadhesive and nonadherent. They may be either hydrophilic (absorb fluids) or hydrophobic (do not absorb fluids). Most are moderately fluid absorptive. They create a moist wound environment and provide thermal insulation of the wound. They are designed for use with pressure ulcers, stasis ulcers, certain types of small burns, donor graft sites, postoperative incisions, and moderately exudative wounds. They may be used as a secondary dressing for wounds with packing. At least two brands add a layer of activated carbon to the dressing in order to help control wound odor. Examples are Allevyn, Epi-Lock, Lyofoam, and Odor Absorbent Dressing.

4. **Hydrocolloids.** Dressings composed of an outer polyurethane layer that covers an inner layer composed of gum-like materials such as guar, karaya, gelatin, or pectin. They protect the wound mechanically from injury; they prevent bacteria from entering the wound; they maintain a moist wound healing environment; and they can be shaped to conform and seal to hard-to-cover parts of the body such as heels, elbows, knees, and sacrum. They thermally insulate the wound. The inner layer *normally* liquefies over the wound surface. The yellowish mass is thick, smelly, and may be difficult to remove completely. However, this can be accomplished with isotonic saline irrigations if it is necessary to see the total wound surface. If another dressing is going to be applied and there is no indication of wound deterioration/infection, then *complete* removal of the gelatinous mass is not necessary. These dressings may be used for a variety of wounds, both acute and chronic, such as partial-thickness wounds, wounds with necrosis or slough, and wounds with light to moderate exudate. They are not indicated in infected wounds because anaerobic organisms will proliferate under them. They encourage the body's autolytic process and, therefore, encourage wound debridement. Examples are Duo-Derm, Restore, Tegasorb, and Comfeel.

5. **Hydrogels.** Water- or glycerin-based amorphous gels, impregnated gauze, or sheet dressings. They may be adhesive or nonadhesive. Most can be used in both clean and infected wounds. They do not have strong adherent properties and require that an appropriate secondary dressing also be used to hold the hydrogel in place. These dressings contain a large amount of water (80–99%). They cool and soothe the wound surface by up to 5 degrees. They are transparent, so the wound can be easily observed. They are not recommended for wounds with much exudate. If used alone, they do not keep bacteria out of the wound. The frequency for dressing change is every one to two days. They are used on partial- and full-thickness wounds and deep wounds with light exudate. They are absorptive, but the rate of absorption is low. They are useful in treating wounds of persons with sensitive skin and in those with significant inflammation where cooling helps to relieve pain and discomfort. Examples are Biolex, NuGel, and Vigilon.

6. **Absorptive products.** Dressings such as calcium alginates and hypertonic saline; absorptive powders, pastes, beads, and granules. Calcium alginates are the newest of these products. Made from brown seaweed, they have a very high ability to absorb wound exudate, help to reduce wound odor, and activate macrophages in the wound. They may be used on partial- and full-thickness wounds with moderate to heavy exudate, wounds with tunneling or sinus tracts, wounds with necrotic tissue and exudate, and both noninfected and infected wounds. They should not be used on wounds with little drainage because they can absorb up to 20 times their own weight in fluid. They will dehydrate the wound bed in a minimally wet wound. Examples are Algosteril, DermaSORB, Kaltostat, and Sorbsan.

Hypertonic saline-impregnated gauze dressings have the ability to "wick" away wound exudate and yet leave a moist environment at the wound surface. Example: Mesalt.

The powders, pastes, beads, and granules differ somewhat in their individual properties. Most absorb wound exudate by drawing fluid away from the wound surface through osmosis. Some can digest necrotic tissue. In general, they form a gelatinous mass when the wound exudate is absorbed. The mass can be irrigated out of the wound with isotonic saline. The major use of all absorptive products is to control the wound exudate in heavily draining wounds. As a class of products, the powders, pastes, beads, and granules are not without problems. Patients may experience local stinging and pain when applied; some can raise the wound pH above normal levels; one has been reported to cause granulomas if not washed thoroughly out of the wound. Examples of these products include: Allevyn Cavity Wound Dressing, Bard Absorption Dressing, Debrisan, Comfeel paste or powder, DuoDerm paste or granules.

7. **Impregnated dressings.** Gauze dressings that are impregnated with antibacterial or bactericidal compounds such as scarlet red, Vaseline, and Xeroflo. Such medicated dressings, designed to be placed directly on the wound, are not without a negative side. They may help to control the bacterial population of the wound, but at the same time exert cytotoxic effects on healing cells. The fibroblast is especially vulnerable to their chemical reactivity.

This brief overview of dressing products can be supplemented by consulting any of the following lists of wound products available: *1995 Wound Care Products Resource* [19], *Nurse's Clinical Guide: Wound Care* [20], Wound care products: A directory [22], or Wound care products [23]. The first of these lists [19] is updated annually and is available through *Advances in Wound Care*.

The AHCPR [6] recommends the following wound dressing guidelines:

- Use a dressing that will keep the ulcer bed continuously moist. Wet-to-dry dressings should be used only for debridement and are not considered continuously moist saline dressings.
- Use clinical judgement to select a type of moist wound dressing suitable for the ulcer. Studies of different types of moist wound dressings showed no differences in pressure ulcer healing outcomes.
- Choose a dressing that keeps the surrounding intact (periulcer) skin dry while keeping the ulcer bed moist.
- Choose a dressing that controls exudate but does not desiccate the ulcer bed.
- Consider caregiver time when selecting a dressing.
- Eliminate wound dead space by loosely filling all cavities with dressing material. Avoid overpacking the wound.
- Monitor dressings applied near the anus, since they are difficult to keep intact.

Pressure reduction/relief devices are usually discussed under prevention of pressure ulcers and will not be discussed here in detail. It is important to remember, however, that patients with pressure ulcers have already proven their high risk. Therefore, they should be placed on an appropriate support surface designed to reduce interface pressure to a level less than capillary closing pressure, which has been generally accepted as 32 mm Hg [24]. This is an arbitrary figure based on research with young, healthy male volunteers. It is highly likely that elderly and/or debilitated patients have capillary closing pressures much lower than this. Capillary closing pressures as low as 12 mm Hg have been reported in the elderly (Krouskop et al. [25].

AHCPR [4, 6] recommendations on support surfaces are as follows:

1. Any individual in bed who is assessed to be at risk for developing pressure ulcers should be repositioned at least every 2 hours if consistent with overall patient goals. A written schedule for systematically turning and repositioning the individual should be used.

2. For individuals in bed, positioning devices such as pillows or foam wedges should be used to keep bony prominences (for example, knees or ankles) from direct contact with one another, according to a written plan.

3. Individuals in bed who are completely immobile should have a care plan that includes the use of devices that totally relieve pressure on the heels, most commonly by raising the heels off the bed. Do not use donut-type devices.

4. When the side-lying position is used in bed, avoid positioning directly on the trochanter.

5. Maintain the head of the bed at the lowest degree of elevation consistent with medical conditions and other restrictions. Limit the amount of time the head of the bed is elevated.

6. Use lifting devices such as a trapeze or bed linen to move (rather than drag) individuals in bed who cannot assist during transfers and position changes.

7. Any individual assessed to be at risk for developing pressure ulcers should be placed when lying in bed on a pressure-reducing device, such as foam, static air, alternating air, gel, or water mattresses.

Use a static support surface if a patient can assume a variety of positions without bearing weight on a pressure ulcer and without "bottoming out."

Use a dynamic support surface if the patient cannot assume a variety of positions without bearing weight on a pressure ulcer, if the patient fully compresses the static support surface, or if the pressure ulcer does not show evidence of healing.

If a patient has large stage III or IV pressure ulcers on multiple turning surfaces, a low-air-loss bed or an air-fluidized bed may be indicated.

When excess moisture on intact skin is a potential source of maceration and skin breakdown, a support surface that provides airflow can be important in drying the skin and preventing additional pressure ulcers.

Pressure ulcers seldom exist in patients who are not suffering from other chronic health problems and debilitation. Prudent care of the patient with a pressure ulcer therefore requires a health care team approach. Those members with special knowledge and skills that are often vital to successful treatment are the physician, nurse, nutritionist, clinical pharmacist, and physical therapist. A team planning approach is essential. The physician determines the goals of medical treatment. He/she decides the treatment plan for both the pressure ulcer wound(s) and the other medical conditions present. If the patient is not to be treated with curative intent, as might be the case with a terminal condition, then the medical plan might be to keep the patient comfortable and turn infrequently. The professional nurse is responsible for planning the daily care of the patient and the wound and for assisting in the determination of a proper support surface. The wound care regimen includes cleansing the wound, assessing it for healing or deterioration, performing conservative sharp debridement (in some states), applying ordered topical medications, and applying dressing. The nurse is further responsible for assessing and managing the nursing care of the patient's general condition and keeping the physician apprised of any changes. The nutritionist determines the dietary treatment indicated, provides the nutrients in a form that can be used by the patient, assesses the adequacy of nutrition, and changes the dietary management if indicated. The clinical pharmacist evaluates the drug therapy needed for successful wound management and recommends

changes if wound healing does not take place within a reasonable time frame (usually two to four weeks). The physical therapist in some states may perform sharp debridement of the wound, provide whirlpool treatments, dress the wound following the treatments, and help with positioning and transfer activities. All of these professionals are needed if optimum treatment of the wound is to be obtained.

ESTABLISHMENT OF NURSING DIAGNOSES RELEVANT TO PRESSURE ULCER MANAGEMENT

The establishment of appropriate nursing diagnoses is essential to the formulation of the nursing care plan for the patient with pressure ulcers. The first step is to obtain a careful nursing history and physical examination. Such an assessment is basic to making informed nursing diagnoses, planning care, administering the care necessary for successful intervention, and evaluating of its effectiveness.

A number of nursing diagnoses have relevance for the patient with established pressure ulcers, whereas others relate to the patient's general physical condition and medical diagnoses. This discussion will be limited to those diagnoses that have a direct bearing on the pressure ulcer itself.

"Impaired skin integrity" [31] is the primary nursing diagnosis for the patient with a partial-thickness pressure ulcer. This is appropriate only for the patient with a stage I or stage II pressure ulcer that is caused primarily by friction. If the pressure ulcer appears as a deeply reddened lesion that involves all layers of the unbroken skin, it is likely to be an incipient stage III or IV ulcer. These are truly *pressure* lesions and involve deeper tissue layers than do the superficial friction-induced skin problems. However, the nurse cannot make this determination until breakdown occurs. Therefore, the diagnosis is still "impaired skin integrity."

"Impaired tissue integrity" [31] is the primary nursing diagnosis for the patient with a full-thickness pressure ulcer. These wounds are of stage III or IV depth. By definition, they involve skin and subcutaneous tissue, and may involve fascia, muscle, and bone. Related factors (those that place the patient at risk for this diagnosis) are unrelieved pressure; friction and shear; impaired physical mobility from paralysis, loss of consciousness, muscle weakness, neurological impairment, depression and/or medications; fluid deficit/excess; altered circulation; nutritional deficit; prolonged surgical procedures; incontinence; and knowledge deficit.

There are a number of nursing diagnoses that are related to the preceding two [31] primary ones. These are:

1. **Potential for infection.** Any chronic wound is at risk for this. All such wounds are colonized with bacteria; therefore, any deterioration in the patient's condition or breakdown in the standard of wound care by personnel allows the bacterial burden to increase to a level that can result in wound infection.

2. **Potential impaired skin integrity.** If the patient has a pressure ulcer or ulcers, the nurse can anticipate that other unbroken areas of the skin are also at risk.

3. **Impaired physical mobility.** If the patient is unable to move without assistance, then the likelihood of unrelieved pressure on weight-bearing surfaces is greatly increased.

4. **Altered tissue perfusion.** Pressure impedes the circulation through the body parts that are weight bearing while the patient is in the bed or chair.

5. **Decreased cardiac output.** Pressure ulcers are demonstrated to occur with frequency in patients who have cardiac problems that compromise circulation and become an additive factor when coupled with prolonged pressure on weight-bearing surfaces.

6. **Altered nutrition.** If the patient is in a state of poor or malnutrition and has low albumin levels (< 3.5), this plays a part in changing the ability of the tissues to withstand pressure.

7. **Body image disturbance.** If the patient is conscious, he/she is aware of the cosmetic alteration produced by the skin wounds that may yield a long-term unsightly result. Some of these wounds involve joints which may result in alterations in gait or other movements.

8. **Anxiety.** The patient may feel that the wound means that he/she is getting worse or will not get well or will die.

9. **Bowel incontinence.** A common occurrence with pressure ulcers that develop in the buttocks area. It contributes its effects by maceration, enzymatic activity, and bacteria.

10. **Total incontinence.** The patient with both urine and bowel incontinence is at risk for the reasons cited in 9. Also, when urine and stool mix, ammonia is created from stool bacterial action on urea. Ammonia changes the pH of skin from acid to alkaline and, thereby, destroys part of its protective barrier function.

11. **Fluid volume deficit.** The dehydrated patient will have dry skin that cracks; this opens the way for further breakdown to occur.

12. **Fluid volume excess.** The patient with edema has greater difficulty in oxygenating the cells because of perfusion problems.

13. **Potential for injury.** The patient confined to bed and chair is at risk because of limited mobility, because his sensorium may be affected, and because of his other medical conditions.

14. **Ineffective family coping: compromised.** The management of these chronic wounds may be too much for family caregivers to physically, emotionally, and/or financially handle.

15. **Sensory alterations.** If the patient is comatose or otherwise unaware of his surroundings, he has no perception of the discomfort that results from unrelieved pressure, and there is loss of the impetus to change position. The paralyzed patient is unable to perceive pain and loses impetus to move as a result of discomfort.

16. **Pain.** Unrelieved pressure activates pain receptors to the extent that discomfort is the first sensation felt. This is followed by pain if the duration of pressure is beyond that of tissue tolerance. The patient who has a pressure ulcer has a *wound*. Wounds are usually painful. If the patient is conscious, he should be questioned about the presence and nature of the pain so that appropriate management can be implemented. If he is confused but restless, it is possible that pain is the cause.

17. **Knowledge deficit.** Patients who are paralyzed must be taught to move at intervals in order to prevent skin breakdown. Patients who are conscious and able to move may be at risk if they are on medications that interfere with their perception of discomfort (narcotics, analgesics, soporifics). They should be reminded to move at intervals. Family members should be taught

wound management techniques and taught how to prevent further skin and soft tissue breakdown.

When the nursing diagnoses have been made, then planning of care can be done. This planning is dependent on many factors. Is the patient condition stable or unstable and progressive? Is it terminal? The nursing care must take into consideration priority of the patient's needs and safety as well as the goals of medical therapy. Therefore, the nursing care plan should include measures to (1) prevent further tissue damage, such as turning at regular intervals and placing the patient on special support surfaces if indicated, (2) provide wound care designed to prevent infection by careful cleansing and application of appropriate dressings, (3) prevent injury to other body systems by turning, coughing, and deep breathing the patient, observing safety precautions, etc., (4) promote patient comfort by giving pain medication if needed and by positioning, (5) promote nutrition through consultation with a nutritionist and ensuring that the recommendations are implemented, (6) control incontinence problems, (7) educate the patient and/or family about how to prevent further tissue damage and how to promote tissue healing, (8) promote rehabilitation to the extent possible, (9) promote attainment of patient independence if possible, (10) assist patient, family, or friends to attain skills necessary for safe wound care after patient is discharged.

Evaluation of the effectiveness of care planning and its implementation is dependent upon setting specific outcome criteria whose achievement by the patient/family is evidence of the plan's success. The following outcome criteria are such indicators for the patient treated with curative intent:

1. The patient will achieve normal wound healing as evidenced by a continued decrease in size of the wound, absence of drainage, absence of temperature elevation, decrease in discomfort, and improvement in subjective sense of well-being.

2. The patient will achieve acceptable nutritional status as evidenced by normal skin turgor, weight within normal range for body build and height, and progression of wound healing. (Laboratory results such as serum albumin and lymphocyte count should be monitored if available).

3. The patient will progress toward attainment of preinjury status as evidenced by improvement in strength, nutritional status, ability to perform activities of daily living, and increasing participation in his own care.

4. The patient or family member will perform correct wound care techniques as demonstrated by his primary nurse prior to discharge to the home setting.

5. The patient or family member will state the signs and symptoms of wound complications such as redness around the wound, pain, swelling, fever, and drainage and will understand the need to report them to the health care provider should they occur.

6. The patient and/or family member will verbalize all discharge instructions about the wound correctly.

Many factors influence the nature of the nursing care plan. Most are familiar to those accustomed to planning nursing care such as patient need, nature of the care setting (hospital, skilled care, home), skill level of the nursing personnel responsible for wound care, and the type of wound, its treatment, and its closure. Other considerations are not as familiar to care planners although they may have significant impact on the care that will be delivered. Chief among these in today's health care environment is economics. Consideration must now be given to formulating a plan that will return the patient to the home situation as rapidly as possible. This means that essential safe care is the priority for the patient rather than optimum care. It means that professional nurses must be conversant with reimbursement policies that drive agency decisions about employment of personnel and purchases of equipment and supplies with which to provide care. These reimbursement policies have a direct effect on the length of patient stay and, therefore, on the kind of care that can be planned and provided. Some reimbursement policies are setting-specific such as wound dressings. Patients in the hospital have more latitude in the types of dressings that can be used to treat their wounds. In the nursing home and home care settings, however, there are very specific guidelines designed to prevent the unnecessary use of costly dressings. This may mean that the best product for wound care is not reimbursable under all circumstances in these settings.

A second major variable in nursing care planning is that of the goal of medical therapy. Nurses are attuned to a medical therapy plan that treats with curative intent or that seeks to maintain the patient's present health level if cure is not realistic. In terminally ill patients neither of these goals is appropriate or possible. Planning nursing care in the terminally ill means that aggressive measures to prevent a worsening of the patient's wound are not indicated. For example, turning every two hours is not indicated in a patient for whom movement is agonizing. The National Pressure Ulcer Advisory Panel states that "pressure ulcers can be an indication of the multi-system failure that accompanies the terminal stages of many disease processes. In these cases, patient comfort should be the primary goal." (NPUAP [26]).

IMPACT OF FEDERAL/STATE POLICIES/ GUIDELINES ON PRESSURE ULCER MANAGEMENT

The United States government influences pressure ulcer care in several ways—some indirect and some direct. An example of each will be given. In 1986 the Omnibus Budget Reconciliation Act (OBRA) called for the Secretary of Health and Human Services to develop a uniform needs assessment instrument with which national data about all Medicare patients in all health care facilities could be collected. In 1989 the needs assessment instrument was ready for use. It included pressure ulcer data. The use of this instrument will provide a data bank for tracking national pressure ulcer cost and prevalence (Maklebust and Sieggreen [27].)

OBRA also created the Agency for Health Care Policy and Research (AHCPR) in 1989 to "enhance the quality, appropriateness, and effectiveness of health care services and access to these services." (AHCPR [4].) The AHCPR set about the issuance of clinical practice guidelines. One of the areas chosen for guideline development was pressure ulcers. In 1992 *Pressure Ulcers in Adults: Prediction and Prevention* was published, followed by *Treat-*

ment of Pressure Ulcers in 1994. These booklets were issued to "assist practitioners in the prevention, diagnosis, treatment, and management of clinical conditions." (AHCPR [4, 6], inside cover.) The intent was that they be *guidelines*, not standards, because it was felt that there was too little scientific data to serve as a basis for standard setting. They were to be an indirect means of influencing care.

Soon after the publication of the AHCPR guidelines, some state regulatory bodies that oversee the operation of skilled nursing care facilities began to use the guidelines to develop criteria for a standard of care. Health care attorneys also began using these publications as the basis for their contention that minimum safe care had or had not been provided to patients who developed pressure ulcers. These are good examples of governmental guidelines being used for purposes other than that for which they were developed.

A federal program that directly impacts pressure ulcer management is Medicare. The Medicare program was established by Title XVIII of the Social Security Act of 1965. Medicare Part A pays for patient services rendered by a hospital, skilled nursing facility, home health agency, and hospice. Part B covers physician's bills, outpatient care, durable medical equipment, prosthetics, and orthotics. With the advent of Medicare coverage, reimbursement for wound care outside the hospital became possible for many elderly patients with chronic wounds. However, it soon became obvious that the approximately 6 million people with chronic wounds in the United States (Wound Ostomy Continence Nursing [28]) were not sufficiently covered.

The Medicare policy for wound care outside the hospital was limited. It paid for *up to two weeks* of surgical wound costs under the following conditions: the wound must have first been surgically debrided by an M.D., and the covered dressing had to be one that actually touched the wound. The patient had to pay for any other supplies—reinforcing dressings, compression dressings, tape, etc. If dressings were needed after two weeks then the patient had to pay *all costs of all supplies*.

By 1992, it had become increasingly obvious that the Medicare wound care provision was too restrictive to allow for the proper handling of a wide variety of chronic wounds. This was true because chronic wounds rarely heal within two weeks, surgical debridement by an M.D. is not always required and is not always available, and many combinations of dressings are used today that did not exist five years ago.

Numerous organizations concerned with wound care became increasingly troubled by Medicare restrictions on wound care outside the hospital setting. They began to lobby to have the *Medicare Carrier's Manual* changed with respect to Section 2079, Surgical Dressings, and Splints, Casts, and Other Devices Used For Reductions of Fractures and Dislocations. The lobbying groups represented caregivers, care sites, and manufacturers of wound care equipment and products. Organizations included in the effort to get Section 2079 changed were the National Pressure Ulcer Advisory Panel, the Wound Ostomy Continence Nurses Society, the National Coalition for Wound Care, the American Health Care Association, the American Society of Consulting Pharmacists, the Council of Nursing Home Suppliers, the Health Industry Manufacturers Association (HIMA), the National Association of Medical Equipment Suppliers, the National Association of Retail Druggists, and the National Association for the Support of Long Term Care.

On March 31, 1994, the revised Section 2079 was issued by the Health Care Financing Administration (HCFA). The new policy provided for coverage of both primary and secondary dressings for surgical wounds for as long as needed by the patient (a pressure ulcer can be considered a surgical wound if debridement has been performed). It also allowed nurses and certain other health care providers to perform various kinds of debridement if medically necessary and if within the scope of the health care provider's legal practice as defined by the state. It further recognized surgical dressing orders from nurses with prescriptive privileges.

After HCFA revised Section 2079, the Durable Medical Equipment Regional Carriers (DMERC), consisting of four regional carriers,* were charged by HCFA to develop and implement policies to guide the use of Section 2079. These policies are issued by each of the four DMERCs and input is still continuing to make them more responsive to patient care needs.

The direct impact of Section 2079 on pressure ulcer management can best be appreciated when one realizes that reimbursement for wound care will not take place unless its provisions are adhered to carefully. Other nongovernmental payers such as private insurers may adopt different policies, but the $161.5 billion Medicare program (fiscal 1994 expenditures) will dominate what is done for the bulk of the 6 million chronic wound sufferers in the United States.

Nurses must be aware of these federal policies as well as those of their own state. These policies will have relevance for (1) ensuring that minimal standards of care for the pressure ulcer patient are being met, (2) ensuring that the care of the pressure ulcer is adequately documented, (3) ensuring that progress or lack of progress in wound healing is carefully documented, (4) justifying the need to change the wound management protocol, and (5) guiding a decision about when the patient needs the services of a physician.

PREVENTION OF AVOIDABLE PRESSURE ULCER LITIGATION

It has been estimated by the RAND corporation that about 1 in 30 people who suffer injury go to court (Asseo [29]). The American Tort Reform Association, citing a 1992 actuarial study, says that such lawsuits cost 2.3% of the gross domestic prod-

---

*Region A: Connecticut, Delaware, Maine, Massachusetts, New Hampshire, New Jersey, New York, Pennsylvania, Rhode Island, Vermont

Region B: District of Columbia, Illinois, Indiana, Maryland, Michigan, Minnesota, Ohio, Virginia, West Virginia, Wisconsin

Region C: Alabama, Arkansas, Colorado, Florida, Georgia, Kentucky, Louisiana, Mississippi, New Mexico, North Carolina, Oklahoma, Puerto Rico, South Carolina, Tennessee, Texas, Virgin Islands

Region D: Alaska, Arizona, California, Guam, Hawaii, Idaho, Iowa, Kansas, Missouri, Montana, Nebraska, Nevada, North Dakota, Oregon, South Dakota, Utah, Washington, Wyoming

uct. Pressure ulcers are responsible for many of the health-related cases that are litigated each year. Because pressure ulcers occur with such frequency in patients with chronic health problems (Miller and Delozier [30] estimate that the national cost for pressure ulcer treatment in the United States is greater than $1.335 billion), all agencies that provide nursing care should be concerned with teaching personnel how to both provide and document a safe standard of prevention and management.

The first step in minimizing litigation risk is to ensure that all personnel involved in giving pressure ulcer care have been adequately in-serviced on a regular basis on safe prevention and management of these wounds. Testing personnel on the contents of the in-service with a minimum cutoff point helps to ensure that no one gives care who does not possess a minimum knowledge base. The agency should keep records of this in-service. All newly hired personnel should be provided in-service about pressure ulcers at the time of hiring and/or should be required to test out of the in-service with a minimum acceptable test score. Yearly programs are recommended because of the speed with which new products are developed and new federal/state regulations occur affecting pressure ulcer care.

Comprehensive records cannot prevent litigation, but they certainly aid in showing whether care rendered met the standard of nursing care expected in the community. Charting should include the following information:

1. It should be stated whether or not the wound was present on admission to the hospital or other agency. This can only be ascertained if a head-to-toe inspection of the skin is done by the professional nurse on admission. If there is no skin problem this should be documented. A patient risk assessment should be done and recorded and appropriate preventive measures begun. If there is redness that does not blanch 30 minutes after finger pressure is removed, it should be recorded as a stage I pressure ulcer *and it should be carefully described*. There are two types of stage I pressure ulcers, as has already been described in the section on Pressure Ulcer Assessment. One is much less serious than the other. If the redness is adequately described, then when breakdown occurs, documentation will show that damage occurred prior to admission.

2. If the pressure ulcer was present on admission, a history of the wound should be obtained. How did it start? How long has it been present? If this is not known, record that the information is not known and why it is not known. Record whether any preventive devices were in use prior to admission; e.g., egg crate mattress.

3. All existent wounds should be described in detail. If the agency policies allow, color photograph(s) of the wound(s) at the time of admission to care should be made and attached to the record. Photographs documenting wound healing or deterioration should be made at regular intervals with detailed descriptions in the Nurses Notes that specifically explain reasons for wound deterioration if known. All photographs in all cases should be made with the same type of camera, the same type of film, and under standard conditions of lighting and distance. The specific location of the wound using anatomic reference points should be given; e.g., "on the (L) buttock over the ischial tuberosity," not "on the (L) buttock." The wound measurements, surface dimensions, depth, and presence of tunneling, sinus tracts, and dead space should be carefully noted, as well as the presence or absence of necrotic tissue and/or drainage, periwound skin condition, and any systemic signs of infection. This should be documented at regular intervals.

4. Pressure ulcers should be staged using the staging system given in the section on Pressure Ulcer Assessment. The agency in-service should ensure that personnel are able to use the staging system correctly.

5. The patient's state of nutrition with respect to skin turgor, height/weight ratio, food and fluid intake, and increased metabolic demands from fever should be recorded. If the patient is in a hospital setting, check laboratory results for albumin and serum lymphocyte levels. If the patient is in the nursing home or the home setting, these data are more difficult to obtain. It is important to take periodic albumin values in these settings.

ROLE OF THE ACUTE CARE NURSE PRACTITIONER/CLINICAL NURSE SPECIALIST IN THE MANAGEMENT OF THE PRESSURE ULCER PROBLEM

This chapter has been devoted to an explanation of nursing management of an individual patient with pressure ulcers. It is obviously in the best interests of patient, health care provider, and agency to prevent these skin wounds whenever possible. To this end, the advanced practice nurse should be active in the development of policies and programs designed to minimize their occurrence and to manage effectively those pressure ulcers that do develop. This can be achieved by performing a carefully planned audit of the institutional prevalence of pressure ulcers to determine both the actual number of ulcers and whether certain units have more of a problem than others. Once that determination is made, steps should be taken to institute a quality assurance program. If the agency does not have a skin care team, it would be advisable to organize one and to then start pressure ulcer policy development. The skin care team can help to evaluate products designed for pressure ulcer prevention and/or management through well-structured clinical research projects. Education of health care personnel and formulation of teaching plans for the patient and family/significant others should be begun and monitored for effectiveness. Lastly, the acute care practitioner/clinical nurse specialist is in a particularly advantageous spot to both identify pressure ulcer problems that could benefit from clinical research studies and to help in the design and implementation of these studies.

REFERENCES

1. Fuhrer, M. J.; Rintala, D. H.; Hart, K. A.; Clearman, R.; and Young, M. E., Depressive symptomatology in persons with spinal cord injury who resided in the community, *Arch Phys Med Rehabil* 1993; 74(3):255–260.

2. Shannon, M. L., and Skorga, P., Pressure ulcer prevalence in two general hospitals, *Decubitus* 1989; 2(4):38–43.

3. Lewis, T., and Grant, R., Observations upon reactive hyperaemia in man, *Heart* (London) 1925; 12:73–120.

4. Panel for the Prediction and Prevention of Pressure Ulcers in Adults, *Pressure Ulcers in Adults: Prediction and Prevention*, Clinical Practice Guideline no. 3., AHCPR Publication no. 92-0047. Rockville, MD: Agency for Health Care Policy and Research,

Public Health Service, U.S. Department of Health and Human Services, May 1992.

5. Barr, J. E., Questions about staging, *Decubitus* 1993; 6(5):6,8,10.

6. Bergstrom, N.; Bennett, M. A.; Carlson, C. E.; et al., *Treatment of Pressure Ulcers*, Clinical Practice Guideline No. 15, Rockville, MD: U.S. Department of Health and Human Services, Public Health Service, Agency for Health Care Policy and Research, AHCPR Publication no. 95-0652. December 1994.

7. Bates-Jensen, B. M., New pressure ulcer status tool, *Decubitus* 1990; 3(3):14–15.

8. Bates-Jensen, B. M.; Vredevoe, D. L.; and Brecht, M. L., Validity and reliability of the pressure sore status tool, *Decubitus* 1992; 5(6):20–28.

9. Cooper, D. M., Wound assessment and evaluation of healing, in R. A. Bryant, ed., *Acute and Chronic Wounds: Nursing Management*. St. Louis: Mosby Yearbook, 1992:69–90.

10. Lazarus, G. S.; Cooper, D. M.; Knighton, D. R.; Margolis, D. J.; Pecoraro, R. E.; Rodeheaver, G.; and Robson, M. C., Definitions and guidelines for assessment of wounds and evaluation of healing, *Arch Derm* 1994; 130:489–493.

11. Ayello, E., Teaching the assessment of patients with pressure ulcers, *Decubitus* 1992; 5(7):53–54.

12. Rodeheaver, G., Controversies in topical wound management, *Ost Wound Mgmt* 1988; Fall:58–68.

13. Rutala, W. A., APIC guidelines for selection and use of disinfectants, *Am J Infect Control* 1990; 18(2):99–117.

14. Neiderhuber, S.; Stribley, R.; and Koepke, G., Reduction of skin bacterial load with use of therapeutic whirlpool, *Phys Ther* 1975; 55(5):482–486.

15. Bohannon, R. W., Whirlpool versus whirlpool rinse for removal of bacteria from a venous stasis ulcer, *Phys Ther* 1982; 62(3):304–308.

16. Ashford, R.; Plant, G.; Maher, J.; and Teares, L. Double-blind trial of metronidazole in malodorous ulcerating tumors, *Lancet* 1984; 2(8388):1232–1233.

17. Witkowski, J., and Parish, L., Topical metronidazole gel: The bacteriology of decubitus ulcers, *Inter J Dermatol* 1991; 30:660–661.

18. Poteete, V., Case study: Eliminating odors from wounds, *Decubitus* 1993; 6(4):43–46.

19. *1995 Wound Care Products Resource*, published by *Advances in Wound Care*. Magazine published by Springhouse in Springhouse, PA.

20. Hess, C. T., *Nurse's Clinical Guide: Wound Care*, Springhouse, PA: Springhouse Corporation, 1995:32.

21. Wound Debridement Task Force, WOCN position statement for conservative sharp wound debridement for registered nurses, *WOCN News* 1994; Aug/Sept:13–14.

22. Hess, C. T., Wound care products: A directory, *Ost Wound Mgmt* 1994; 40(3):70–94 passim.

23. Krasner, D., Wound care products, *Ost Wound Mgmt* 1991; 23:47–60.

24. Landis, E. M., Micro-injection studies of capillary blood pressure in human skin, *Heart* 1930; 15:209.

25. Krouskop, T. A.; Garber, S. L.; and Cullen, B. B., Factors to consider in selecting a support surface, In D. Krasner, ed., *Chronic Wound Care*, King of Prussia, PA: Health Management Publications, 1990:142–151.

26. National Pressure Ulcer Advisory Panel, *Statement on Pressure Ulcer Prevention*, Buffalo, NY: NPUAP, 1992:5.

27. Maklebust, J. A., and Sieggreen, M., *Pressure Ulcers: Guidelines for Prevention and Nursing Management*, West Dundee, IL:S-N Publications, 1991:175.

28. Wound Ostomy Continence Nursing (WOCN), *Wound Care Alert*, Spring, 1994.

29. Asseo, L., Notions of America awash in lawsuits, awards just folklore, some experts say, *Houston Post* March 8, 1995.

30. Miller, H., and Delozier, J., *Cost Implications of the Pressure Ulcer Treatment Guideline*, Columbia, MD: Center for Health Policy Studies, 1994, Contract no. 282-91-0070, 17p, sponsored by AHCPR.

31. North American Nursing Diagnosis Association, *Taxonomy I Revised*. St. Louis: NANDA, 1990.

14

THE DIABETIC FOOT: A COMPREHENSIVE APPROACH

Bok Y. Lee, M.D., V. J. Guerra, M.D., and Robert E. Madden, M.D.

INTRODUCTION

Diabetes mellitus is a disease characterized by hyperglycemia resulting from impaired insulin secretion and/or effectiveness. It is associated with risks for diabetic ketoacidosis or nonketotic hyperglycemia, hyperglycemic-hyperosmolar coma and a group of late complications including retinopathy, nephropathy, atherosclerotic coronary and peripheral arterial disease, and peripheral and autonomic neuropathies. Diabetes mellitus has diverse genetic, environmental, and pathogenic origins [1].

In the United States diabetes affects approximately 12 million people of all ages. The presence of infections in the diabetic foot is an especially important clinical problem because lower extremity infections are one of the most common reasons for hospital admission in the diabetic patient. Typically, diabetic patients with lower extremity infections are in their fifth decade, have had diabetes for approximately 18 years, and, although most are type II diabetics, they generally require insulin for blood glucose control. The average hospital stay for a diabetic with a foot infection is more than one month, with 44% of these patients being hospitalized for more than three months. This resulted in direct medical costs that exceeded $14 billion in 1988. New Jersey alone reported hospital costs of $19,670,000 for diabetics requiring amputation [2].

The hospital cost for amputations in the United States is probably about $1.2 billion, not including prostheses, rehabilitation, loss of income, and, frequently, lost jobs. Loss of family income as a result of patient death adds to these expenses. Without doubt, the problem of foot infections in the diabetic patient population is costly to both the patient and society. Consequently, health care expenditures and medical efforts must be directed at patient education, prevention, early detection, and prompt treatment of foot infections [2–4].

PHYSIOLOGY

Each day, during locomotion the feet are exposed to continuous pressures, and it is not surprising that foot infections are a frequent problem in the diabetic. The foot must not only support the body but must also absorb the impact forces of walking and running, adjust to uneven surfaces, provide leverage for propulsion, and accommodate the transverse rotational forces associated with knee and hip motions. A 150-pound, active individual takes more than 10,000 steps per day and distributes more than 120 tons of force between his two feet for every mile traveled. The foot must withstand a tremendous amount of repetitive compressive, torsional, and shear forces every day. The thickened epidermis and dermis situated on loculated fatty tissue of the plantar foot pad effectively cushion these high-stress impact forces. The normal plantar surface can be viewed as a specialized anatomic region that absorbs the impact forces of locomotion while protecting the underlying soft tissues and bony structures. Consequently, factors that lead to alterations of the normal transmission of the forces of locomotion or to loss of sensation, as may occur in the diabetic foot, clearly potentiate the risk of local tissue injury [5, 6].

PATHOPHYSIOLOGY

Diabetic foot infections often result in major (below- or above-knee) amputation. Although only 3% of diabetics are amputees, 50% of all nontraumatic major amputations of the lower extremities are performed on diabetics [7]. Previously, the natural history of the diabetic undergoing a below- or above-knee amputations was poor, with two-thirds of the patients in some series dying within five years of their amputation [8]. Therefore, attention must be directed toward understanding the pathophysiologic changes predisposing a diabetic patient to foot infections in order to prevent amputations and the subsequent poor prognosis. Ischemia and neuropathy are the major predisposing factors for the development of diabetic foot infections [7, 8].

In vitro and in vivo studies demonstrate increased tissue oxygen utilization during acute episodes of hyperglycemia [9, 10]. This phenomenon appears to be due to the preferential shunting of glucose through the sorbitol pathway instead of the glycolytic pathway, which results in decreased mitochondrial pyruvate utilization and decreased energy production. This process has been termed hyperglycemia-induced pseudohypoxia [10]. The oxidation-reduction imbalance can be seen in poorly controlled diabetics as well as in nondiabetics experiencing acute episodes of hyperglycemia lasting longer than four hours and is associated with elevated intracellular levels of fructose, sorbitol, and lactate. Increased levels of these metabolic products correlate with impaired neural, skeletal, and smooth muscle function, as well as increased capillary permeability. The potential clinical relevance of this event is that inhibitors of key enzymes of the sorbitol pathway (aldose reductase and sorbitol dehydrogenase) can limit neural, skeletal, and smooth muscle dysfunction in acute but not chronic hyperglycemia. This metabolic blockade of oxygen utilization in poorly controlled diabetics may explain why these patients experience a greater degree of tissue loss than nondiabetics after relatively mild ischemic episodes. These findings might also explain why diabetics are more prone to develop foot ulcerations than nondiabetics with comparable foot transcutaneous oxygen tensions. Additionally, the increased capillary permeability resulting from pseudohypoxia is believed to accelerate atherogenesis by allowing atherogenic proteins and fatty acids access to the subendothelial space. This metabolic information suggests that control of hyperglycemia is important in both the treatment of foot infection and the healing of ulcerations in the diabetic [9–11].

The wound healing abnormalities in patients with diabetes mellitus are the result of several factors. When carbohydrates are not available to cells for normal aerobic metabolism, oxidation of amino acids for caloric needs results in amino acid and protein depletion. When glycogenolysis and gluconeogenesis fail to provide glucose to meet the energy requirements for fibroblasts and leukocytes, they become dysfunctional, and impaired wound healing results. In addition, the impaired healing appears to be related not only to the abnormal glucose mechanism but also directly to insulin. It has been demonstrated that topical application of insulin improves skin healing in mice. Other studies have shown that uncontrolled diabetic rats exhibit improved wound healing with the administration of vitamin A [11]. Interestingly, hyperglycemia interferes with ascorbate transfer into fibroblasts and leukocytes, which also impairs the healing response. In fact, high ascorbate intake in rats increases collagen production in streptozotocin-induced diabetic rats [11].

Impaired fibroblast and endothelial cell proliferation, epithelization, decreased collagen deposition, and reduced collagen strength are also characteristics of these streptozotocin-induced diabetic animals. In diabetic animals, beta fibroblast growth factor (β-FGF) reduces the degree of impairment of wound healing. Experimentally, many of these effects can be reversed by insulin and good glucose regulation if achieved after wound healing [12]. Regarding increased susceptibility to infection, there has been a myriad of studies describing the poor inflammatory response in diabetic patients [13]. Abnormalities range from the inability of polymorphonuclear leukocytes to kill bacteria to T cell defects [13]. In clinical practice, this means one must be extraordinarily aggressive surgically, excising necrotic tissue and using broad spectrum antibiotics until the invasive organisms are identified; then appropriate antibiotic therapy should be given.

HYPERCOAGULABLE STATES

We have observed that a considerable number of diabetic patients who undergo surgery for either amputations or vascular reconstructive procedures experience a hypercoagulable state. Many patients who have received heparin, have a poor response to heparin or have rebound phenomenon. Unfortunately, the current available laboratory techniques used to determine the coagulation status or the adequacy of each patient's heparin effect are not ideal for ensuring the agent's efficacy and safety or the actual global status of the coagulation process. They are semiquantitative at best, and there are inherent errors in the accuracy and specificity of their results, such as those from thromboplastin time, activated clotting time, and thrombin clotting time. In addition, the lack of a readily available, direct chemical assay for measuring heparin concentrations has limited the collection of pharmacokinetic data. Therefore, most of the patients who are given heparin and are monitored using routine coagulation tests are in poor control.

We use the Surgical Analyzer, which is a hemostatic functional measurement instrument of the global coagulation process. The instrument uses an attached recorder to capture a continuous "signature" of the entire clotting process. Automated analysis shows the time of initial fibrin formation through fibrin gelation, full clot development, contraction, and lysis. The instrument is a useful tool for measuring clot formation, platelet function and anticoagulant effect. The instrument has an axially vibrating probe immersed to a controlled depth into a cuvette containing a small sample of blood. The viscous drag (viscous impedance) of the probe by the blood is sensed by the transducer. The electronic circuitry quantifies the drag as a change in electrical output. The signal is transmitted to a time-based strip chart recorder, which provides a "signature" of the clot formation, clot contraction, and clot lysis processes. Two values are obtained: (1) SonACT time (onset) is defined as the time for the first fibrin strands to form and is mediated by the extrinsic and intrinsic clotting mechanisms. SonAct time, normal value is 85–130 seconds. (2) Clot RATE is defined as the rate at which fibrin mass is generated and demonstrates the speed at which fibrinogen is being transformed to fibrin. The acceptable range of rate of nonheparinized samples is 15–35%. The "signature" also permits measurement of the clot retraction time, normal values are less than 30 minutes, and measures the platelet retraction process. The results obtained by the Surgical Analyzer have been compared to thromboelastography, which also evaluates the global hemodynamics of blood using three values. The direct-writing thromboelastograph is an instrument with a stylus that traces the thromboelastogram on heat-sensitive paper. The thromboelastogram is obtained by the oscillation of a cuvette containing 0.3 cc of blood. The thromboelastogram gives three main values: (a) reaction time (r-time), normal: 8–12 minutes; (b) k-time, normal: 4–8 minutes, and (c) maximum amplitude (ma), normal: 50 mm. We established normal values of the Surgical Analyzer in patients under general anesthesia (SonACT time 80–130, Clot RATE 15–40%) and then we measured the coagulation status in patients undergoing arterial reconstructive procedures with the thromboelastograph (Figure 14-1) and the Surgical Analyzer (Figure 14-2) in patients undergoing arterial reconstructive procedures.

We have found that the Surgical Analyzer provides: (1) improved hemostasis management in surgery, (2) reduced usage of donor blood products, (3) faster identification of surgical versus nonsurgical bleeders (results are obtained in 5–10 minutes), (4) accurate and inexpensive heparin anticoagulation management, and (5) quick and easy screening for

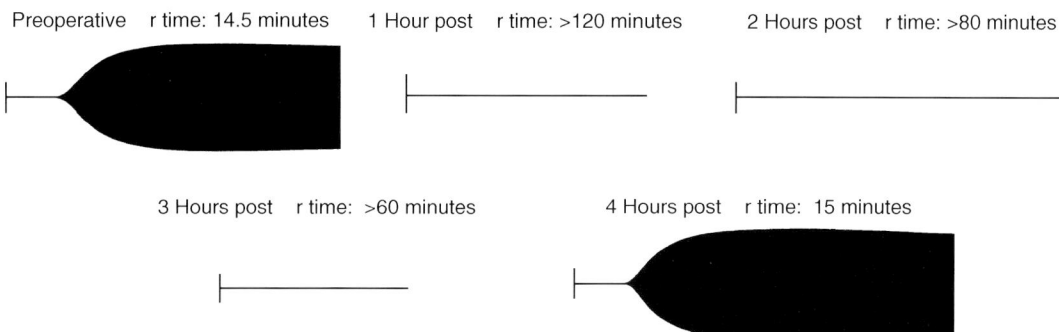

Heparin - 70 u/kg
Preoperative r time: 14.5 minutes
1 Hour post r time: >120 minutes
2 Hours post r time: >80 minutes
3 Hours post r time: >60 minutes
4 Hours post r time: 15 minutes

Figure 14-1. Thromboelastograph tracings of a patient undergoing a vascular reconstructive procedure. Baseline tracing showing a normal coagulation tracing. After bolus administration of 70 μ/kg of heparin there is straight line tracing at first hour and second hour showing anticoagulation effect. Third hour still depicting effect, and rebound phenomenon in the fourth hour.

Clot
Signal
Time (minutes)
100
90
80
70
60
50
40
30
20
10
0
0 2 4 6 8 10 12 14 16

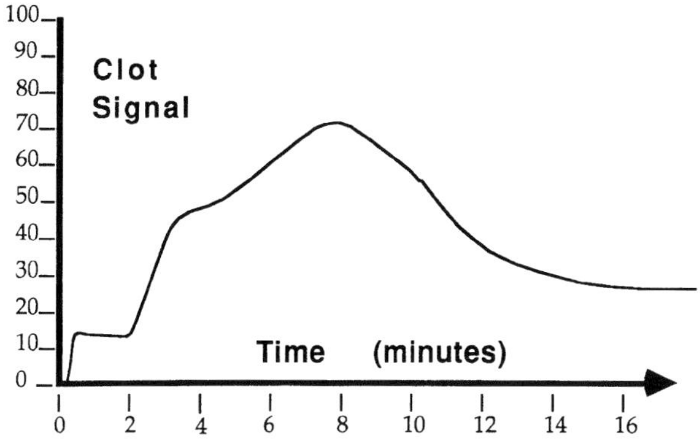

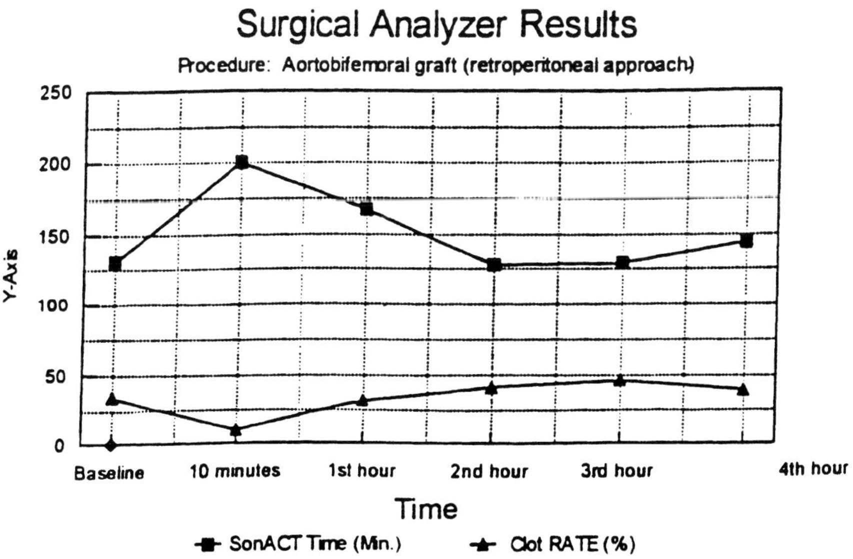

Surgical Analyzer Results
Procedure: Aortobifemoral graft (retroperitoneal approach)
Y-Axis
250
200
150
100
50
0
Baseline
10 minutes
1st hour
2nd hour
3rd hour
4th hour
Time
SonACT Time (Min.)
Clot RATE (%)

Figure 14-2. Surgical Analyzer Tracings. The first graphic shows a typical normal tracing and the results during arterial reconstructive procedure.

hypercoagulable states. Heparin has been shown to produce the following effects on the Surgical Analyzer signature: (a) the sample has a longer SonACT time, (b) the gel formation phase occurs more slowly, and (c) clot retraction is very slow or not even observed, which is indicative of reduced platelet activity.

Although our purpose has been to find a reliable method to assess heparinization, we have also found the Surgical Analyzer to be useful in assessing patients with hypercoagulable states. We have found that diabetic patients who undergo amputation or foot debridement for treatment of foot infections experience a transient hypercoagulable status during the operation detected in at least 30% of the cases. Therefore, it seems reasonable to find a strategy that protects these patients who have a hypercoagulable status that could cause further damage to the vascular tree [14–21].

ROLE OF SUBSTANCE P IN DIABETICS WITH PERIPHERAL VASCULAR DISEASE

Substance P is a small peptide (Arg-Pro-Lys-Pro-Gln-Gln-Phe-Phe-Gly-Leu-Met-NH$_2$) derived from a single gene of preprotakinin A found in both unmyelinated C fibers and thinly myelinated Aδ afferent sensory fibers. In vitro and in vivo studies [23, 24] have shown that substance P modulates neurogenic pain sensation and acute and delayed inflammatory reaction, and stimulates proliferation of smooth muscle cells. Based on our own studies, we have identified for the first time substance P in the ventral root sympathetic ganglia and chain, in 20 patients with severe arterial insufficiency and/or nonhealing diabetic ulcers who underwent lumbar sympathectomy. Our data suggests that substance P is involved in the pathophysiology of chronic inflammatory reaction at the molecular level in diabetic patients with atherosclerotic occlusive disease. At the molecular level, lumbar sympathectomy may play an important role in the management of chronic inflammatory reactions, local plasma extravasation, endothelial cell proliferation, impaired wound healing and immune response, perhaps by reducing an afferent-efferent sympathetic reflex to injury which perpetuates the local inflammatory response. [22–24].

ANATOMY

All the arterial supply of the foot is derived from the popliteal artery. At the lower border of the popliteus muscle the popliteal artery divides into anterior and posterior tibial arteries. The anterior tibial artery penetrates the upper part of the interosseous membrane and enters the anterior compartment of the leg. Distally it lies between the tibialis anterior and the extensor muscles. At the ankle the anterior tibial artery lies more medially and crosses the ankle joint anteriorly, becoming the dorsalis pedis artery. The dorsalis pedis artery usually lies lateral to the extensor hallucis longus muscle. In the space between the first and second metatarsal, the dorsalis pedis artery generally divides into a deep plantar and dorsal metatarsal branch. The peroneal artery arises from the posterior tibial about 2.5 cm below the lower border of the popliteus, passes obliquely towards the fibula, and descends along its medial crest in a fibrous canal between tibialis posterior and flexor hallucis longus. It is then behind the tibiofibular syndesmosis and divides into calcanean branches, which ramify on the lateral and posterior surfaces of the calcaneus. The posterior tibial artery accompanies the tibial nerve. The artery lies between the tibialis posterior and flexor digitorum muscles and the soleus muscle and tendon of the calcaneus. In the plantar space the posterior artery divides into the medial and lateral plantar arteries. These arteries accompany the medial and lateral plantar nerves. The plantar arch is formed by anastomosis between the medial and lateral plantar arteries, with a branch from the dorsalis pedis artery at the first intermetatarsal space. Small dorsal digital arteries arise from an inconstant dorsal arcuate branch of the dorsalis pedis artery. The plantar digital vessels arise from the plantar arch. The plantar arch varies in detail, but in healthy individuals it provides abundant opportunity for collateral circulation in the distal foot. The arterioles of the skin form an internal vascular belt at the junction between subcutaneous tissue and dermis. Arising from this internal vascular belt are dermal plexi that are intimately interconnected, forming a reticular network of vessels of different sizes. From this network, arboreal terminal branches form a subpapillary plexus with capillary loops in the dermal papillae, which integrate a number of papillae

Table 14-1. Compartments of the Foot

Compartment	Muscles
1. Central	Adductor hallucis, quadratus plantae, flexor digitorum brevis, and flexor digitorum longus
2. Medial	Flexor hallucis longus, flexor hallucis brevis, and abductor hallucis
3. Lateral	Flexor digiti minimi brevis and abductor
4. Interosseous	Interossei muscles (7)

into vascular districts that are also interconnected [25].

There are four compartments of the foot: medial, central, lateral, and interosseous (Table 14.1 and Figure 14-3). The first three are on the sole of the foot and are called the plantar compartments. The floor of the plantar compartments consists of the rigid plantar fascia, and the roof is formed by the metatarsal bones and the interosseus fascia. The medial compartment is separated from the central compartment by the medial intermuscular septum, which extends from the medial calcaneal tuberosity to the head of the first metatarsal. This compartment contains the muscles associated with the great toe: the abductor hallucis, the flexor hallucis brevis, and the flexor hallucis longus. (The first limit is the shaft of the first metatarsal bone.) The medial intermuscular septum is incomplete, as it is perforated by the flexor hallucis longus passing into the central compartment. The flexor hallucis longus also has a slip connecting it to the flexor digitorum longus and the peroneus longus. The medial intermuscular

septum is also breached distally where the oblique head of the adductor hallucis passes from the central to the medial compartment. Proximally, the septum is breached by the lateral plantar neurovascular bundle. Its deep attachments are the navicular bone, posterior tibial tendon, medial cuneiform bone, and lateral side of the first metatarsal bone [26].

The central compartment contains the flexor digitorum brevis, quadratus plantae, flexor allucis longus, peroneus longus tendon, posterior tibial tendon, lumbricals, and adductor hallucis [27, 28]. Jones [29] includes the lateral head of the flexor hallucis brevis in the central compartment. The medial intermuscular septum forms the medial boundary of the central compartment. Similarly, the lateral intermuscular septum forms the lateral boundary. The central component of the plantar fascia forms the superficial border, and the metatarsal bones and interossei fascia provide the deep border. The central compartment is triangular in shape (its apex being proximal) and is divided into several fascial spaces. The medial *intermusculal* septum separates the intrinsic muscles of the great toe from the soft tissue structures of the central compartment: the extrinsic flexor tendons of the toes, medial and lateral plantar nerves and plantar vascular arches, and intrinsic muscles of the second through fourth toes.

In the lateral compartment are the muscles associated with the fifth toe: the abductor digiti quinti, the flexor digiti quinti brevis, and the adductor of the fifth toe. The medial boundary of the lateral compartment is the lateral intermuscular septum,

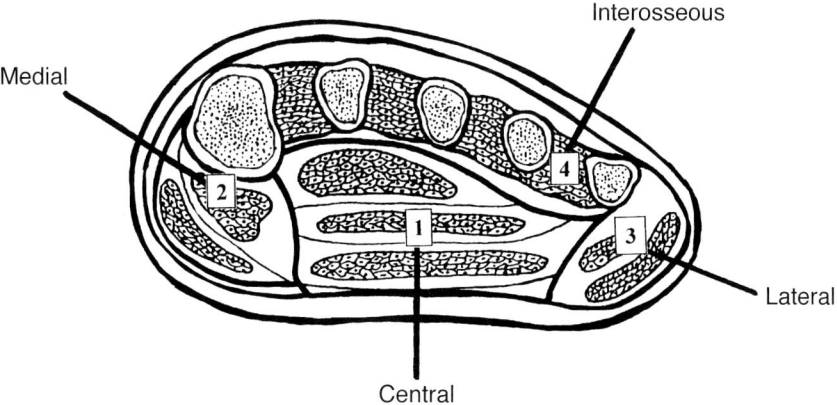

Figure 14-3. Cross-section of the four compartments of the foot.

which arises from the plantar aponeurosis and extends from the medial tubercle of the calcaneus to the medial side of the head of the fifth metatarsal. The septum is found in the interval between the abductor digiti quinti brevis and flexor digitorum brevis. The lateral intermuscular septum is incomplete, as it is breached by the lateral plantar artery and nerve where they exit the central compartment through the second layer, midway between the calcaneus and the fifth metatarsal, to enter the lateral compartment, and later when they reenter the central compartment approximately 2.5 cm distal to the base of the fifth metatarsal entering the fourth layer [30].

The interosseous compartment is bound by the interosseous fascia and the metatarsals, and contains the seven interosseous muscles [30, 31].

Because these four deep compartments are bounded by rigid fascial and bony structures, edema associated with an acute infection may induce a rapid elevation in compartment pressures, resulting in ischemic necrosis of the confined tissues.

Studies done by Goldman, who injected fluid into the compartment, showed that the lateral compartment has the least potential space, the central compartment has the largest potential space, and the medial compartment has a potential space greater than that of the lateral but less than that of the central [32].

In the face of infection, bacterial spread from one compartment to another may take place at the proximal calcaneal convergence or by direct perforation through the intercompartmental septa. However, because each compartment is bound by rigid fascial separations in the medial-to-lateral and dorsal-to-plantar directions, the lateral or dorsal spread of infection is a late sign of infection. Based on the anatomy of the foot, deep space foot infections frequently show little plantar or dorsal foot abnormality. Therefore, a patient presenting with mild swelling of the foot but toxic systemic symptoms must be evaluated for an occult deep space infection. The deep potential spaces or compartments of the foot can allow a spread of bacteria from the plantar surface or web spaces of the foot to the ankle and lower leg region [33–35].

COMPARTMENT SYNDROME

Compartment syndrome is a well-described clinical entity that results from increased pressure within a myofascial compartment. Mubarak and Hargens [36] introduced the concept of compartment syndrome of the foot and focused on the interossei compartment. They presented a possible treatment by decompression done with longitudinal incisions of the dorsum of the foot. Later, Whitesides [37] anecdotally described isolated compartment syndrome of the foot secondary to burns and direct trauma, and recommended decompression by the medial approach of Henry. The signs and symptoms of compartment syndrome of the foot appear to be similar to that of compartment syndromes in general—a degree of pain that is out of proportion to the injury appears to be the first symptom. An early clinical sign reported by Bonutti and Gordon [38] was paresthesia in the distribution of the digital nerves of the toes, especially to pinprick, two-point discrimination and light touch. Pain with passive dorsiflexion of the toes is also an important sign, although direct trauma may cause similar symptoms. Pallor, paresthesia, and a palpable tense compartment have also been reported. We believe that intracompartmental pressure of the foot is important, not only because of increased interstitial pressure, but also because of the increased gravitational effect sustained by the foot.

We have measured the pressure of the foot compartments using the Stryker catheter and with a noninvasive device. We have developed a noninvasive viscoelastic measurement device consisting of an instrumented hand-held probe, an electronic surface unit, and an X-Y plotter for data display. The hand-held probe has a center indenter mounted at the end of a force transducer (Figure 14-4). This device measures displacement and force, which gives the change in tissue volume, as muscle and fascia sheets form an enclosed space with a constant pressure and tissue compliance (Figure 14-5). The results obtained with this device give an accurate measurement of the interstitial pressure of the compartments of the foot. The results obtained with the viscoelastic measurement device have been com-

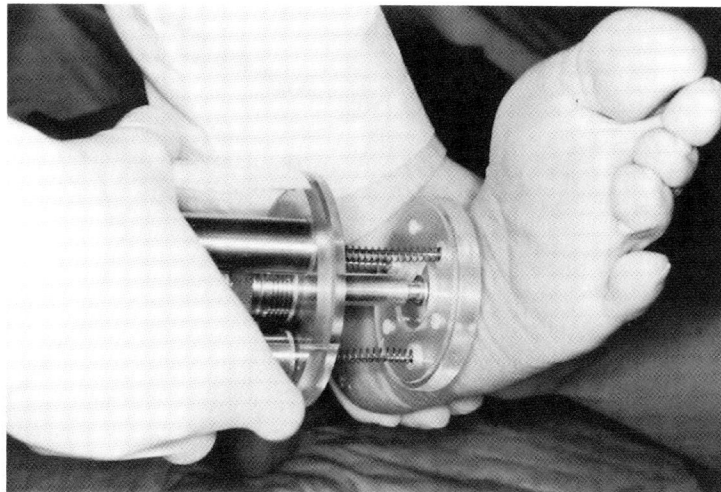

Figure 14-4.   Application of viscoelastic measurement device to the central compartment of the foot.

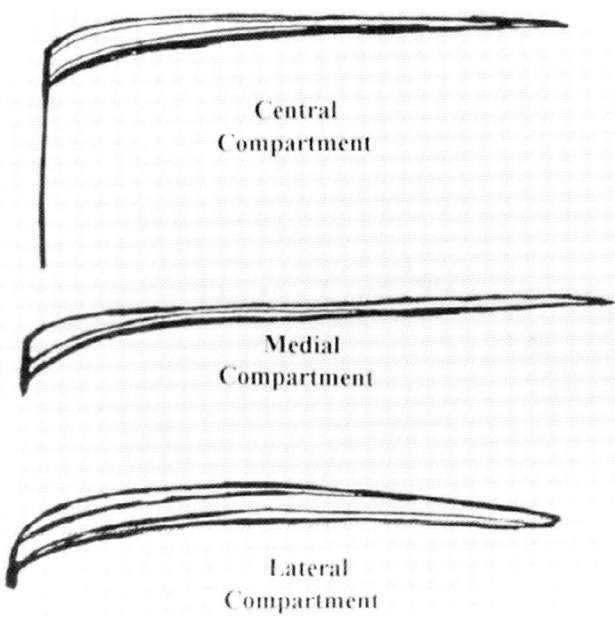

Figure 14-5.   Viscoelastic displacement curves for the three compartments of the plantar surface of the foot.

pared to those of the Stryker catheter, and they have correlated well. We believe that the compartment pressures of the foot play an important role in foot infections, reperfusion injury, and trauma, and may also be an important factor in neurotrophic ulcers [36–38].

ATHEROSCLEROSIS

It is believed that alterations in glucose metabolism are followed by alterations in lipid metabolism. It is no wonder that a diabetic patient has his or her share of common aortoiliac and femoral popliteal atherosclerosis. The development of peripheral arterial disease can be documented in more than 50% of long-term diabetics. In a study of diabetics diagnosed within a single year, it was noted that in 22% of patients lower extremity vascular calcifications were apparent in plain radiographs and that 13% lacked one or more ankle pulses. Atherosclerosis manifests at an earlier age in diabetics and tends to involve distal and smaller peripheral vessels. For example, multisegmental occlusive patterns occur more commonly below the popliteal region in diabetics than in age-matched control subjects, and the metatarsal arteries are occluded in as many as 60% of diabetics. In contrast, the incidence of aortoiliac occlusive disease tends to be similar in diabetic and nondiabetic patients. Because of the frequent association of atherosclerotic peripheral disease with diabetes, as well as the increasingly encouraging results of vascular reconstruction in this patient population, the presence of reconstructable peripheral vascular disease should be considered in diabetic patients with extremity soft tissue infections.

There are no pathognomonic capillary or arteriolar lesions associated with diabetes. Intimal thickening of the basement membrane, originally attributed to diabetics, is also found in 23% of nondiabetics. This microcapillary angiopathy seems to be variable in its tissue penetration from one patient to another, and its role in the development of foot capillary vessel alterations is questionable. Therefore, one should not assume that vascular reconstructive procedures in the diabetic are doomed to failure. In diabetics, a metabolic form of tissue ischemia related to hyperglycemia probably contributes to the development of infection and increased susceptibility to tissue injury.

TIBIAL ATHEROSCLEROSIS

The diabetic has a propensity to develop arteriosclerotic lesions in the small arteries below the knee and the foot. These lesions are not of the same microangiopathy as those associated with blindness and renal failure. Rather, they are histologically typical atherosclerotic lesions involving arteries less commonly involved in patients without diabetes. If a patient presents with a necrotic forefoot and has a popliteal pulse, the chances are overwhelming

that he or she is a diabetic, as other conditions such as Buerger's disease and collagen vascular diseases affecting these arteries are exceedingly rare [35, 39, 40].

DIABETIC PERIPHERAL NEUROPATHY

Peripheral neuropathy clearly predisposes the patient to injury, which potentiates the risk of bacterial invasion and infection. Peripheral neuropathies are found in as many as 55% of diabetics, and the incidence of neuropathies increases with the duration of the disease. The clinical spectrum and presentation of diabetic neuropathies vary greatly; initial symptoms are paresthesias, unpleasant dysesthesias, or hypersensitivity to touch. In some patients these initial symptoms progress to complete loss of sensation. Whether the neuropathy is due to progressive distal axonopathy or focal compressive neuropathy, the results are decreased plantar sensation, intrinsic muscle atrophy, and lack of autonomic glandular and vasomotor responses. Skin insensitivity limits the patient's ability to respond to foot trauma. Intrinsic muscle atrophy produces tendon imbalances that expose the metatarsal heads to excessive trauma and shift the weight-bearing portion of the foot from protected to unprotected portions of the plantar surface. Ultimately, repetitive unprotected trauma results in bony and ligamentous rearrangements that lead to further tissue inflammation and breakdown. Autonomic dysfunction plays a significant role in diabetic foot infection, as the lack of autonomic innervation to the foot results in scaly, cracked, dry skin, decreased vasomotor tone, and edema, all of which predispose to foot infection.

The exact mechanisms and relationships of the metabolic disturbances observed in diabetics to the subsequent development of neural dysfunction are still being debated [41–46]. However, an important role for linolenic acid, a prostaglandin precursor, appears likely, based on multicenter studies demonstrating that the treatment of diabetics with prostaglandin E_1 or high doses of γ-linolenic acid stabilizes and occasionally improves mild diabetic peripheral neuropathy [46]. Additionally, some evidence suggests that a subgroup of diabetic patients with polyneuropathy have unsuspected concomitant compressive neuropathy that may benefit from surgical decompression. Because the development of peripheral neuropathy plays a major role in the pathogenesis of diabetic foot infections, efforts to diagnose the type of neuropathy and therapy directed at preventing, limiting, or reversing diabetic neuropathy are of major importance. Peripheral neuropathy may be mild or severe. If mild, modification of the weight-bearing surface is effective. If severe, one should give early attention in therapeutic attempts to recreate a functional limb [41–46].

PERFORATING ULCERS OF THE FOOT

Perforating ulcers of the foot are of major clinical significance, as they can lead to complications such as sepsis, protein wasting, soft tissue and bone necrosis, and eventual amputation. The management of perforating ulcers remains a complex problem. Overzealous surgical intervention has its associated complications. At times, failure of the surgery can lead to an even larger area of ulceration. Difficulty in the management of perforating ulcers is compounded by the inability to accurately assess the pathogenesis of perforating ulcers. Ulcerations on the plantar surface of the foot are usually associated with specific disease such as diabetes mellitus, syringomyelia, syphilis, and severe peripheral neuropathy. Perforating ulcers are associated with trauma or local pressure that initiates tissue breakdown with associated repetitive mechanical injury. In the neuropathic patient, this problem is further compounded by the relative or absolute insensitivity of the foot. As a result, small lesions in the foot may go unrecognized by the patient and become large ulcers.

Clinically, ulceration begins as a flattened callous beneath a small joint or bone, particularly in the metatarsal region, which is subject to point pressure. With repeated trauma, deformity of the bony structure, ischemia, or subcutaneous neurosis develops, clinically showing as swelling, hematoma, and inflammation. The inner portion of the ulcer may slough with or without exudate and fistulae may form. Fibrotic and sclerotic changes surrounded by a dense circumferential epidermis occur

in the distal connective tissue. Subsequent soft tissue breakdown can lead to exposure of the bone and joint surfaces, which may become secondarily infected.

Perforating ulcer was described as early as 1818 by Mott. He observed the thick, hard cuticle surrounding the plantar ulcer, as well as the insensitivity of the foot. It was not until 1852, when Nealton reported an unusual condition in the bony structure of feet leading to ulceration and when Vesignie coined the term *plantaire mal perforant*, that this ulcer received universal attention. However, it was in 1872 that Duplay and Morat reported these lesions to be neuropathic in origin and substantiated this concept by producing similar changes in the skin of denervated limbs of animals. In 1884, Treves reported ulcerations of the foot in ataxic individuals who had not experienced any alteration of sensation. Treves believed ulcer development to be secondary to the normal pressure associated with standing and movement, and that once the ulcer became infected, the infection followed the course of least resistance to the bone. The following year Kirmission reported diabetes as an associated condition with perforating ulcers of the foot. Fifty years later, Jordon described the first diabetic Charcot's joint. Ulceration was observed beneath the metatarsophalangeal joint with sensation intact at the periphery of the ulcer. Surgical dissection into the deeper structures beneath the ulcer could be made without pain to the patient. In 1953, Martin reported an incidence of 22% of neurotrophic joints in diabetic patients attended at Kings College Hospital. Martin stated that diabetic neuropathy was responsible for the associated soft tissue, joint, and bone changes leading to perforating ulceration. In such patients, it was believed, damage to nonmyelinated nerve fibers occurred earlier than to myelinated nerves, thereby lowering tissue resistance and predisposing the skin to more extensive trauma. Cutaneous ulcer's association with neuropathic arthropathies led a number of authors, notably Hodgsen, Pugh, and Young in 1948, to suggest that infection leading to osteomyelitis was the direct cause of bone changes, independent of any associated nervous disorder.

In 1964, Classen [47] presented the results of conservative and surgical treatment in 45 cases of plantar perforating ulcers of the foot. Healing was complete in those patients who had amputation of a metatarsal head, amputation of a toe with the metatarsal head, or amputation of the joint. One of eight patients who were treated conservatively healed. In 1972 Friedman and associates studied the peripheral vasoconstrictor capacity in patients with diabetic neuropathy by measuring reflex skin temperature changes in the foot [47]. Skin temperature measurements showed vasomotor tone to be totally absent in only 1 of 19 patients tested. It was concluded that adrenergic sympathetic function is usually preserved in the lower extremity, even in those patients with severe diabetic neuropathy, and that most patients with this condition lack the protective effect of "autosympathectomy" for their distal cutaneous circulation. Friedman and associates recommended that neuropathic diabetics not be automatically excluded from lumbar sympathectomy when they have significant arterial occlusive disease. Edmonds and associates in 1982 reported blood flow to be abnormal in neurotrophic subjects, even in those limbs without ulceration [47]. In patients with neurotrophic joints, there were marked increases in diastolic flow as well as a sharp decrease in pressure from ankle to toe. Edmonds et al. concluded the neurotrophic foot to be more susceptible to abnormal mechanical stress, which eventually could lead to the neurotrophic joint and perforating ulcer. Based on the etiology and pathomechanics, and the emphasis on locating plantar perforating ulcers of the foot and the status of the peripheral circulation, surgical treatment has been redirected toward correcting the structure underlying the ulceration, using procedures that augment blood flow to the distal part of the extremity [47].

PATHOMECHANICS

Weight distribution on the foot and the function of the great toe during pushoff are major factors in the development of ulcers on the plantar aspect of the foot. Force plate analysis has shown that, before toe-off, weight is transferred to the medial side of the foot, which subjects the plantar surface of the great toe to heavy weight bearing and stress at the

time of pushoff. Ctercteko and associates measured vertical forces acting on the feet of diabetic patients with neurotrophic ulceration and found proportionally less force transmitted through the toes than in normal individuals [47]. They also showed a medial shift of the force transmitted through the metatarsal heads. All ulcers in the metatarsal region were located at the site of maximum loading. The general vertical force distribution pattern on the plantar surface of the feet of diabetics varied in important aspects from normal. The diabetic group had reduced toe loading, which was probably a reflection of neuropathic paresis of the long and short flexors and intrinsic muscles of the toes. The reduction of toe loading resulted in heavier loading in the metatarsal region. Normally 70% of toe loading is transmitted through the hallux. Ctercteko suggests that when toe loading is reduced, the load previously taken by the hallux is transferred back onto the first metatarsal head [47]. Barrett and Mooney and Stokes and associates reported similar results, showing definitively that ulcers do occur at the site of maximum vertical force [47].

The relationship between pressure and plantar ulceration can be appreciated when mechanical stresses are classified in four ways: First, a necrotic blister can become an ulcer *by friction* of the skin between bone, shoe, and ground. Second, *impact* by the body's weight at heel contact produces repeated tissue damage, ulceration, and scar formation. Third, *thrust* during walking or running causes intermittent and concentrated pressures, especially under the metatarsal heads before toe-off. If sufficient, these pressures can crush cells or rupture capillaries. Because skin is more resistant to trauma, the subcutaneous tissue is more readily affected with a deep focus of necrosis or hematoma production. With repeated high pressures and an accumulation of necrotic tissue, fistula formation may ensue. Fourth, *shear* of the skin during walking, especially over the metatarsal region, can tear previously scarred tissue because of loss of elasticity. In those individuals with relative or absolute insensitivity of the foot, a long walk is more likely to produce ulceration than a number of short walks under similar conditions. When the sole of the foot is subjected to a long succession of mildly traumatic steps, the effect may be cumulative, making the tissue more susceptible to serious damage.

CLINICAL FINDINGS

More than 60 patients have been referred for perforating ulcers of the foot that had not responded to conservative treatment. Clinical findings included perforating ulceration on the plantar surface of the foot, usually under the metatarsophalangeal joints. The most frequent site was the first metatarsal. The base of the ulcerations contained dermal connective tissue with fibrotic and sclerotic changes surrounded by dense circumferential epidermis margin. Infection was characteristically low grade. Noninvasive assessment of the peripheral vascular system was measured by using Doppler segmental systolic pressure profile, external magnetic flowmetry, digital photoplethysmography, and thermistor thermometry. In patients who demonstrated vascular disease, arteriography was done to locate lesions of pathological significance. Patients with impaired circulation of the distal extremities not amenable to direct arterial surgery were considered for lumbar sympathectomy, using the following criteria for patient selection: an ischemic index greater than 0.35, pulsatile calf flow greater than 30 ml/min, with an absence of an ankle/toe temperature gradient and an ankle/room temperature gradient greater than 1.20°C. In all patients, radiographic examination of the feet was done, which demonstrated one or more of the following findings: (1) absorption of bone, (2) penciling of the metatarsal shaft, (3) fracture of the metatarsal head, (4) destruction and obliteration of joints, (5) disarticulation of phalanges, and/or (6) periosteal thickening remote from the ulcer site. The chief distinguishing difference between diabetics and nondiabetics was neuropathy. Although diabetic neuropathy was frequently accompanied by pain and paresis, the loss of pain sensation allowed the foot to endure repeated trauma. Clinical findings were therefore a result of complications stemming from a combination of microangiopathy and neuropathy. Commonly, these patients present with infected ulcer, either primary or superimposed on the vascular or neurotrophic lesion [47].

INFECTIONS

In the presence of impaired blood supply or sensation, minor trauma to the foot can result in a serious foot infection. Unfortunately, in many patients, lack of meticulous attention to foot hygiene and use of poorly fitting shoes are major preventable factors in the development of infection. Diabetic foot infections range from local fungal infections of the nail to severe necrotizing limb- or life-threatening infections. Early diagnosis and prompt definitive treatment may be delayed because of lack of foot sensation, the patient's poor eyesight, or failure of the physician who initially sees the patient to accurately diagnose the extent of the infectious process. Because the development of infection or delayed wound healing is often multifactorial, and because diabetics have a high incidence of reconstructable vascular disease, all diabetics presenting with a foot infection must be evaluated for the presence of vascular disease [48, 49].

Loss of skin integrity resulting from a puncture, laceration, or abrasion can be the initiating factor in the development of a foot infection; however, foot infections in the diabetic usually originate at the nail plates or the interdigital web spaces. In one study, 60% of foot infections started in the web spaces, 30% started around the nails, and 10% were secondary to puncture wounds [35]. The high incidence of web space and toe infections is related to the increased moisture level in the web space and the presence of excessive amounts of keratin and other debris around the nail plates. These environmental factors promote bacterial overgrowth and thereby predispose to infection. The clinical presentation of a diabetic with a foot infection ranges from mild episodes of acute cellulitis to life-threatening episodes of necrotizing fasciitis.

Diabetic foot infections are classified as acute

and chronic. Acute infections include localized cellulitis, septic arthritis of metatarsophalangeal joints, necrotizing cellulitis or fasciitis, deep space infections, and gangrene (clostridial and nonclostridial). Chronic infections include neurotrophic ulcers and osteomyelitis.

Acute cellulitis beginning in the web space, if left untreated, spreads along the tendons and lumbricals associated with each toe and can quickly lead to a deep space infection or, less commonly, to acute necrotizing cellulitis or fasciitis. In fact, toe and web space infections that progress to advanced deep space infections are associated with the highest rate of major limb amputations. Acute necrotizing cellulitis or fasciitis and deep compartment infections are characterized by systemic signs and symptoms of infection, including spiking fever, malaise, nausea, and the development of ketoacidosis. Clinically, necrotizing cellulitis more commonly involves the dorsum of the foot. In deep space infections, however, a loss of the plantar surface contour and skin crease occurs, and the presence of dorsal foot swelling is variable.

Deep space infections generally involve only the central compartment of the foot, but because of the anatomy of these space compartments, a high index of suspicion concerning bacterial spread from the central to the lateral or medial compartment must be maintained. Destruction of the interosseous fascia allows bacteria to spread from the central to the lateral or medial compartment, and the migration of the bacteria along the long flexor tendons leads to infection in the calf and lower regions. The small vessel thrombosis that accompanies deep space infections leads to progressive tissue ischemia and necrosis. With progressive inflammation, the accumulating tissue edema results in elevation of deep compartment pressures, contributing to ischemic necrosis of the intrinsic muscles of the foot. The development of bullous lesions on the plantar aspect of the foot is a late sign and signals the loss of plantar vessel patency, and the presence of massive plantar tissue necrosis.

The presence of gas between the tissues on radiography can be due to clostridial infections or the milking of air into the tissues by continued walking. In this circumstance, Gram staining of the exudate or infected tissue is critical in differentiating clostridia from other bacterial pathogens and in choosing appropriate antibiotic coverage as well as the extent and type of surgical intervention. Clostridial infection, although uncommon, tends to present with acute systemic toxicity and a rapidly ascending course [35].

DIFFERENTIAL DIAGNOSIS

In the diabetic patient presenting with an acutely inflamed foot, a differential diagnosis must be made among gouty arthritis, Charcot's joint and infection. Gouty arthritis causes inflammation around the metatarsophalangeal joint of the great toe. The lack of systemic toxicity, presence of elevated serum uric acid levels, and uric acid crystals on aspiration of the joint aid in distinguishing gouty arthritis from acute infection. Charcot's joint occurs in as many as 2.5% of diabetics and is related to repetitive traumatic injury to the insensate foot. The joints characteristically involved in this acute inflammatory process are the metatarsophalangeal, metatarsotarsal, intertarsal, and interphalangeal joints. The presence of acute erythema, edema, and joint effusions may cause a Charcot's joint to be mistaken for a foot infection, especially when a Charcot's joint is associated with a foot ulcer. However, in contrast to patients with foot infections, patients with a Charcot's joint do not show signs of systemic toxicity and white blood cell counts, and erythrocyte sedimentation rates are not elevated [49–53].

DIAGNOSTIC METHODS

A careful neurologic examination includes assessment of vibratory sense, proprioception, and light touch. The proximal extent of the neuropathy should be documented. It is common for only the forefoot to have significant neuropathy, while the hindfoot and lower leg have normal sensation.

Noninvasive vascular tests frequently underestimate the extent and severity of arterial insufficiency in diabetic patients. Bilateral ankle/brachial indices via Doppler are useful, but their accuracy in the presence of calcified vessels is severely limited. The readings can be falsely high. Other noninvasive studies include transcutaneous oximetry. These should be used only as a complement to bedside evaluation and clinical judgment. In selected patients with significant limb-threatening ischemia (ankle/brachial index < 0.5, rest pain, or ischemic tissue necrosis), arteriography of the lower extremity including the foot vessels should be performed. [54].

We have used noninvasive electromagnetic flowmetry in the assessment of patients with peripheral arterial disease. This technique is capable of distinguishing three relatively discrete clinical zones (femoral, popliteal, and posterior tibial) by quantitating the peak pulsatile flow of blood through the thigh and the calf. As previously reported, the obtained peak pulsatile flow values are comparable to ischemic indices for grading the degree of ischemia. The use of electromagnetic flowmetry has enabled us to select the proper operative procedure by providing information about arterial flow (proximal, site of the lesion, and status of the runoff) [55–57].

Currently, adapted from fluid flowmetry in industrial applications, magnetic resonance flowmetry has been applied clinically. The basic principle of nuclear magnetic resonance (NMR) flowmetry can be simplified by relating the NMR signal of blood flow as follows. (1) magnetization is induced as the hydrogen nuclei (N) tendency in the blood to align along the direction of an applied magnetic field; (2) blood is magnetized and the amount of magnetism (M) is detected, and the flow rate of magnetized blood is measured; (3) magnetization is measured by making the hydrogen nuclei resonate (R) and then applying the principle of magnetic induction: a changing resonating magnetic field creates an electric voltage in the detector, accounting for the R. Blood flow measurements using NMR have been in close agreement with those obtained using other plethysmographic techniques. The examination is performed without physical contact, so evaluation of extremities having fresh or open wounds or of burn patients can be done. Perhaps more important, calcified vessels do not interfere with the accuracy of measurements, making MRI of particular value in diabetic patients [58, 59].

Plain radiographs of the foot are not very reliable in detecting osteomyelitis because of the high incidence of false-positive and false-negative studies [54]. False-negative studies are relatively common for several reasons. First, lytic lesions due to infection must cause a greater than 30% bone density loss (based on the density of normal bone) to be demonstrated on plain radiographs. Furthermore, the infection must be present for longer than seven to fourteen days before these subtle radiographic changes can be demonstrated. The bone density of the diabetic is often reduced, and the presence of osteopenic bone further decreases the ability of plain radiographs to detect osteomyelitis [35]. For this reason, radionuclide studies are often used to confirm or rule out osteomyelitis. Currently, the three-phase bone scan using technetium 99, methylene diphosphonate, and gallium 67 citrate is the most accurate and sensitive. The intense uptake of technetium 99 diphosphonate followed by an intense uptake of gallium 67 is highly suggestive for osteomyelitis. Failure to intensely localize gallium 67 suggests a localized inflammatory process. Indium 111 oxyquinolone leukocyte scan has recently been shown to detect osteomyelitis with a sensitivity of 89% and to be a reliable method for following the effectiveness of antibiotic therapy. The combined use of the three-phase bone scan and the indium 111 leukocyte scan have a sensitivity of 100% and a specificity of 81% [54]. Computerize tomography is a superior examination for detecting the presence of sequestra. Although the MRI has been used to diagnose osteomyelitis, no comparison has been made with radionuclide scans [60].

CASE REPORTS

CASE 1

A forty-two-year-old, insulin-dependent, diabetic black male was admitted with the chief complaint of a perforating ulcer on the sole of the left foot of one week's duration. The ulcer developed from a callus that was present four months prior to admission. Examination of the left foot showed a thick callus surrounding the plantar ulcer with dirty granulation and purulent discharge (Figure 14-6). Routine noninvasive vascular studies showed nor-

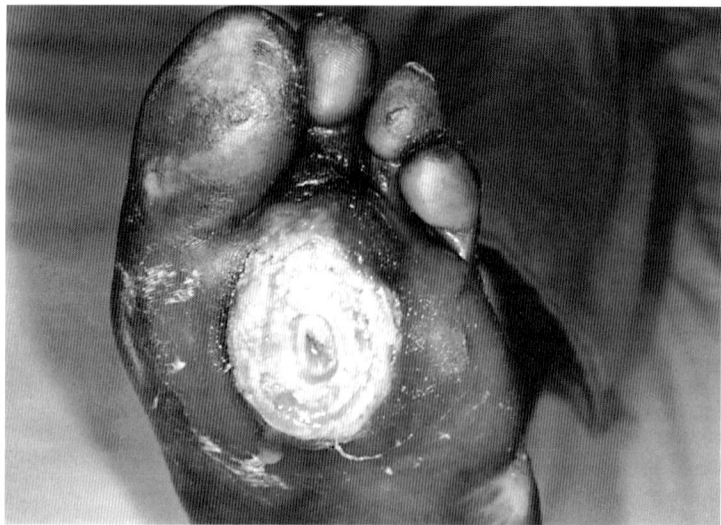

Figure 14-6. Forty-two year-old diabetic black male presented with perforating ulcer on the sole of the left foot with purulent discharge.

mal blood flow to the lower extremities. Arteriography demonstrated no significant arterial occlusive disease. Skin thermistor thermometry evaluation, however, showed evidence of reduced tissue perfusion at the foot with a room/toe temperature gradient of 7.75°C. Radiographic examination of the left foot showed absorption and penciling of the distal two-thirds of the second and fifth metatarsal bones with disruption of the articular surface and partial dislocation of the second proximal phalanx (Figure 14-7). To increase blood flow to the left lower extremity, a left lumbar sympathectomy was performed. A follow-up examination at six months demonstrated increased skin temperatures at the left calf, ankle, and toe levels, compared to those of the right extremity, with a 1.25°C improvement in the left room/toe temperature gradient. Examination of the left foot showed partial healing of the ulcer. Following this increased tissue perfusion in the sympathectomized limb, debridement of the callosity over the sole of the left foot and excision of the base of the phalanx of the left great toe through a small dorsal incision were performed to alleviate pressure necrosis. Long-term follow-up digital photoplethysmography was decided on. This was

done, and thermistor thermometry demonstrated a sustained increase in tissue perfusion and digital temperatures of the sympathectomized limb. At ten years follow-up, the ulceration on the plantar surface of the foot remained healed (Figure 14-8).

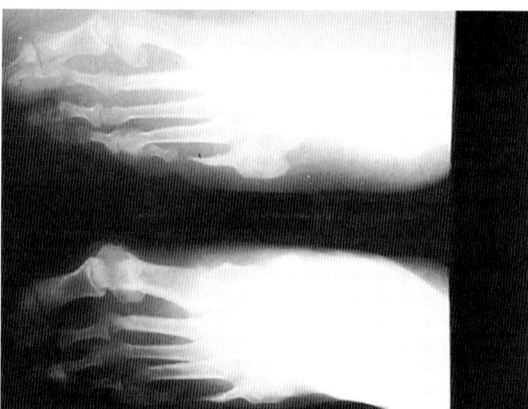

Figure 14-7. Radiograph examination of left foot shows absorption and penciling of the distal two-thirds of the second and fifth metatarsal bones with disruption of the articular surface and partial disarticulation of the second proximal phalanx.

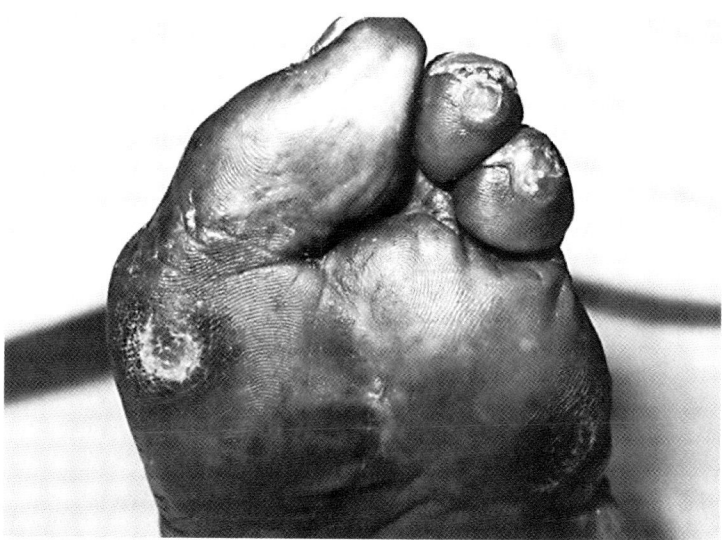

Figure 14-8. At ten years follow-up, perforating ulceration on the sole of the left foot remains healed.

CASE 2

A fifty-three-year-old white male was admitted with cellulitis, infection, and progressive gangrene of the left foot. The patient had been diabetic for the past fifteen years and controlled with insulin. Physical examination showed swelling of the left foot and ankle with tenderness and multiple sinuses and discharge. The distal phalangeal and metatarsal regions were deformed from a distal tendon repair performed three years previously. Routine noninvasive external magnetic flowmetry demonstrated good pulsatile flow at the thigh and calf bilaterally, and segmental Doppler ischemic indices were exaggerated distally (Figure 14-9). Digital photoplethysmography demonstrated reduced photoplethysmographic waveforms at the toes bilaterally, and Doppler ankle/metatarsal systolic pressure showed exaggerated pressures indicative of the presence of calcified small vessel disease (Figure 14-10). Arteriography demonstrated good visualization of the major vessels of the lower extremities with good distal runoff into the popliteal and tibial arteries with no significant arterial occlusive disease to the ankle level (Figure 14-11). Radiographic study of the left foot showed osteomyelitis and advanced bony absorption, characteristic of diabetes mellitus (Figure 14-12). Multiple debridements and incisions and drainage of the left foot did not significantly improve the foot, and the patient underwent a left lumbar sympathectomy. Follow-up radiographic examination of the left foot showed actual reconstruction of the remaining bony fragment involving the phalanx of the great toe. The right foot, however, demonstrated a significant distortion of the first, second, third, and fourth toes with fusiform deformity. Active osteomyelitis involving the metatarsal bones was present (Figure 14-13). Ulceration was present on the plantar surface of the right foot (Figure 14-14). A right lumbar sympathectomy was recommended, but the patient refused and was discharged. Two years later the patient was readmitted with extensive necrosis of the sole of the right foot and extensive purulent discharge and exposure of the tarsal and metatarsal bones. He then underwent a right lumbar sympathectomy and subsequent extensive debridement of the right foot with excision of the metatarsal and cuneiform bone. Following skin graft, postoperative healing was excellent (Figure 14-15). At eight years follow-up, thermistor thermometry studies demonstrated a sustained increase in digital temperatures and tissue perfusion at the toes.

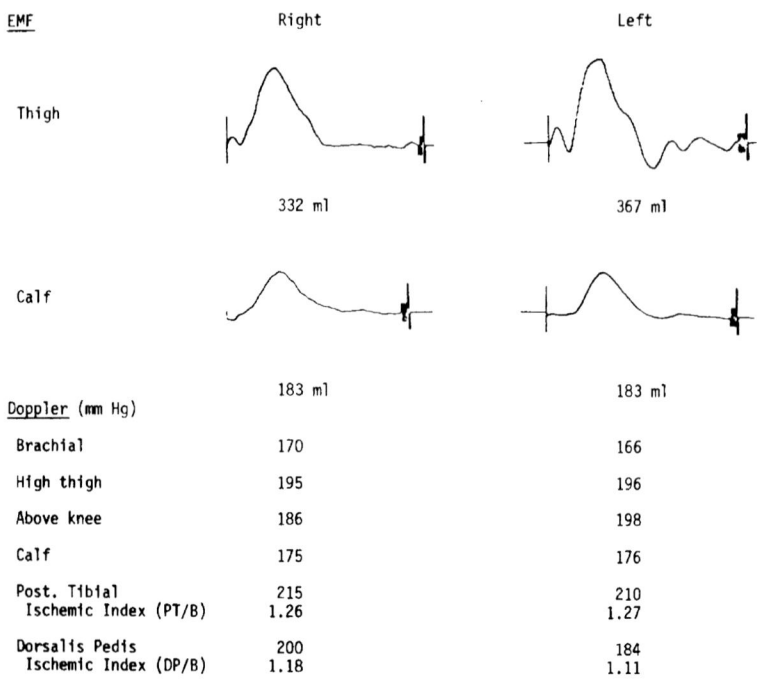

W. Mc. Age 53 Male
Non-Invasive Electromagnetic Flowmeter and Doppler Blood Pressure

Figure 14-9. External noninvasive electromagnetic flowmetry and Doppler segmental systolic pressures in a fifty-three-year-old man showing no significant arterial occlusive disease to the level of the ankle. However this does indicate calcification of distal arteries.

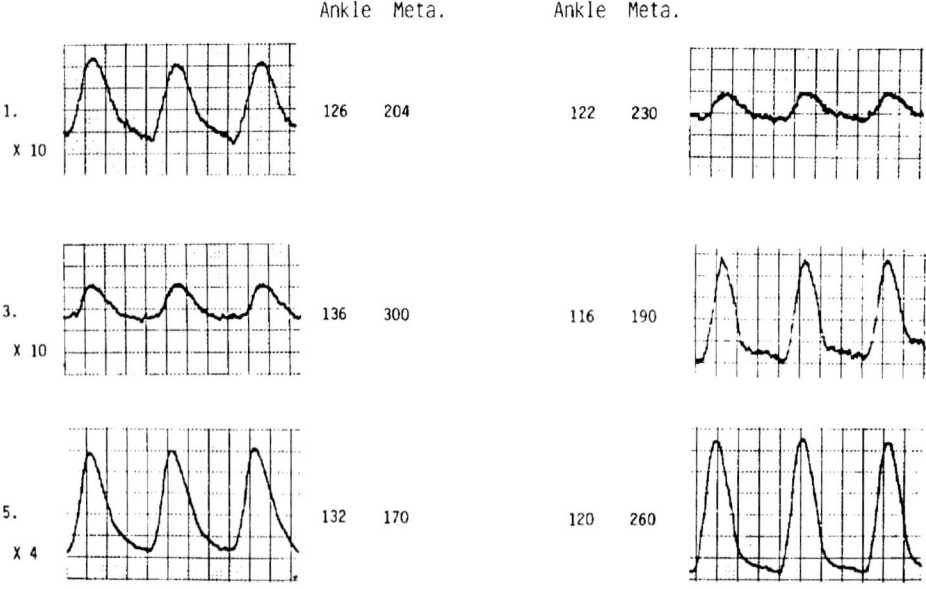

W.Mc. Age 53 Male

Photoplethysmographic Waveforms and Ankle/metatarsal Systolic Blood Pressure.

Figure 14-10. Bilaterally reduced toe photoplethysmographic waveforms and exaggerated ankle/metatarsal pressure in a fifty-three-year-old man demonstrate the presence of small vessel disease indicative of calcified arteries.

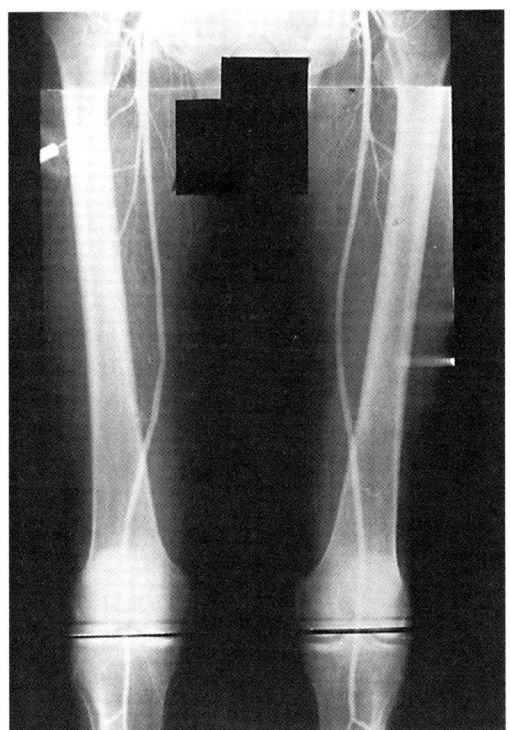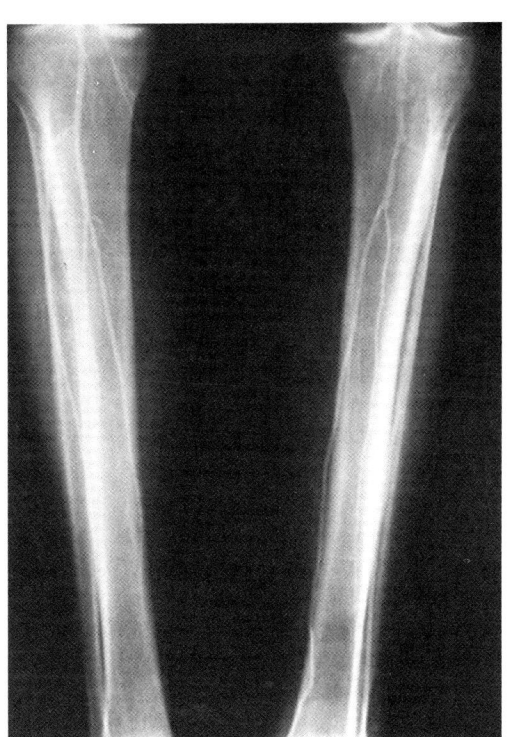

Figure 14-11 (a) and (b). Arteriography shows no evidence of arterial occlusive disease.

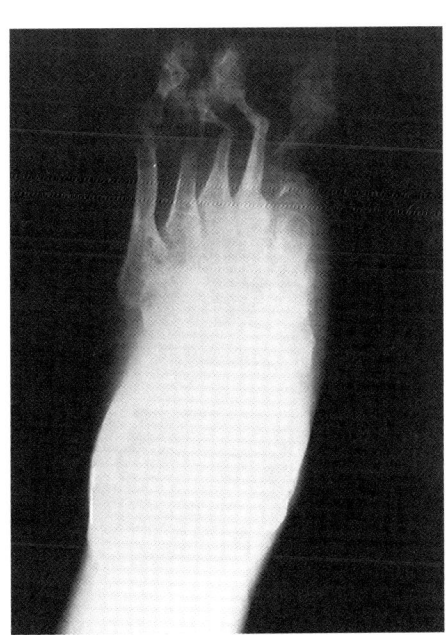

Figure 14-12. Radiographic examination of the left foot shows osteomyelitis and advanced bony absorption characteristic of diabetes mellitus.

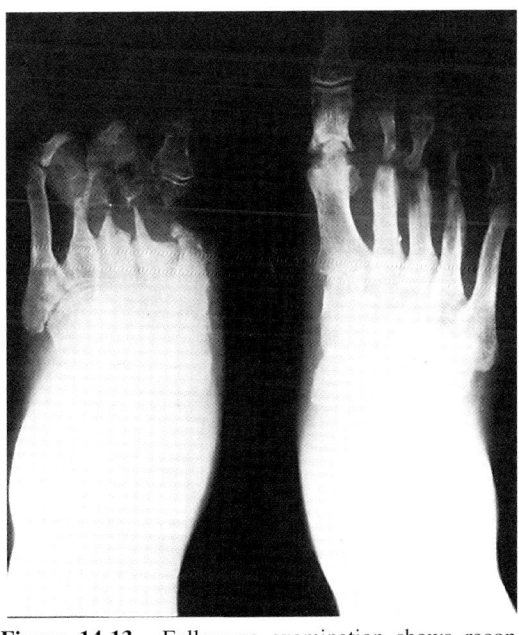

Figure 14-13. Follow-up examination shows reconstruction of the remaining bony fragment involving the phalanx of the left great toe. Right foot shows distortion of the first, second, third, and fourth toes associated with osteomyelitis.

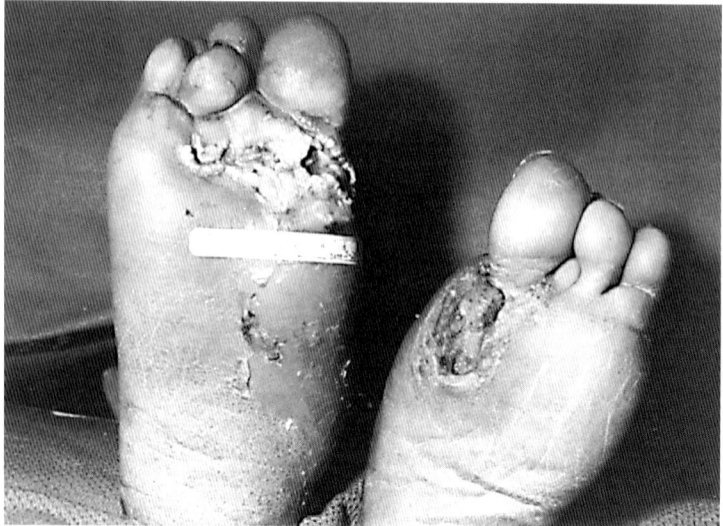

Figure 14-14.   Presence of perforating ulcers on the plantar surface of both feet (preoperatively).

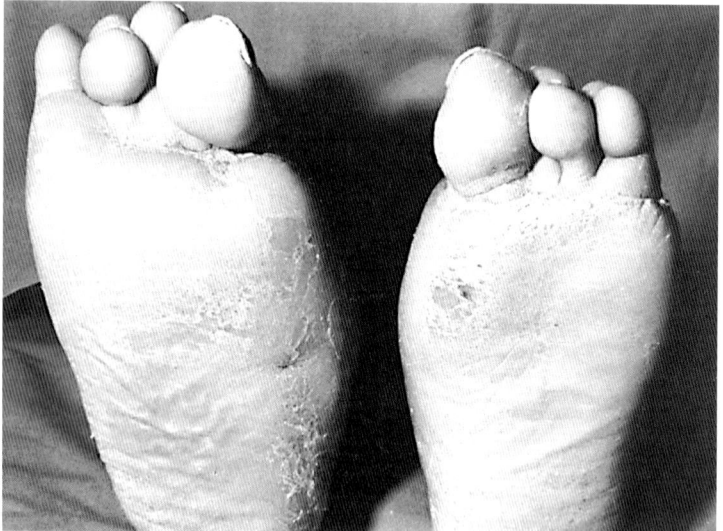

Figure 14-15.   Postoperatively both feet show excellent healing.

CASE 3

A thirty-eight-year-old, diabetic white male was admitted with neurogenic ulcerations on the plantar aspect of the great toe and sole of the left foot (Figure 14-16). Neurological findings of the lower extremities were dissociated impairment of sensa-

tion for pain and temperature, while touch and other sensory modalitis were intact. Motor power was well preserved with proprioception at the toes. Fasciculations were present in the gastrocnemius bilaterally. Electromyography demonstrated no delay in nerve conduction. Radiographic examination of the spine were unremarkable. A lumbar myelogram,

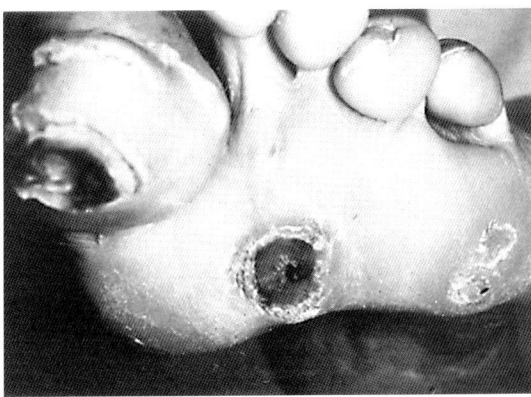

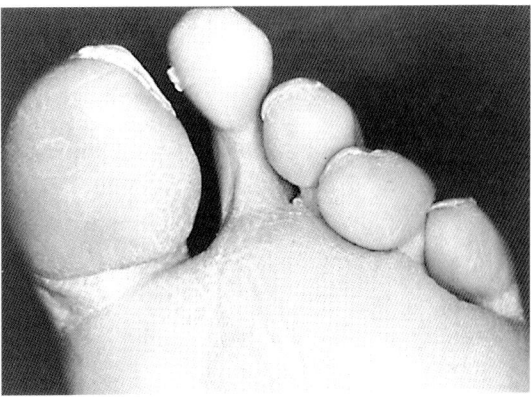

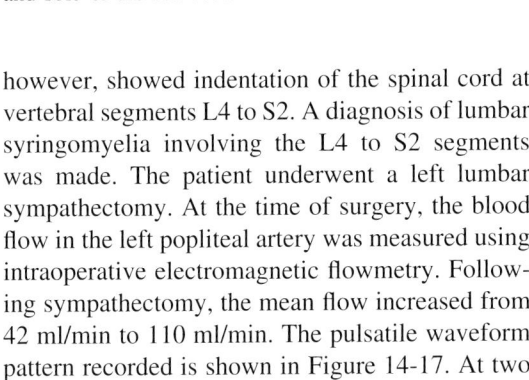

Figure 14-16. (Preoperatively) patient presented with perforating ulcers on the plantara aspect of the great toe and sole of the left foot.

Figure 14-18. Two months postoperatively, perforating ulcers of the left foot are completely healed.

however, showed indentation of the spinal cord at vertebral segments L4 to S2. A diagnosis of lumbar syringomyelia involving the L4 to S2 segments was made. The patient underwent a left lumbar sympathectomy. At the time of surgery, the blood flow in the left popliteal artery was measured using intraoperative electromagnetic flowmetry. Following sympathectomy, the mean flow increased from 42 ml/min to 110 ml/min. The pulsatile waveform pattern recorded is shown in Figure 14-17. At two months postoperatively, the ulcers on the left foot were completely healed (Figure 14-18). In this case,

lumbar sympathectomy alone sufficiently augmented blood flow to promote healing of the neurogenic ulcers.

CASE 4

A seventy-five-year-old male with a history of insulin-dependent diabetes for over fifteen years presented with a right foot infection and complaining of severe pain. On examination, the foot appeared swollen, with increased local temperature and areas of necrosis in the dorsum of the foot. X-rays did not show the presence of gas. The ankle/

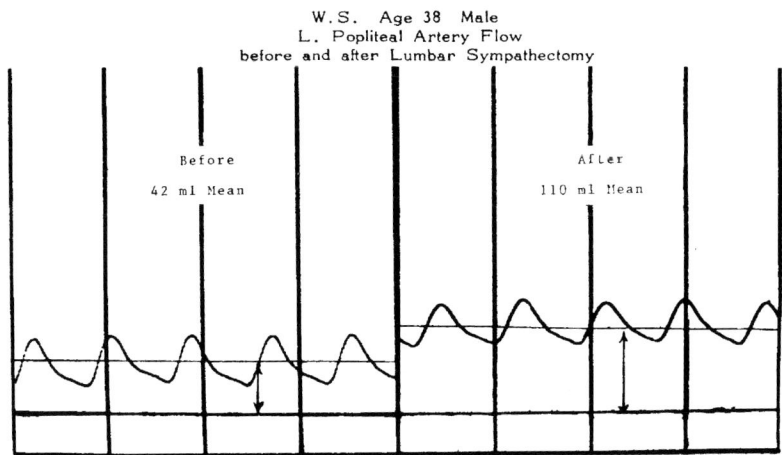

Figure 14-17. Intraoperative electromagnetic flowmetry of a thirty-eight-year-old man demonstrates an increase in blood flow during lumbar sympathectomy.

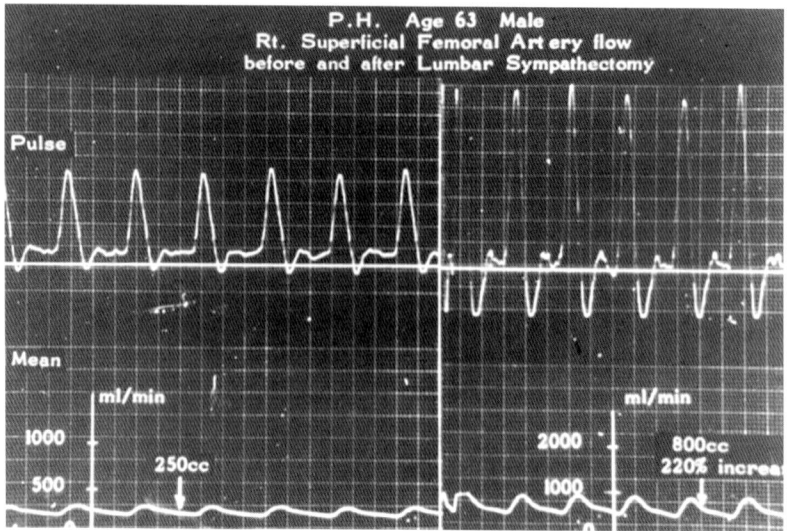

Figure 14-21. Intraoperative electromagnetic flow studies of the superficial femoral artery showed a 220% increase in flow immediately following sympathectomy from 250 ml/min to 800 ml/min.

brachial indices were normal, as was a CT scan of the foot. The clinical diagnosis was necrotizing fasciitis. The patient underwent extensive debridement (Figure 14-19 Color Plate 1). In the postoperative period he received intensive local wound care, including application of topical collagenase and local and systemic antibiotics. After resolution of infection, skin grafting was employed with early good results. At six months follow-up, the foot was in good condition with only a limited dorsiflexion deformity.

CASE 5

A sixty-five-year-old white male had been seen at another facility and was scheduled to undergo a below-knee amputation, which he refused (Figure 14-20 Color Plate 1). He had been a diabetic for the past ten years controlled with insulin. Physical examination showed a swollen right foot with necrotic areas in the dorsolateral aspect of the foot as well as on the fourth and fifth toes. The entire area was erythematous. X rays did not show the presence of gas, but lytic lesions were observed in the fourth and fifth distal phalanges. Systolic segmental Doppler pressures were within the normal range. The patient underwent local wound care and received systemic antibiotics. He underwent a

right lumbar sympathectomy. Intraoperative electromagnetic flow studies of the superficial femoral artery showed a 220% increase in flow immediately following the sympathectomy from 250 ml/min to 800 ml/min (Figure 14-21). The patient underwent amputation of only two toes instead of a below-knee amputation (Figure 14-22). Five years postoperatively, digital temperatures showed a marked difference in the sympathectomized limb compared to the contralateral (nonsympathectomized) extremity, and the Doppler systolic pressures were

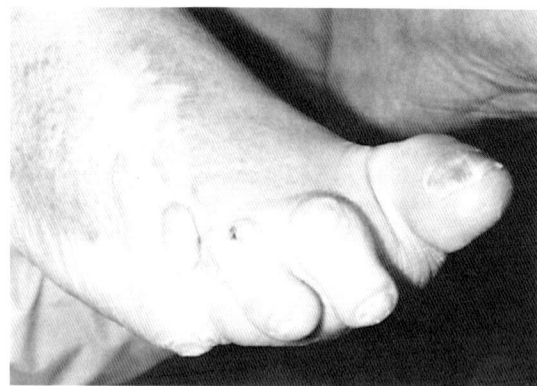

Figure 14-22. Postoperative sympathectomy showing complete healing of huge ulcerations of dorsum of right foot.

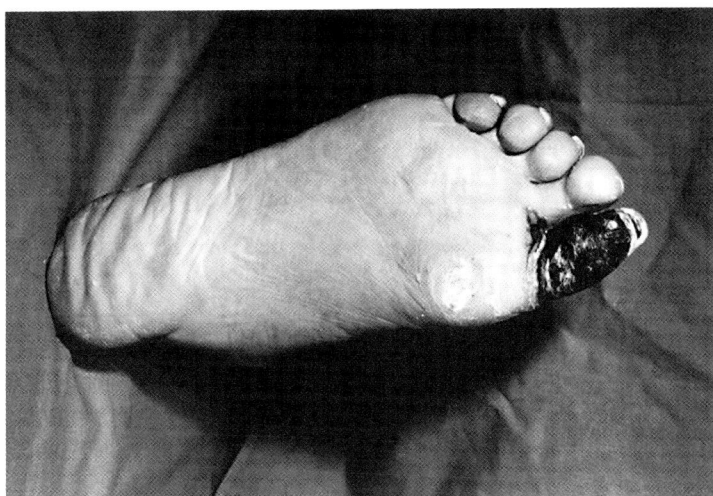

Figure 14-23. Gangrenous right great toe and necrotic area on the dorsum of the foot.

within normal limits. The sympathectomy effect was present nine years later, and the patient died of a myocardial infarction ten years postsympathectomy.

CASE 6

A sixty-eight-year-old male, in long-term noninsulin-dependent diabetes, presented with a gangrenous right great toe and a necrotic area on the dorsum of the foot (Figure 14-23). Angiography showed a patent common femoral artery with occlusion of the superficial femoral artery and reconstitution of the popliteal artery with two vesels runoff. After thorough assessment, the patient underwent a right femoropopliteal bypass using a reversed saphenous vein graft. Four months later, because of an ischemic ulcer on the anterolateral aspect of the middle third of the leg, another angiogram was performed which showed a patent right bypass and an occlusion of the left superficial femoral artery with a patent posterior tibial artery (Figure 14-24). Subsequently, the patient underwent a left femoro-posterior tibial bypass using an in situ saphenous vein graft and a concomitant ipsilateral lumbar sympathectomy. An intraoperative angiogram showed a patent graft with good visualization of the distal runoff and good communication with the dorsalis pedis artery (Figure 14-25). Photoplethysmography results and digital tempera-

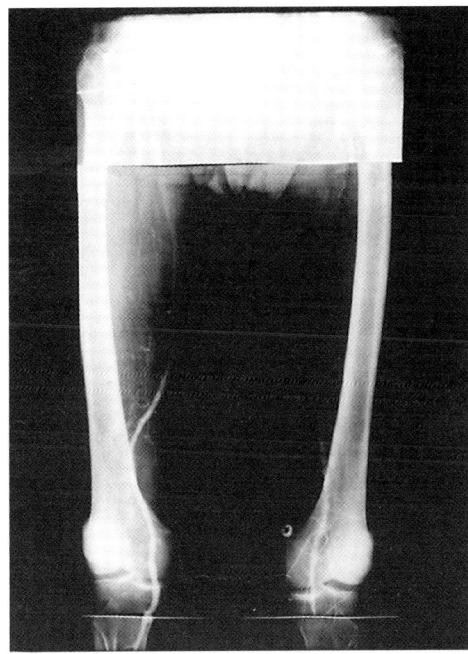

Figure 14-24. Angiogram showing a patent right bypass and occlusion of left superficial femoral artery with a patent posterior tibial artery.

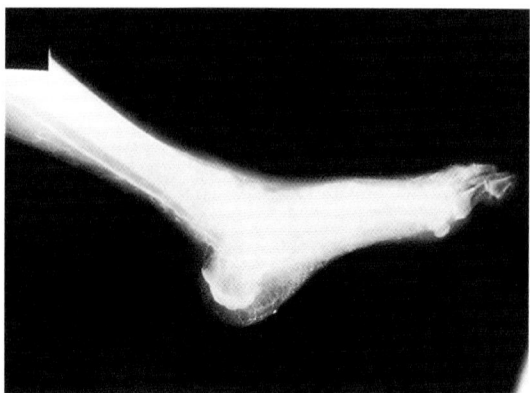

Figure 14-25. Intraoperative angiogram showing a patent graft, adequate anastomosis, and good distal runoff with communication with the dorsalis pedis artery.

tures improved in the sympathectomized extremity compared to the extremity with a bypass graft alone (Figure 14-26). After debridement of the necrotic area and a skin graft, the ulcer healed (Figure 14-27). Twelve years later the patient had a viable left lower extremity and had undergone a right below-knee amputation (Figure 14-28).

CASE 7

A sixty-year-old white, male, insulin-dependent diabetic presented complaining of severe pain with a swollen, erythematous left foot infection. Systolic Doppler pressures were within normal limits. X-rays showed neither gas nor bone involvement. The

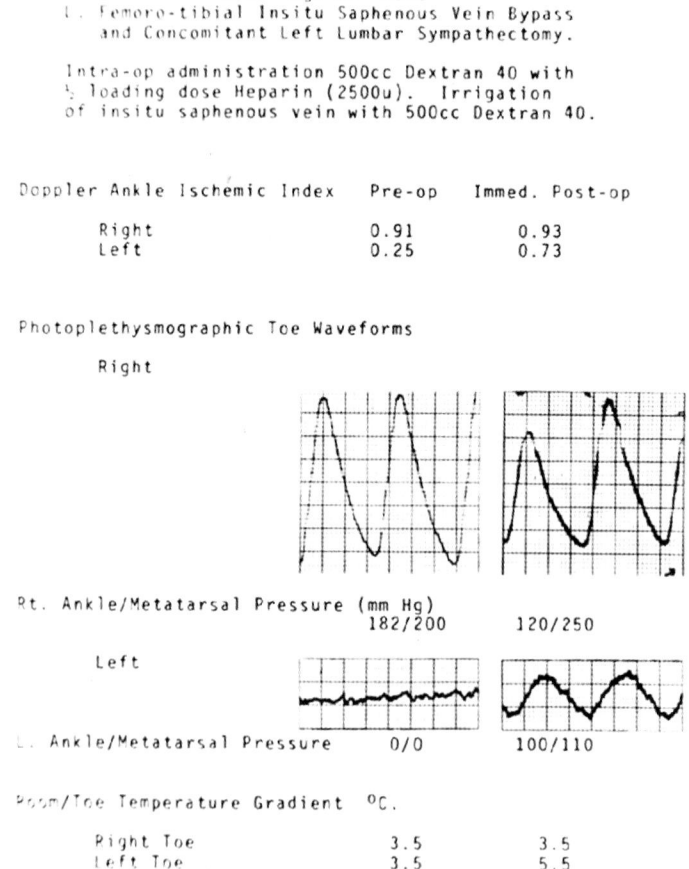

Figure 14-26. Noninvasive vascular studies after the patient underwent a femoro-posterior tibial bypass graft and concomitant sympathectomy.

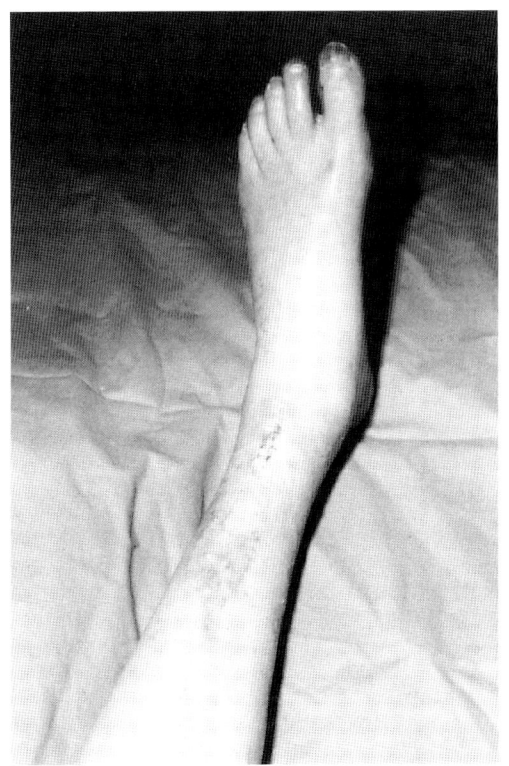

patient was placed on antibiotics, but continued to have severe pain especially on dorsiflexion and the foot continued to be swollen and tense. The patient subsequently underwent a fasciotomy using a modified medial approach of Henry for decompression of the medial, central, interosseous, and lateral compartment of the foot (Figure 14-29 Color Plate 1). Abundant pus was obtained from the medial and central compartments. Intensive local wound care and systemic antibiotics were employed in the postoperative period. One month later, the patient received a skin graft with good healing. At one year follow-up, the fasciotomy wound is completely healed with no residual pain (Figure 14-30 Color Plate 1).

TREATMENT

An analysis of the problem must be made, and intermediate goals and outcomes must be established. Control of diabetes, which may be worsened by foot infection, is of clinical importance. Surgical intervention may be necessary for debridement of the necrotic tissue or even amputation of an irreversibly gangrenous digit. Although a major de-

Figure 14-27. After a skin graft, the foot lesion healed completely.

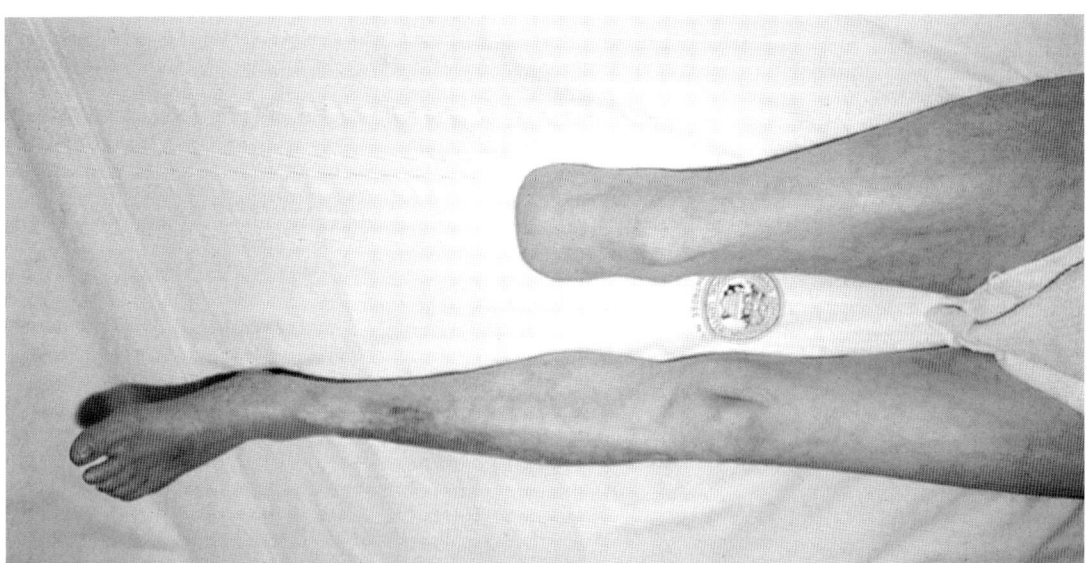

Figure 14-28. Right lower extremity: right femoro-infrapopliteal bypass (only) without lumbar sympathectomy ended in right below-knee amputation five years postoperative.

bridement followed by minor debridement at the bedside or in the clinic may be satisfactory, advanced infections will require multiple major debridements or definitive amputation. This is different than the approach required for pure ischemia.

ANTIBIOTIC THERAPY

Diabetic soft tissue infection can spread very quickly and lead to gangrene or osteomyelitis. The infections are usually mixed infections, and the most severe involve a greater number and variety of Gram-negative aerobes and anaerobes. Empiric therapy for diabetic foot infections should begin with a broad-spectrum antibiotic. The microbial population is influenced by the patient's local environment (e.g., home, nursing home, hospital, farm, occupation) [61]. The Gram-positive cocci are primarily *Staphylococcus aureus* as well as groups D and B streptococci. Gram-negative organisms are commonly *Escherichia coli, Klebsiella, Enterobacter aerogenes, Proteus mirabilis*, and *Pseudomonas aeruginosa*. Anaerobic species include *Bacteroides fragilis*, peptostreptococci, and clostridial species. The anaerobes can outnumber the aerobes 10 to 1, and systemic bacteremias are most commonly associated with *B. fragilis* and *S. aureus* infections [60]. Despite the polymicrobial nature of diabetic foot infections, they can be treated on an outpatient basis using short- and long-acting cephalosporins, fluorinated quinolones such as ciprofloxacin and oral clindamycin. These have been demonstrated to be effective in diabetic foot infections. However, inpatients with diabetic foot infections are treated in a different manner, using intravenous antibiotics (Table 14-2). Ticarcillin with clavulanate as well as ampicillin with sulbactam are considered to be the first choice in the case of the superficial ulcer. Second-choice antimicrobials include cefoxitin, cephamycin, ceftizoxime, ciprofloxacin, and either clindamycin or metronidazole. For systemic sepsis, ticarcillin with clavulante or ampicillin with sulbactam are first antibiotic choice as are cephalosporins, aztreonam, and clindamycin. An aminoglycoside can be added to a third-generation cephalosporin. As a second choice in systemic sepsis, intravenous ciprofloxacin and either metronidazole or clindamycin may be used [61, 62].

Table 14-2.   Initial Antimicrobial (Empiric) Therapy of Diabetic Foot Infections

Type of Infection	Common bacterias	First-choice antimicrobial therapy	Second choice of antimicrobials and/or addition
Superficial ulcer	*S. aureus, S. epidermidis*, enterococci, Gram-negative aerobes, *Proteus, Pseudomonas*, anaerobes	Ticarcillin / clavulanate Ampicillin / sulbactam	Cefoxitin or other cephamycin, ceftizoxime, ciprofloxacin, and either clindamycin or metronidazole
Sepsis	*S. aureus, S. epidermidis*, enterococci, Gram-negative aerobes, *Proteus, Pseudomonas*, anaerobes	Ticarcillin / clavulanate, Ampicillin / sulbactam, Imipenem / cilastatin Third-generation cephalosporin or aztreonam with clindamycin Aminoglycoside, aztreonam, or third-generation cephalosporin with ampicillin and clindamycin	Ciprofloxacin and either clindamycin or metronidazole

WOUND CARE

Wound care after a major surgical debridement should provide an ideal environment for tissue healing. Meticulous cleaning of the wound with normal saline or isotonic soaps is done along with periodic sharp debridement of exudates and the application of antibiotic ointment dressings. Occlusive dressings enhance the ingrowth of delicate granulation tissues and wound closure.

TOTAL CONTACT WALKING CAST

The application of a cast over the wound aids in wound healing by (1) redistributing the weight-bearing load over the entire lower leg and plantar surface, (2) immobilizing the limb to decrease the spread of bacteria, (3) protecting the wound from further direct trauma, (4) improving the microcirculation by reducing interstitial edema, and (5) eliminating the need for patient participation in local wound care. The total contact plaster cast is applied with a minimum of padding around each maleolus, the anterior tibia, and the bony prominences of the first and fifth metatarsal heads. Following application of the padding, a contour plaster cast with a walking platform bottom is applied. Usually, the cast is changed weekly until the wound is healed. In patients with excessive wound exudate, the cast is changed more frequently. Wound healing time averages six to eight weeks with this technique [62].

TREATMENT OF NEUROTROPHIC ULCERS

Neurotrophic ulcers can be divided into the following four clinical groups: (1) uncomplicated ulcers with a granulating bed, (2) uncomplicated ulcers with localized areas of necrotic debris, (3) locally infected ulcers, and (4) infected ulcers with extension of the infection into the deep spaces of the foot. Uncomplicated ulcers usually have minimal drainage. The treatment of an uncomplicated neurotrophic ulcer with a granulating tissue bed consists of debridement of the surrounding callus followed by the application of a total contact plaster cast. Neurotrophic ulcers with necrotic debris or local infection require more extensive surgical debridement, which commonly includes the plantar fascia, flexor tendons, the volar plate of the metatarsophalangeal joint, and the head of the metatarsal bone. If, after the debridement of necrotic and infected tissue is complete, the metatarsophalangeal joint is open, the metatarsal head and cartilaginous surface of the proximal phalanx should be excised. Infections extending into the deep spaces of the foot require extending the incision longitudinally along the plantar surface to provide adequate drainage and debridement. During the dissection, intact vascular structures and viable muscle should be preserved. However, because tendons often undergo rapid necrosis owing to their tenuous blood supply, they must be completely debrided to control the infectious process. In all cases, debridement should extend down until bleeding tissue is reached.

AMPUTATION

When considering an amputation, whether it is a toe or an above-knee amputation, the goals must be to: (1) control infection and remove all necrotic tissue, (2) optimize rehabilitation by performing the lowest level of amputation consistent with wound healing, (3) avoid exacerbation of other disabilities by a high-level amputation, and (4) have an adequate blood supply for wound healing.

Amputation of the lower extremity is a frequent consequence of peripheral vascular disease, peripheral neuropathy, and infection in the diabetic foot. Patients with peripheral vascular disease comprise approximately 80% of the amputees in the Western world, and 75% of these amputees are diabetic [63].

The metabolic cost of walking is increased and the self-selected walking speed decreased with more proximal level amputations. These factors become critical in the diabetic patient who has concomitant multiple system disease and a limited cardiopulmonary reserve, as compared with traumatic amputees. To optimize the independence of these patients, it is essential to perform amputations at the most distal level feasible, with the potential to walk after amputation [64, 65].

The *biologic amputation level* is the most distal functional amputation level with a reasonable (85–90%) potential to be healed. This is determined by clinical examination and a measure of adequate vascular inflow, tissue nutrition, and immunocompetence. For amputations of the foot and ankle, the following criteria must be met: (1) the heel pad must be free of open lesions, (2) there should be no gross pus at the amputation site, and (3) there should be no local soft tissue infection; i.e., cellulitis at the level of surgery. When ascending soft tissue cellulitis is present, this must be resolved with antibiotics, local surgery, or a combination of both, because primary wound closure will not be successful in the presence of ascending cellulitis. Impending gangrene should be evaluated by a vascular surgeon whose highest priority is limb salvage. An open partial foot amputation has frequently been performed to decompress an infection, removing gangrenous tissue, prior to performing vascular reconstruction and a definitive secondary functional amputation [35].

The Doppler-determined ankle/brachial pressure ratio (ankle/brachial index or ABI) is an important predictor of wound healing [66]. The ABI has been popularized by Wagner, who has suggested that wound healing rates approach 90% when adequate inflow is present [67]. Measurement of transcutaneous oxygen partial pressure (TcPO$_2$) currently predicts a wound healing rate of approximately 90% when it is greater than 30 mmHg, 70% when it is between 20 and 29 mmHg, and less than 50% when it is below 20 mmHg [68]. At present, using different light reflectance technology, the muscle oxygen of patients with peripheral vascular disease is being assessed [69, 70].

TOE AMPUTATION

Toe amputation should be performed in diabetic patients with persistent toe ulcerations, gangrene limited to the toe, osteomyelitis of the distal and middle phalanx, or a septic interphalangeal joint. Usually, the amputation is performed after medical treatment has been instituted to control the infection. The level of amputation is determined by the level infection in the phalanx and the level of uninvolved and viable skin. The maximum amount of proximal toe that can be salvaged is to the base of the proximal phalanx. However, if the capsule of the metatarsophalangeal joint must be entered, then the amputation should be performed proximally to

the neck of the metatarsal to avoid exposure of the articular cartilage. Frequently, such wounds are not closed initially but are allowed to granulate under a topical occlusive dressing or a cadaveric skin graft. Later, a split-thickness skin graft may be used to close the wound. If the wound is closed primarily, this should be done without skin tension, and a closed system drain should be used [34, 35].

RAY AMPUTATION

When the necrotic process involves the base of the toes, a Ray amputation of the metatarsal bone is necessary. An amputation more proximal than the metatarsal neck may be performed to facilitate adequate soft tissue coverage of the bone. If several toes are involved, they may be resected individually, either at the metatarsal necks or more proximal at the base of the metatarsals. A transmetatarsal amputation has no advantage over multiple Ray amputations. Both of these foot amputations require only a simple foam shoe insert for ambulation and differ little in their ability to preserve foot function [34, 35].

TRANSMETATARSAL AMPUTATION

A transmetatarsal amputation may have to be performed for foot salvage when the infection involves multiple toes or the metatarsal phalangeal joints, or when inadequate distal soft tissue is available for bony coverage. An intact plantar foot pad is necessary because the amputation will be reflected dorsally, placing the suture line on the dorsum of the foot and the thick pad on the stump end. Amputations of each metatarsal sometimes need to be varied at the osteotomy level in order to have a tension-free skin closure or to preserve sufficient tissue for wound closure over the bone. The skin incision should allow maximal preservation of excess skin and any tension on the wound closure mandates that the wound be left open to heal by secondary intention or subsequent skin grafts [34, 35].

MAJOR AMPUTATION

Major amputations are often necessary in patients with overwhelming sepsis or deep compart-

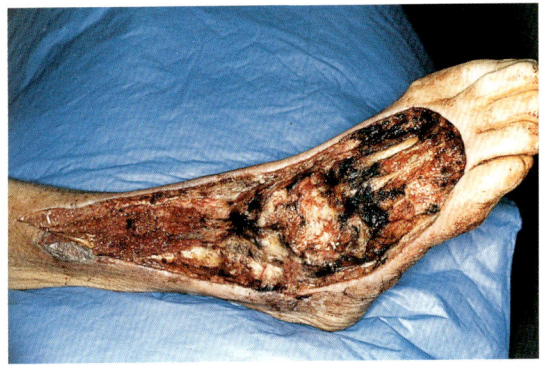

Figure 14-19. Right foot with necrotizing fascitis involving its dorsum, after debridement.

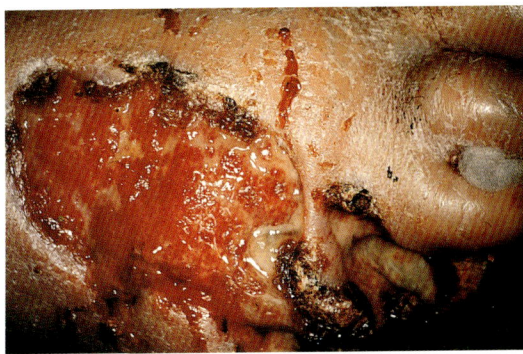

Figure 14-20. Gangrenous changes of the right foot.

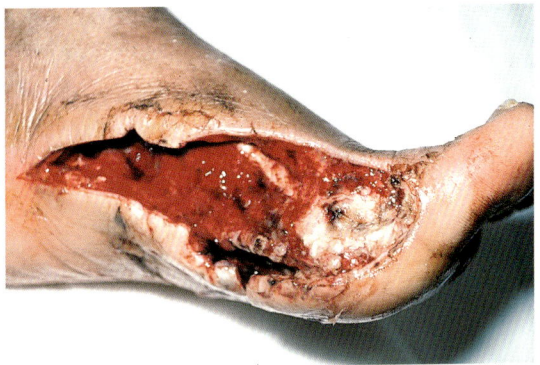

Figure 14-29. Modified medial approach of Henry for decompression of the four compartments of the foot.

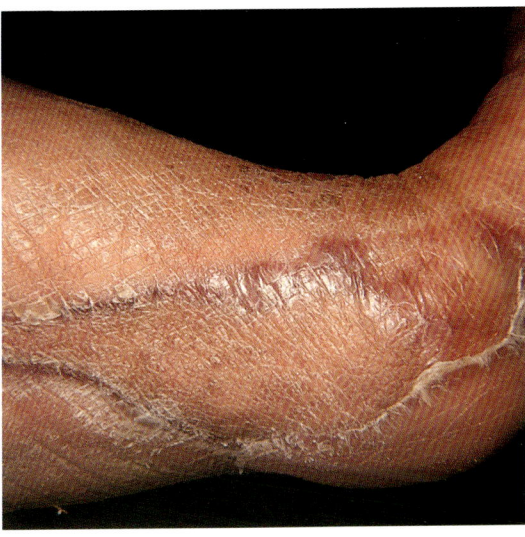

Figure 14-30. Complete healing of fasciotomy with no residual pain at one year follow-up.

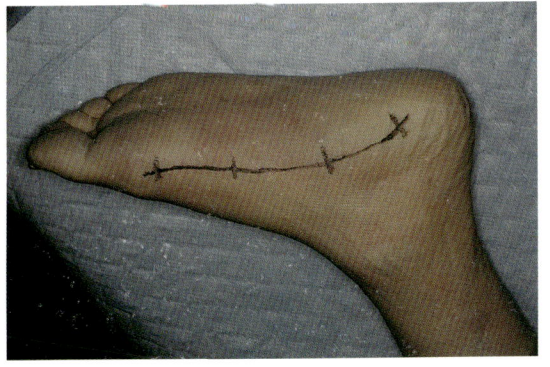

Figure 16-2. A plantar medial incision is shown, dividing the skin and superficial fascia at the inner side of the foot, from the ball of the great toe to the heel. This follows the length of the plantar surface of the first metatarsal and curves up to cross the tuberosity of navicular bone. The limits of the incision are the tuber calcanei and the head of the first metatarsal.

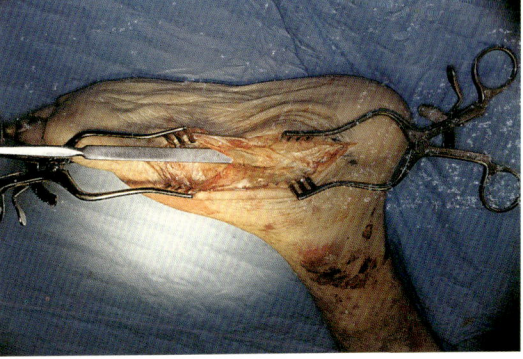

Figure 16-3. This figure shows that the medial extension of the plantar aponeurosis is incised longitudinally to decompress the medial compartment.

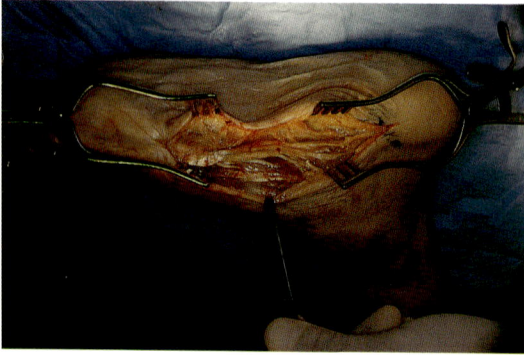

Figure 16-4. The abductor hallucis tendon is identified at the inner side of the first metatarsal. This tendon is mobilized, taking care to leave intact adjoining fleshy fibers of flexor hallucis brevis.

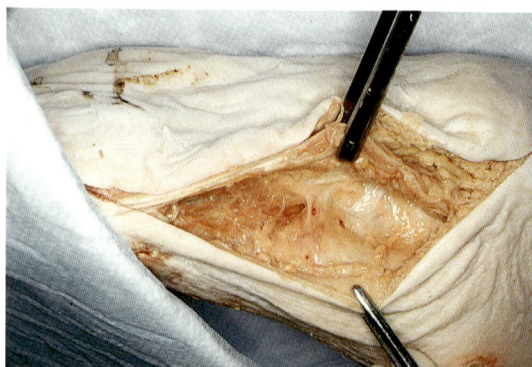

Figure 16-5. This figure shows that the abductor hallucis muscle is retracted inferiorly. When this is done, a partial screen of fascia is observed.

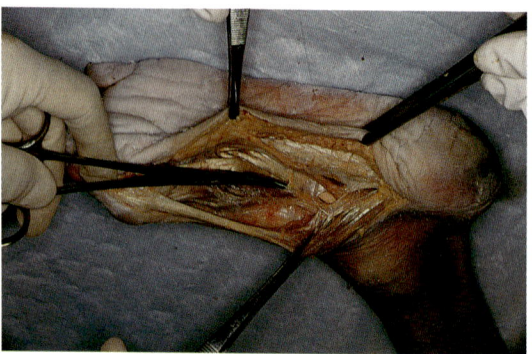

Figure 16-6. The master knot is shown. The master knot is an aponeurotic band attached approximately 1 cm lateral to the tuberosity of the navicular.

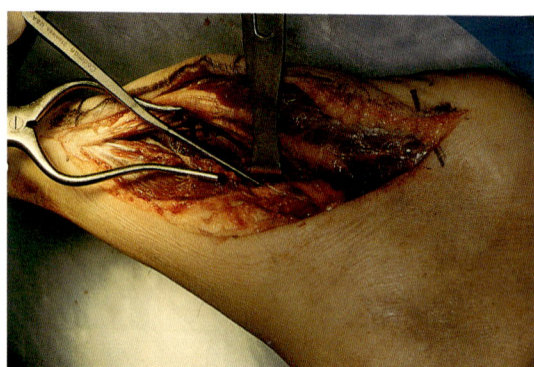

Figure 16-7. The medial intermuscular septum is exposed and open longitudinally, decompressing the central compartment.

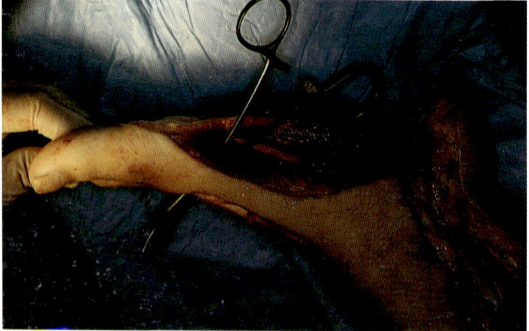

Figure 16-8. The interosseous compartment is decompressed by longitudinally incising the plantar interosseous fascia superior to the quadratus plantae muscle. Note that in this case, additional dissection has been done to decompress the interosseous fascial compartment via the dorsum of the foot. The plantar medial incision is also extended more proximally above the level of the ankle.

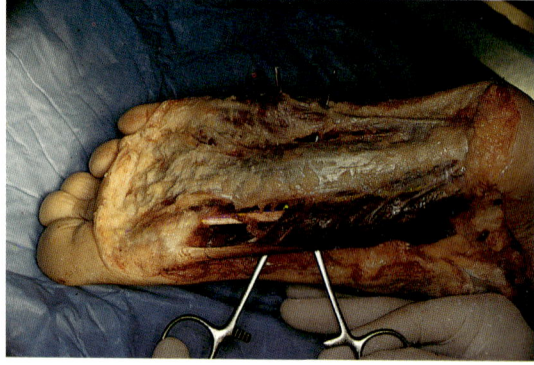

Figure 16-9. Dissection between the lumbrical muscles and the flexor digitorum brevis muscle allows incision of the lateral intermuscular septum and decompression of the lateral compartment. In this case, an amputated foot has been dissected in which the plantar skin flap has been removed, in order to better illustrate the dissection.

Color Plate 2

Figure 17-1 (a). A typical sacral pressure sore with chronically scarred tissue heaped at the margin.

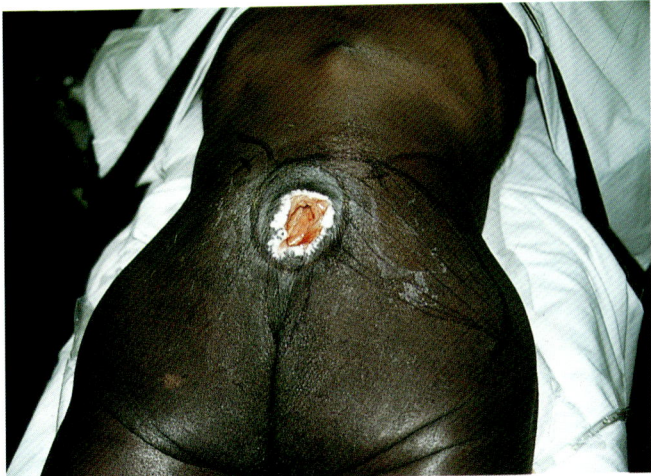

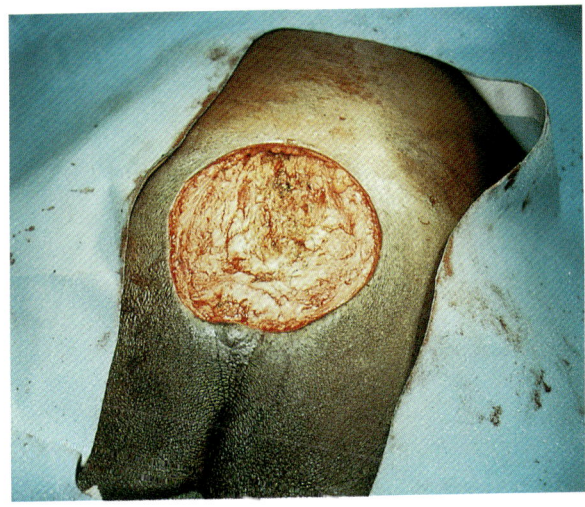

Figure 17-1 (b). The "true" defect after excision of the ulcer including a wide margin of indurated skin. The created wound contains only clearly surgical planes without granulation tissue or bursa lining to allow for primary healing.

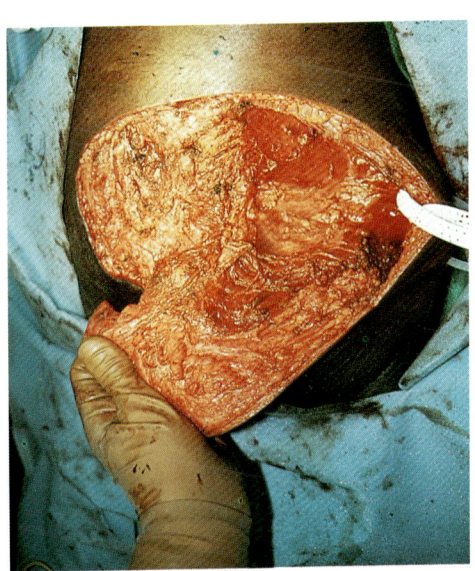

Figure 17-1 (c). A large, inferiorly based, gluteus maximus myocutaneous flap is incised and elevated. This is supplied by both the superior and inferior gluteal vessels.

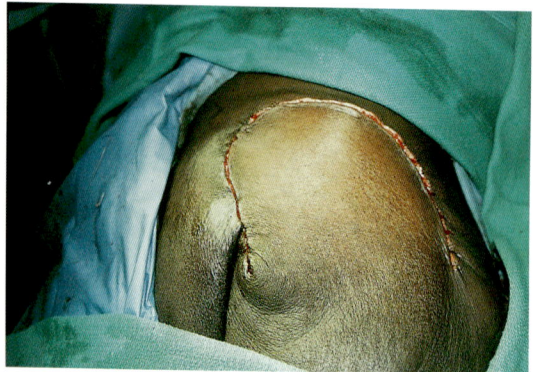

Figure 17-1 (d). Flap rotated into defect.

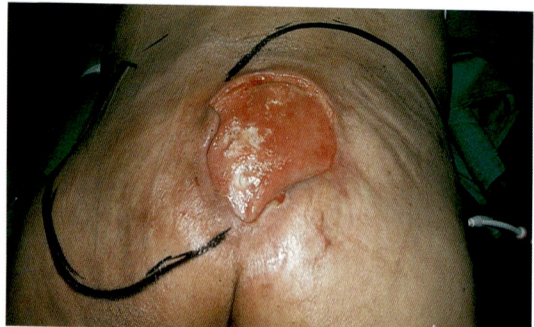

Figure 17-2 (a). A larger sacral pressure sore prior to excision. Bilateral gluteus maximus myocutaneous rotation flaps are outlined. One is superiorly based, the other inferiorly based.

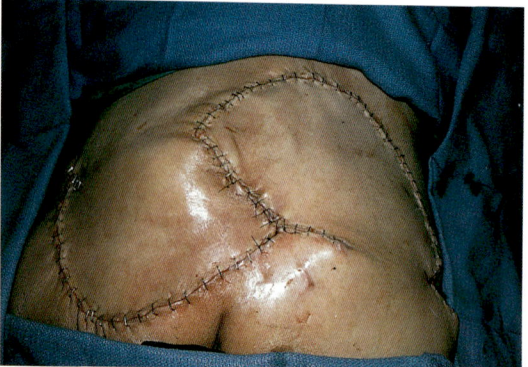

Figure 17-2 (b). Wound closed with bilateral rotation in "yin-yang" fashion.

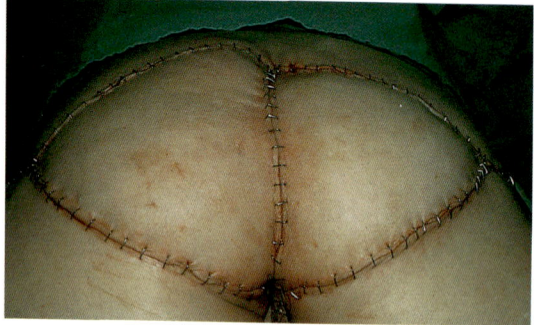

Figure 17-3. A similarly large sacral pressure sore closed by bilateral gluteus maximus myocutaneous advancement flaps. Each flap is incised in a V-shape. After both flaps are advanced medially to fill the defect, the lateral donor regions are closed in linear fashion, resulting in a final Y-shaped closure.

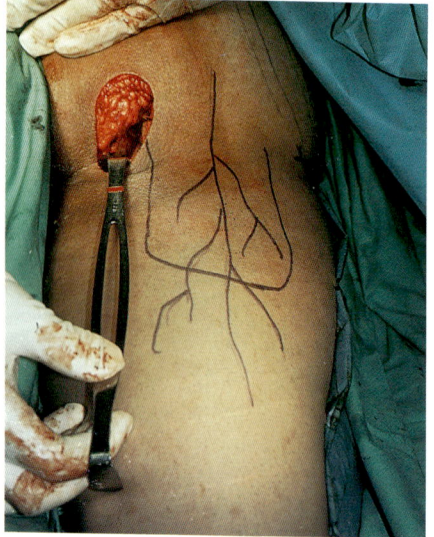

Figure 17-5 (a). An ischial pressure sore after excision. The gluteal thigh flap is outlined, centered about the posterior thigh extension of the inferior gluteal vessels.

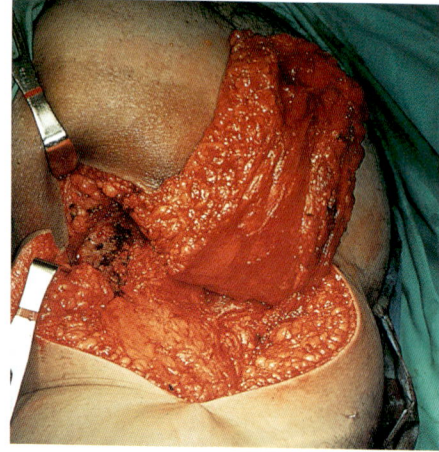

Figure 17-5 (b). The flap is elevated deep to the muscle fascia to ensure that it contains the vessels.

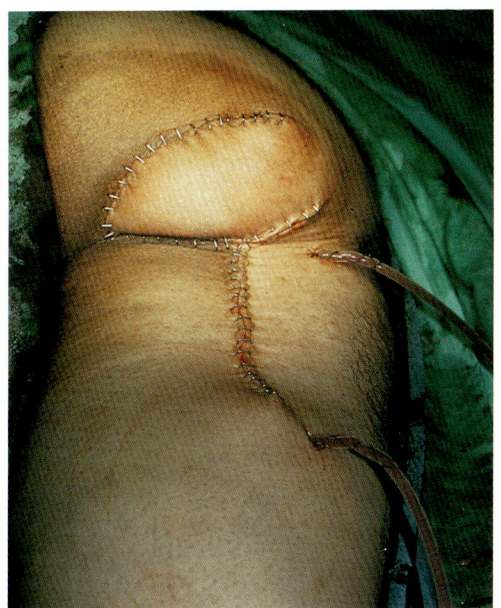

Figure 17-5 (c). Gluteal thigh flap rotated into defect with primary closure of donor site.

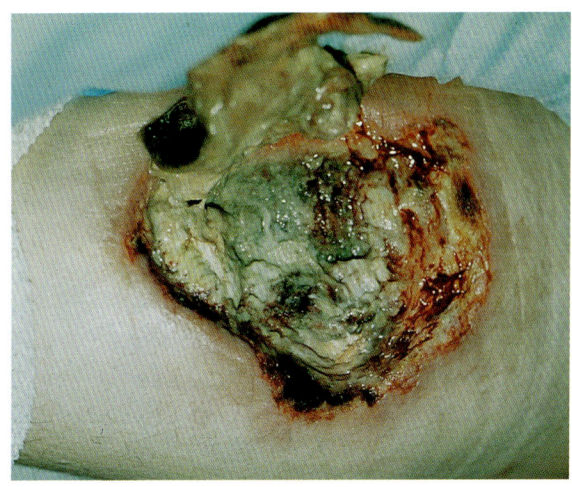

Figure 18-1 (a). Extensive trochanteric pressure ulcer.

Figure 18-1 (b). Multiple extensive recurrent pressure ulcers.

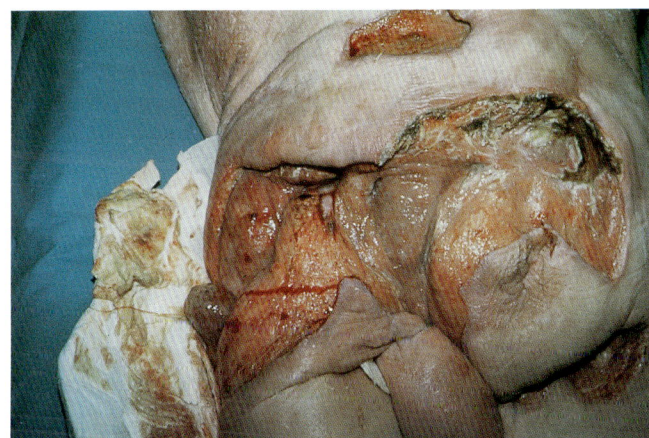

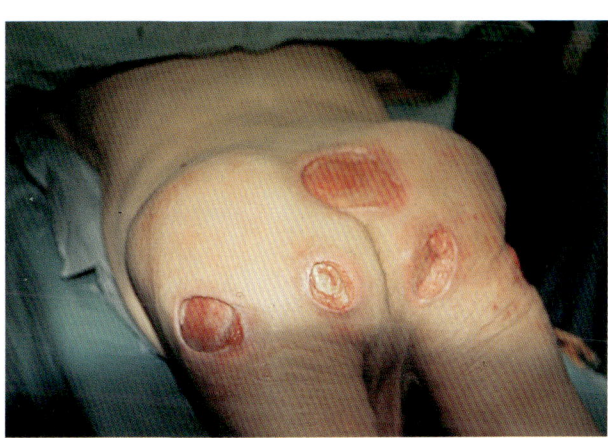

Figure 18-1 (c). Bilateral trochanteric, bilateral ischial, and sacral pressure ulcers.

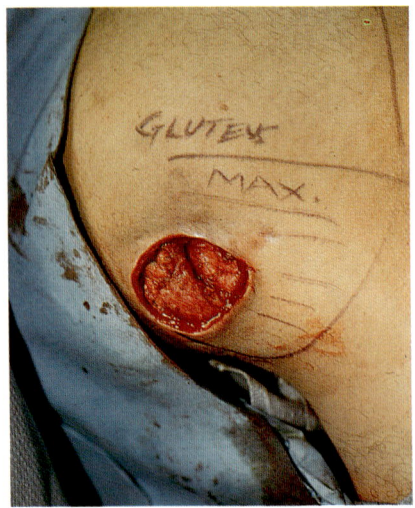

Figure 18-2 (a). Debrided ischial pressure ulcer with a superiorly based gluteus maximus myocutaneous flap outlined.

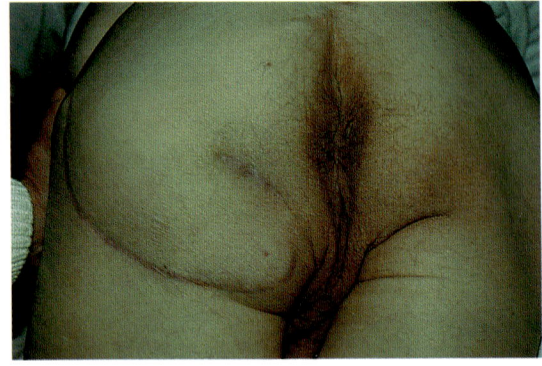

Figure 18-2 (b). A three-month postoperative result of gluteus maximus myocutaneous flap transfer to cover an ischial.

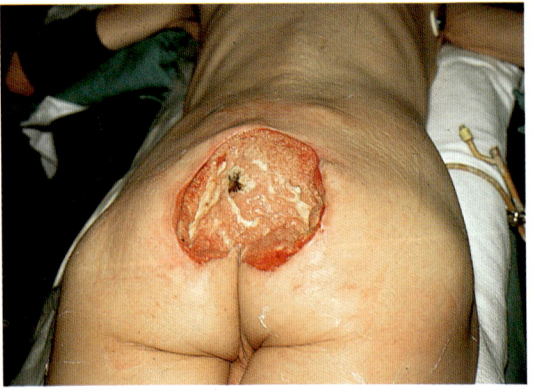

Figure 18-3 (a). A typically shallow sacral pressure ulcer.

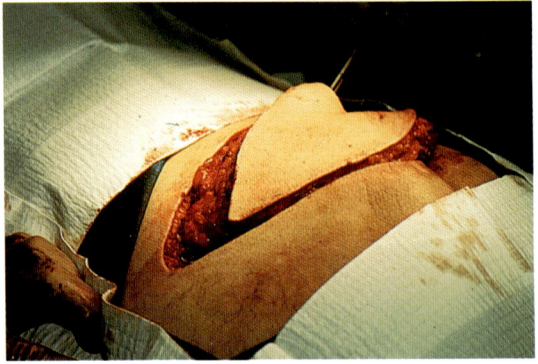

Figure 18-3 (b). A V-Y advancement of a heart-shaped gluteus maximus myocutaneous flap to cover a sacral pressure ulcer.

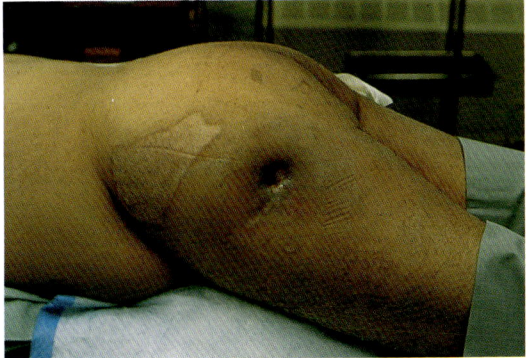

Figure 18-4 (a). A typical early trochanteric pressure ulcer with a small cutaneous defect.

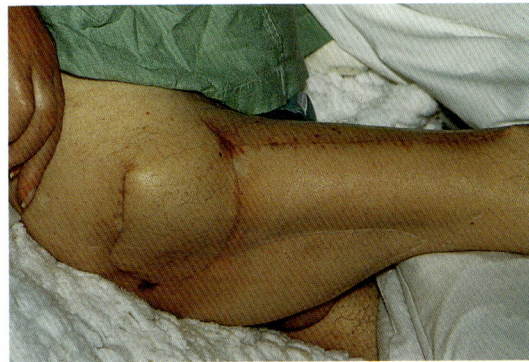

Figure 18-4 (b). A tensor fascia lata myocutaneous flap transposed to cover a large trochanteric ulcer and a recurrence of an ischial ulcer.

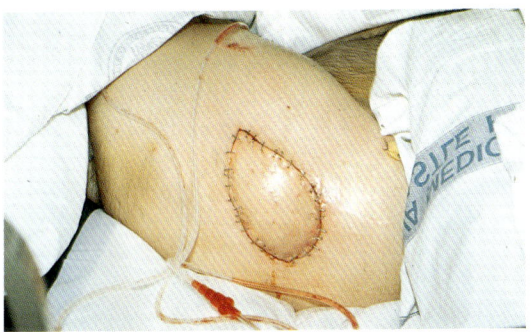

Figure 18-4 (c). A rectus femoris myocutaneous island flap transferred for a trochanteric defect.

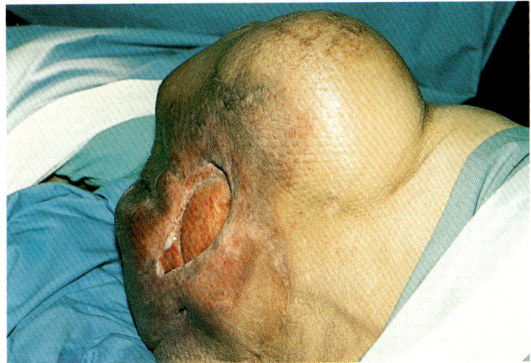

Figure 18-5. An example of a recurrent sacral pressure ulcer with a tissue expander in position under the gluteus maximus muscle.

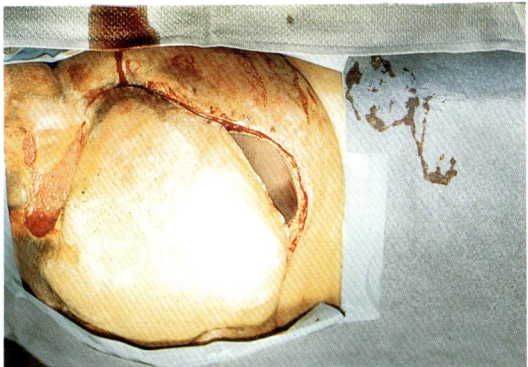

Figure 18-6 (a). An expanded gluteus maximus myocutaneous flap with expander in situ for a recurrent ischial pressure sore.

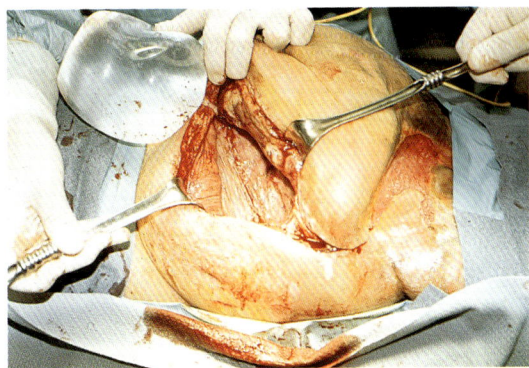

Figure 18-6 (b). An expanded gluteus maximus flap with expander removed and flap being raised.

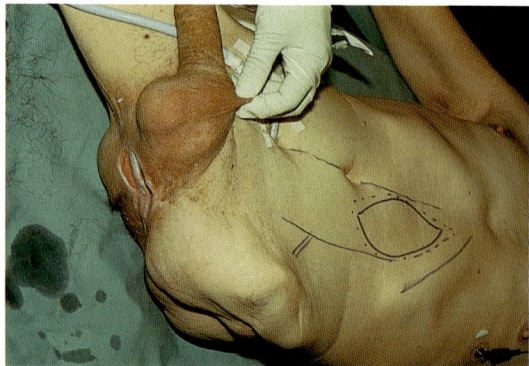

Figure 18-7 (a). An ischial pressure sore in an amputee with perineal extension. An outline of the proposed inferiorly based abdominis flap is seen on the abdomen.

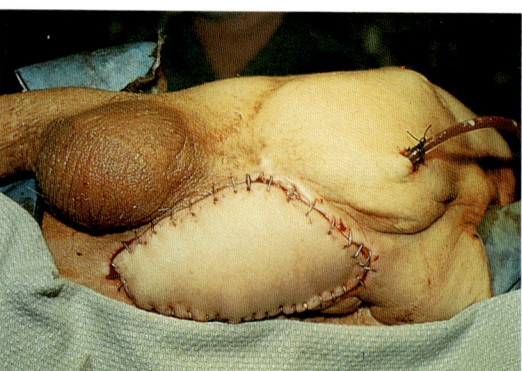

Figure 18-7 (b). The inferiorly based rectus abdominis myocutaneous flap raised and transferred as an island and inset in the ischial and perineal wound.

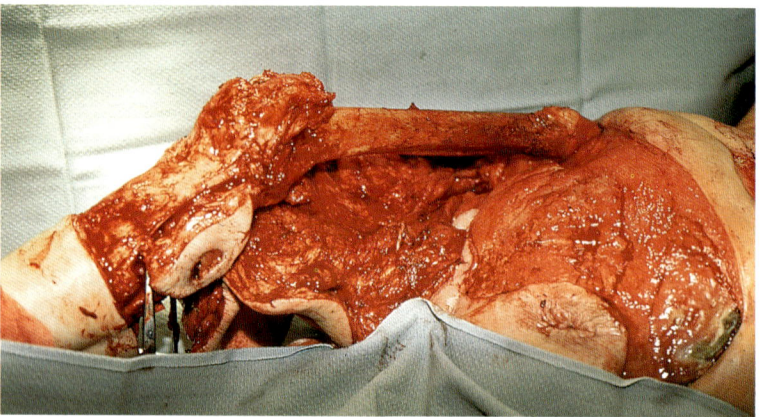

Figure 18-8 (a). Extensive, recurrent, confluent ulceration of the sacral, ischial, and trochanteric area with fillet flap of thigh operative procedure in process.

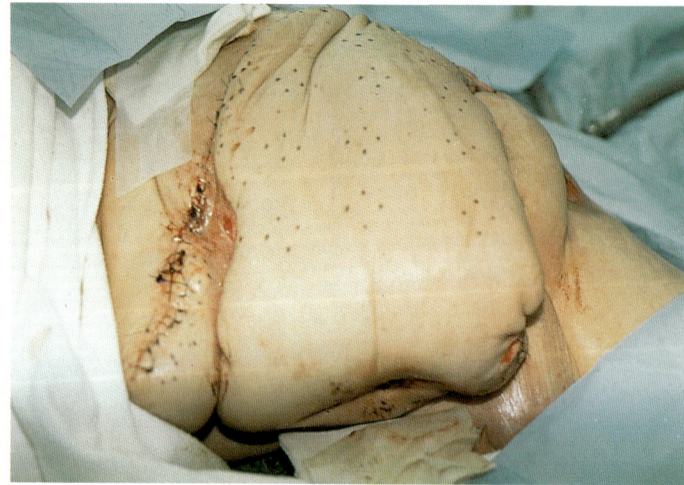

Figure 18-8 (b). Fillet flap of thigh used as a salvage procedure to cover an extensive confluent area of ulceration.

ment abscesses with extensive forefoot gangrene or impending tissue loss. Below-knee amputations are the most commonly performed amputations. Although through-the-knee amputations are easy to perform, they are less desirable because of the difficulty of fitting a prosthesis with an appropriate knee. The level of amputation is based on the extent of necrosis, inflammation, and infection, in addition to an evaluation of the patient's vascular status. The longer the stump the better the anticipated rehabilitation results; therefore, every effort should be made to preserve extremity length consistent with prosthesis fitting. This may require that the amputation, whether above or below the knee, be staged, with the initial operation performed to control the infectious process and subsequent procedures performed to achieve wound closure at a later date. In the case of a staged below-knee operation, the posterior flap should be left as long as possible at the initial operation and then trimmed at the time of definitive closure to give a tension-free closure of the skin and a soft muscular pad at the stump end [34].

ARTERIAL RECONSTRUCTIVE SURGERY

The decision to perform vascular surgery depends on the severity of the vascular lesions, the risk associated with surgery, and the potential for rehabilitation. Advanced age per se does not preclude surgical intervention. Modern revascularization procedures are tailored to individual requirements based on a thorough preoperative assessment. With aggressive preoperative cardio vascular monitoring, revascularization can be as safe as a major amputation and less costly. At three years after the bypass, , 87% of patients with autogenous vein bypass grafts to the foot vessels continue to have patent arteries, and 92% did not require amputation. In patients with extensive tissue loss or gangrene of the foot, restoration of pulsatile blood flow to the foot is required for healing. Aggressive arterial reconstruction, including bypass grafts to the foot vessels, allows debridement of soft tissue and resection of osteomyelitic bone without amputation. The attempts of revascularization for limb salvage in diabetic patients as reported by Dalsing et al. have shown a prevention of amputation in 70% of patients for one year and 60% for three years [71]. This result, together with a low operative mortality rate (1.7%), justifies an aggressive attempt at limb salvage. Various factors such as outflow resistance, pedal arch anatomy and graft material influence the results of distal bypasses. Graft material is the most important factor influencing patency. The PTFE grafts have a higher failure rate compared to vein or composite sequential grafts. The site of distal anastomosis was not a factor influencing graft patency in some reported series [72, 73]. Anastomosis to the anterior tibial, posterior tibial, or peroneal artery had the same chance for success [74].

Endovascular techniques (balloon angioplasty and atherectomy) may restore the patency of proximal arteries with limited occlusive disease but are generally contraindicated for limb threatening occlusion of infrainguinal arteries [75–77].

LUMBAR SYMPATHECTOMY

Lumbar sympathectomy is useful in increasing blood flow in both diabetic and nondiabetic patients. We suggest resection of more than two ganglia; specifically, the second, third, and fourth, in the case of more distal atherosclerotic occlusive disease. This will improve blood flow to the digits. The main indication for sympathectomy will be a diffuse distribution of atherosclerotic occlusive disease not amenable to arterial reconstructive procedures. We have an eight-year cumulative limb salvage rate of 71%, with a 51% cumulative toe salvage rate. Clinical data and noninvasive vascular studies support the role of sympathectomy in diabetic patients. Our findings suggest that sympathectomy promotes healing through increased blood flow in the presence of limited areas of pregangrene or actual gangrene of the toes, but not with extensive involvement of the toes. Lumbar sympathectomy increases skin blood flow, muscle oxygen content, improves claudication, promotes wound healing, and decreases the level of amputation [78]. There have also been reports concerning the value of sympathectomy in ischemic rest pain, ischemic ulceration, and wet gangrene, particularly digital gangrene. Lumbar sympathectomy has also been proven useful when performed before or during arterial reconstructive surgery [78, 79].

DECOMPRESSIVE FASCIOTOMY

The association of infection and neuropathy will lead to a delay in the diagnosis of a deep diabetic foot infection. An increase in the compartment pressure occurs with infection involving the compartment and the presence of a previously deteriorated arterial circulation. Once increased pressure has developed in the foot compartments, the only effective mode of treatment is decompression. Surgical intervention should be performed in those cases of foot infection with clinical signs of compartment syndrome, such as loss of motor power or sensation of the foot. An increase in tissue pressure above 30 mm Hg is an absolute indication for fasciotomy.

A review of the orthopedic literature reveals various recommendations regarding the surgical techniques used to decompress the osseofascial compartments of the foot. Mubarak and Hargens recommended two longitudinal dorsal incisions [36]. Hansen, Bonutti and Bell, and Wright and associates suggested a plantar medial incision [80]. Myerson compared the use of these two approaches in experimental and clinical studies and found a double dorsal longitudinal approach to be technically easier [81]. The plantar medial approach provides more rapid decompression of compartment pressure and can be extended proximally to allow exploration of the neurovascular bundle and its branches on the medial side of the foot and ankle. Myerson stated that the plantar medial approach is the most effective way to treat compartment syndromes not associated with fractures [36, 80, 81]. We believe that the medial approach to the compartments of an infected diabetic foot with increased compartment pressure is the best approach because it allows decompression of all four compartments with a single incision, and additionally, pressure points are avoided (see Chapter 16).

PREVENTIVE PROCEDURES

Operative procedures designed to reduce mechanical trauma to the foot, wound or plantar surface reduce the risk of plantar ulcerations and the development of infections. These might include metatarsal osteotomies or removal of metatarsal heads. Bunions and clawtoe deformities should be surgically corrected before pressure-related complications occur. Fixed clawtoe deformities are corrected by resecting the base of the proximal phalanx of the great toe. Resection of the metatarsal head through a dorsal approach allows healing of the plantar ulcer by relieving the plantar prominence. Likewise, a dorsal wedge osteotomy of the adjacent metatarsal shaft near its base subsequently prevents the formation of an adjacent plantar ulcer [82, 83].

PROGNOSIS

Cutaneous ulcers are among the most common reasons for hospital admission in the diabetic patient. A diabetic foot infection represents a failure by the patient and his management team to understand and correct the multifactorial conditions that predisposed the patient to this problem. Efforts directed toward prevention of foot lesions are much more likely to meet with success than is therapy of the established foot sore. This preventive approach is likely to lead to a reduction in the incidence of major amputations and thereby improve the quality of life and life expectancy.

Understanding the pathophysiology associated with the diabetic foot is essential to the care of the diabetic patient. When there is a failure in skin integrity, prompt assessment of vascular, neural, soft tissue, and wound status enhances the possibility of a successful clinical outcome. The complexity of the management of a diabetic requires the knowledge and skill of a multidisciplinary team—an internist, podiatrist, rehabilitation specialist, prosthetist, dietitian, and social worker in addition to a surgeon interested in caring for the complications of diabetic feet. The goals of a multidisciplinary approach are to optimize local wound care, provide correct footwear, improve glucose control, educate the patient concerning diet and life style changes, and identify the presence of peripheral neuropathies and reconstructable arterial lesions. The goals will also include improvement in circulation when necessary through arterial reconstruction and/or sympathectomy. This combined team approach has been documented to substantially reduce the incidence of major and minor amputations in the diabetic [84, 85].

REFERENCES

1. Berkow, R., Disorders of carbohydrate metabolism, in R. Berkow, ed., *The Manual Merck*. Rahway, NJ: Merck Research Laboratories, 1992:1106–7.

2. Hughes, C. E.; Johnson, C. C.; Bamberger, D. M.; et al., Treatment and long-term follow-up of foot infections in patients with diabetes or ischemia: A randomized, prospective, double blind comparison of cefoxitin and ceftisoxime, *Clin Ther* 1987; 10 (Suppl A):36.

3. Keen, H.; Payan, J.; Allawi, J.; et al., Treatment of diabetic neuropathy with gammalinolenic acid, *Diabet Care* 1993; 16:8.

4. Larson, U., and Anderson, G. B. J., Partial amputation of the foot for diabetic or arteriosclerotic gangrene. Results and factors of prognostic value, *J Bone Joint Surg* 1978; 60:126.

5. Wright, D. G.; Desai, S. M.; and Henderson, W. H., Action of the subtalar and ankle joint complex during the stance phase of walking, *J Bone Joint Surg* 1964; 46:361.

6. Bojsen-Moller, F., Anatomy of the forefoot: Normal and pathologic, *Clin Orthop* 1979; 142:10.

7. Bouton, A. J. M., Detecting the patient at risk for diabetic foot ulcers, *Pract Cardiol* 1983; 9:135.

8. Penn, I., The impact of diabetes mellitus on extremity ischemia, in R. F. Kempczinski, ed., *The Ischemic Leg*, Chicago: Year Book Medical Publishers, 1985:56–69.

9. Strandness, D. E., Jr.; Priest, R. E.; and Gibbons, G. E., Combined clinical and pathologic study of diabetic and nondiabetic peripheral arterial disease, *Diabetes* 1964; 13:366.

10. Tilton, R. G.; Daughtery, A.; Sutera, S. P.; et al., Myocyte contracture, vascular resistance vascular permeability after global ischemia in isolated hearts from alloxan-induced diabetic rabbits, *Diabetes* 1989; 38:1484.

11. Cameron, N. E., and Cotter, M. A., Impaired contraction and relaxation in aorta from streptozotocin-diabetic rats: The role of polyol pathway, *Diabetologia* 1992; 35:1011.

12. Kelman, I., and Diegelmann, R. F., Wound healing, in L. J. Greenfield, et al., eds., *Surgery: Scientific Principles and Practice*, Philadelphia; J. B. Lippincott, 1993:100–101.

13. Wozniak, A.; McLennan, G.; Betts, W. H.; Murphy, G. A.; and Scicchitano, R., *Immunology* 1989; 68:359–64.

14. Tuman, K. J.; Spiess, B. D.; McCarthy, R. J.; and Ivankovitch, A. D., Comparison of viscoelastic measures of coagulation after cardiopulmonary bypass, *Anesth Analg* 1989; 69:69–75.

15. Martin, P.; Horkay, F.; Rajah, S. M.; and Walker, D. R., Monitoring of coagulation status using thromboelastography during pediatric open heart surgery, *Int J Clin Monit Comput* 1991; 8:183–187.

16. Lee, B. Y.; Ostrander, L. E.; and Madden, J. L., Optimum heparinization during vascular reconstructive surgery, *Contemp Surg* 1988; 33:37–41.

17. Cruickshank, M. K.; Levine, M. N.; Hirsh, J.; Roberts, R.; and Siguenza, M., A standard normogram for the management of heparin therapy, *Arch Intern Med* 1991; 151:333–337.

18. Van den Besselaer, A. M. H. P.; Meeuwisse-Braun, J.; and Bertina, R. M., Monitoring heparin therapy: Relationships between the activated partial thromboplastin time and heparin assays based on ex-vivo heparin samples, *Thromb Haemostas* 1990; 63:16–23.

19. Cipolle, R. J.; Uden, D. L.; Gruber, S. A.; Jossart, G. H.; et al., Evaluation of rapid monitoring system to study heparin pharmacokinetics and pharmacodynamics, *Pharmacotherapy* 1990; 10:367–372.

20. Lee, B. Y.; Thoden, W. R.; Del Guercio, L. R. M.; and McCann, W. J., Monitoring coagulation dynamics with thromboelastography, *Contemp Surg* 1984; 24:19–24.

21. Lee, B. Y.; Talia, S.; Trainor, F. S.; Kavner, D.; and McCann, W. J., Monitoring heparin therapy with thromboelastography and activated partial thromboplastin time, *World J Surg* 1980, 4:323–330.

22. Tsigos, C.; Diemel, L. T.; White, A.; Tomlinson, D. R.; Young, R. J., Cerebrospinal fluid levels of substance P and calcitonin-gene-related peptide: Correlation with sural nerve levels and neuropathic signs in sensory diabetic polyneuropathy, *Clin Sci* 1993; 84:305–11.

23. Caufield, J. P.; el-Lati, S.; Thomas, G.; and Church, M. K., *Lab Invest* 1990; 63:502–10.

24. Payan, D. Y., Neuropeptides and inflammation: The role of substance P, *Ann Rev Med* 1989; 40:341–52.

25. O'Neal, L. W., Surgical pathology of the foot and clinicopathological correlations, in M. E. Levin,

L. W. O'Neal, eds., *The Diabetic Foot*, St. Louis: C. V. Mosby, 1983:162–200.

26. Draves, D. J., and Sarrafian, S. K., *Anatomy of the Foot and Ankle. Descriptive, Topographic, and Functional*, Philadelphia: J. B. Lippincott, 1983.

27. Draves, D. J., *Anatomy of the Lower Extremity*, Baltimore, MD: Williams & Wilkins, 1957.

28. Gleckman, R. A., and Roth, R. R., Diabetic foot infections: Prevention and treatment, *West J Med* 1985; 142:263.

29. Jones, F. W., *Structure and Function as Seen in the Foot*, Baltimore, MD: William & Wilkins, 1944.

30. Kamel, R., and Sakla, B. F., Anatomical compartments of the sole of the human foot, *Anat Rec* 1961; 140:57–64.

31. Myerson, M., Acute compartment syndromes of the foot, *Bull Hosp Dis Orthop Inst* 1987; 47:251–61.

32. Goldman, F. D., Deep space infections in the diabetic patient, *J Am Podiatr Med Assoc* 1987; 77:431–43.

33. Brand, P. W., Pressure sores. The problem, in R. M. Kennedi, J. M. Cowden, eds., *Bedsore Biomechanics*, Baltimore, MD: University Press, 1976:19–23.

34. Griffiths, H. J., Diabetic osteopathy, *Orthopedics* 1985; 8:401.

35. Bridges, R. M., and Deitch, E. A., Diabetic foot infections. Pathophysiology and treatment, *Surg Clin N Am* 1994; 74:537–555.

36. Mubarak, S. J., and Hargens, A. R., Compartment syndromes and Volkmann's contracture, Philadelphia: W. B. Saunders, 1981.

37. Whitesides, T. E., in *Disorders of the Foot*, M. H. Jahss, ed , Philadelphia: W. B. Saunders, 1982: 1201–1203.

38. Bonutti, P. M., and Gordon, R. B., Compartment syndrome of the foot. A case report, *J Bone Joint Surg* 1986; 68:1449–51.

39. Penn, I., The impact of diabetes mellitus on extremity ischemia, in R. F. Kempczinski, ed., *The Ischemic Leg*, Chicago: Year Book Medical Publishers, 1985:56–69.

40. Haimovici, H., Peripheral arterial disease in diabetes mellitus, in M. Ellenberg, H. Rifkin, eds., *Diabetes Mellitus: Theory and Practice*, New York: McGraw-Hill, 1970:890–911.

41. Ferrier, T. M., Comparative study of arterial disease in amputated lower limbs from diabetics and nondi-abetics (with special reference to foot arteries), *Med J Aust* 1967; 1:5.

42. Edmonds, M. E., and Watkins, P. L. J., Management of the diabetic foot, in J. P. Dyck, P. K. Thomas, E. H. Lamberg, et al., eds., *Diabetic Neuropathy*, Philadelphia: W. B. Saunders, 1987:212.

43. Penn, I., The impact of diabetes mellitus on extremity ischemia, in R. F. Kempczinski, ed., *The Ischemic Leg*, Chicago: Year Book Medical Publishers, 1985:56–69.

44. Thomas, K., and Eliason, S. G., *Diabetic Neuropathy*, 2nd ed., Philadelphia: W. B. Saunders, 1984: 1773–1810.

45. Erdman, W. A.; Tamburro, F.; Jayson, H. T.; et al., Osteomyelitis: Characteristics and pitfalls of diagnosis with MR imaging, *Radiology* 1991; 180:533.

46. Hoshi, K.; Mizushima, Y.; Kiyokawa, S.; et al., Prostaglandin E1 incorporated in lipid microspheres in the treatment of peripheral vascular diseases and diabetic neuropathy, *Drugs Exp Clin Res* 1986; 12:681.

47. Lee, B. Y., and Brancato, R. F., Perforating ulcers of the foot, in Lee, B. Y. ed., *Chronic Ulcers of the Skin*, New York: McGraw-Hill, 1985:111–132.

48. Leichter, S. B., et al., Clinical characteristics of diabetic patients with serious pedal infections, *Metabolism* 1988; 37 (Suppl 1):22.

49. Sinha, S.; Munichoodappa, I.; and Kozak, G. P., Neuro-arthropathy (Charcot joints) in diabetes mellitus (clinical study of 101 cases), *Medicine* 1972; 51:191.

50. Dellon, E. L., Treatment of symptomatic diabetic neuropathy by surgical decompression of multiple peripheral nerves, *Plast Reconstr Surg* 1992; 89:689.

51. Park, H. M., et al., Scintigraphic evaluation of diabetic osteomyelitis. Concise communication, *J Nucl Med* 1991; 23:1246.

52. Eisenberg, B.; Wrege, S. S.; Altman, M. I.; et al., Bone scan: Indium-WBC correlation in the diagnosis of osteomyelitis of the foot, *J Foot Surg* 1989; 28:532.

53. Erdman, W. A.; Tamburro, F.; Jayson, H. T.; et al., Osteomyelitis: Characteristics and pitfalls of diagnosis with MRI imaging, *Radiology* 1991; 180:533.

54. Sapico; What, L. J.; Allen, S. D.; Henry, M.; et al., Diabetic foot infections: Bacteriologic analysis, *Arch Intern Med* 1986; 146:1935.

55. Lee, B. Y.; Trainor, F. S.; Kavner, D.; and Madden, J. L., A clinical evaluation of a noninvasive electromagnetic flowmeter, *Angiology* 1975; 26:317–327.

56. Lee, B. Y.; Trainor, F. S.; Thoden, W. R.; Kavner, D.; and Madden, J. L., Use of noninvasive electromagnetic flowmetry in the assessment of peripheral arterial disease, *Surg Gynecol Obstet* 1980; 150:342–346.

57. Lee, B. Y.; Thoden, W. R.; Trainor, F. S.; and Kavner, D., Noninvasive evaluation of peripheral arterial disease in the geriatric patient, *J Am Geriatr Soc* 1980; 28:352–360.

58. Hinton, P. A.; Nelson, J. R.; and Kroeker, R., Measuring arterial blood flow by nuclear magnetic resonance, in S. J. Kominsky, ed., *Medical and Surgical Management of the Diabetic Foot*, St. Louis: Mosby, 1994:61–70.

59. Rice, K. L., Magnetic resonance flowmetry: Clinical applications, *J Vasc Tech* 1994; 18:277–285.

60. Ingram, C.; Eron, L. J.; Goldenberg, R. I.; et al., Antibiotic therapy of osteomyelitis in outpatients, *Med Clin N Am* 1988; 72:723.

61. Gibbons, G. W., and Freeman, D. V., Diabetic foot infections, in R. J. Howard, R. L. Simmons, eds., *Surgical Infectious Diseases*, 2nd ed., Norwalk, CT: Appleton and Lange, 1988:601.

62. Williams, G. M., The diabetic foot, in J. L. Cameron, *Current Surgical Therapy*, 4th ed., St. Louis, MO: Mosby Year Book, 1992:761–765.

63. Skolnick, A. A., Foot care program for patients with leprosy may also prevent amputations in persons with diabetes, *JAMA* 1992; 267:2288.

64. Pinzur, M. S., Amputation level selection in the diabetic foot, *Clin Orthop* 1988; 229:2236.

65. Sage, R.; Pinzur, M. S.; Cronin, R.; Preuss, H. F.; and Osterman, H., Complications following midfoot amputation in neuropathic and dysvascular feet, *J Am Podiatr Med Assoc* 1989; 79:227.

66. Lee, B. Y.; McCann, W. J.; et al., Noninvasive assessment of wound healing potentials with determination of amputation level, *Contemp Surg* 1980; 19:20.

67. Wagner, F. W., Jr., Management of the diabetic neurotrophic foot: Part II. A classification and treatment program for diabetic, neuropathic, and dysvascular foot problems, in R. R. Cooper, ed., *AAOS Instructional Course Lectures*, vol. 28, St. Louis, MO: C. V. Mosby, 1979.

68. Pinzur, M. S., Amputation level selection in the diabetic foot, *Clin Orthop*, 1993; 296:68–70.

69. Ostrander, L. E.; Cui, W.; and Lee, B. Y., The clinical use of green light photoplethysmography, *Surgical Forum*, 520–522 1989.

70. Cui, W.; Ostrander, L. E.; and Lee, B. Y., In vivo reflectance of blood and tissue as function of light wavelength, *IEEE Trans Biomed Eng* 1990; 37: 632–639.

71. Dalsing, M. C.; White, J. V.; Yao, J. S. T.; Podrazik, R.; Flinn, W. R.; and Bergan, J. J., Infrapopliteal bypass for established gangrene of the forefoot or toes, *J Vasc Surg* 1985; 2:669–77.

72. O'Mara, C. S.; Flinn, W. R.; Neiman, H. L.; Bergan, J. J.; and Yao, J. S. T., Correlation of foot arterial anatomy with early tibial bypass patency, *Surgery* 1981; 89:743–52.

73. Ascer, E.; Veith, F. J.; Morin; et al., Quantitative assessment of outflow resistance in lower extremity arterial reconstruction, *J Surg Res* 1984; 37:8–15.

74. Gibbons, G. W.; Marcacio, E. J., Jr.; Burgess, E. M.; et al., Improved quality of diabetic foot care, 1984 vs 1990: Reduced length of stay and costs, insufficient reimbursement, *Arch Surg* 1993; 128:576–81.

75. Gupta, S. K., and Veith, F. J., Inadequacy of diagnosis related group (DRG) reimbursements for limb salvage lower extremity arterial reconstructions, *J Vasc Surg* 1990; 11:348–57.

76. Pomposelli, F. B., Jr.; Jepsen, S. J.; Gibbons, G. W.; et al., A flexible approach to infrapopliteal vein grafts in patients with diabetes mellitus, *Arch Surg* 1991; 126:724–9.

77. Caputo, G. M.; Cavanagh, P. R.; Ulbretch, P. R.; Gibbons, G. W.; and Karchmer, A. W., Assessment and management of foot disease in patients with diabetes, *N Engl J Med* 1994; 331:854–860.

78. Lee, B. Y.; Madden, J. L.; Thoden, W. R.; and McCann, W. J., Lumbar sympathectomy for toe gangrene: Long-term follow-up, *Am J Surg* 1983; 145:398–401.

79. Lee, B. Y.; Thoden, W. R.; Madden, J. L.; et al., Long-term follow-up of bypass procedures with and without sympathectomy, *Contemp Surg* 1982; 20: 51–55.

80. Bonutti, P. M., and Bell, G. R., Compartment syndrome of the foot: A case report, *J Bone Joint Surg* 1986; 68A:1449–1451.

81. Myerson, M. S., Experimental decompression of the fascial compartment of the foot: The basis for fasciotomy in acute compartment syndromes, *Foot Ankle* 1988; 8:308–314.

82. Jacobs, R. L., Hoffman procedure in the ulcerated diabetic foot, *Foot Ankle* 1982; 3:142.

83. Frykberg, R. G., Podiatric problems in diabetes, In G. P. Kozac, C. Campbell, C. S. Hoar, Jr., et al., eds., *Management of Diabetic Foot Problems*, Philadelphia: W. B. Saunders, 1984:S-67.

84. Edmons, M. E.; Bludell, M. P.; Morris, M.; et al., Reduction in the number of major and minor amputations: Impact of a new combined foot clinic, *Diabetologia* 1984; 27:272.

85. Levin, M. E., and O'Neal, L. W., *The Diabetic Foot*, 4th ed., St. Louis, MO: C. V. Mosby, 1988:1–50.

15

ULCERATIONS OF THE FOOT

Thomas M. De Lauro, D.P.M.

INTRODUCTION

Foot ulcerations are extremely common, as demonstrated by some very current findings. In a recent survey of inpatients with pressure ulcerations, the heel was second only to the sacrum in terms of frequency of involvement [1]. Diabetic foot ulcerations and their complications account for more hospital days than all other diabetic complications combined [2]. Unlike ulcerations of other body areas, foot involvement interferes with ambulation, the activities of daily living, and one's personal independence.

INITIAL ASSESSMENT

Even before considering etiologies, a fairly accurate assessment of a foot ulceration's healing potential can be made on the basis of a cursory examination. For the most part, these ulcers are either (a) painless, accompanied by good macro and microvascular circulations, with a granulating base, or (b) painful, nongranulating, and associated with poor proximal and local vasculature. Obviously, the latter group carries a more grave prognosis than the former.

Foot ulcerations that are painless and granulating are most often due to neurotrophism or venous stasis. On the other hand, painful, nongranulating ulcers are usually secondary to decreased arterial inflow at the macrocirculatory (e.g., caused by atherosclerosis, arterial emboli) or microcirculatory levels. As a cause of foot ulceration, microcirculatory disease can be subdivided into vascular, cytologic, and noncytologic components consistent with **Virchow**'s hypercoagulation triad. *Vascular* microcirculatory disease is implicated in decubital ulcers, connective tissue diseases (e.g., scleroderma), vasculitic syndromes, diabetic microangiopathy, thromboangiitis obliterans, and vasospastic syndromes. *Cytologic* microcirculatory disease includes those conditions in which cellular morphology and/or number are abnormal, such as sickle cell anemia, polycythemia vera, thrombocytosis, leukemia, thalassemia, hereditary spherocytosis, and Felty's syndrome. *Noncytologic (or fluid)* microcirculatory disease occurs in macroglobulinemia, cryoglobulinemia, hypergammaglobulinemia, and paroxysmal hemoglobinuria. Further discussion of many of these entities, the role of the laboratory, and therapeutic options may be found in the following pages.

A final consideration during the initial assessment would be ulcer staging. Although Wagner's [3] system and that of the National Pressure Ulcer

207

Advisory Council were designed for diabetic and decubital ulcers, respectively, enough similarity exists between them that Wagner's approach may be utilized. The system classifies ulcers as follows: grade O (no open skin lesion present but breakdown is possible because of skeletal deformity and sensory neuropathy), grade I (a skin lesion is present but without penetration to tendon, bone, or joint structures), grade II (ulceration extends to tendon, bone, or joint), grade III (in addition to ulceration, deep abscess formation exists with tendon involvement, plantar space infection, osteomyelitis, or infectious arthritis), grade IV (ulceration exists with digital or forefoot gangrene), and grade V (ulceration exists with gangrene involving the entire rearfoot). The coexistence of lymphangitis or lymphadenopathy, fever, or a history of chills signal the need for inpatient care. An entire section of this chapter, therefore, devotes itself to dealing with infected ulcerations.

ETIOLOGIC DIFFERENTIAL DIAGNOSIS

Once the initial assessment of healing potential has been completed, etiologic considerations begin [4]. The great majority of these are vascular (arterial and/or venous) in nature, but metabolic diseases, neurotrophism, neoplasms, drugs, trauma, and infectious diseases are also etiologic possibilities. Because any foot ulcer may become infected, distinguishing between infected wounds and those of infectious etiology will be given special consideration.

VASCULAR

Arterial

Atherosclerosis.   The pathogenesis of atherosclerosis is widely believed to begin with aortic fatty streaks that ultimately transform to fibrous atherosclerotic plaques in both the aorta and the peripheral arterial tree. Partial or complete occlusion of an artery can then occur via plaque-initiated thrombosis or intraplaque hemorrhage. Evidence of atherosclerosis in one vessel warrants a search for other potentially affected vessels.

The typical patient with atherosclerotic foot ulcers is a man over forty-five years of age. Early in the course of the disease, the patient may relate a history of intermittent claudication, and in the end-stage illness, a history of rest pain. The ulcers themselves usually occur on the tips of the digits (periungually or subungually) or over other bony prominences (e.g., the dorsal aspect of the proximal or distal interphalangeal joints in hammertoes or clawtoes/mallettoes, respectively; over the lateroplantar aspect of the fifth metatarsal head in patients with tailor's bunions; over the dorsomedial aspect in patients with hallux valgus). The ulcers are usually painful, have a pale necrotic base, and demonstrate little inflammatory reaction in the periulcer skin (Figure 15-1).

In terms of differential diagnosis, atherosclerotic ulcers should be considered before those of thromboangiitis obliterans (Buerger's disease), because atherosclerosis is more common. Thromboangiitis obliterans affects small-to-medium-sized vessels, whereas atherosclerosis affects larger arteries. Buerger's disease patients are usually younger than forty years of age, and relate a history of heavy cigarette smoking, thrombophlebitis, and paresthesias, all of which are often absent in patients with atherosclerosis.

Unlike the insidious onset of atherosclerosis, arterial emboli have an acute onset and are accompanied by a history or physical evidence of cardiac disease or aneurysm.

Venous stasis ulcers have a good granulating base, occur more often on the medial lower one-third of the leg, demonstrate venous stasis changes in periulcer skin, and are rarely painful.

Livedo reticularis ulcers exhibit livedo skin patterns and usually *normal* pulsations.

Finally, hypertensive ischemic ulcers occur on the lateral malleolus or posterior leg, and are surrounded by a violaceous rim. Pulsations are usually normal, and the patient is hypertensive.

Thromboangiitis obliterans (Buerger's disease, TAO).   In contrast to atherosclerosis, TAO affects the peripheral (and sometimes visceral) arteries and veins of young men who smoke cigarettes heavily. Clinicians must not forget that women may also be afflicted with TAO. Pathologically, nonsuppurative inflammatory changes without giant cells are noted

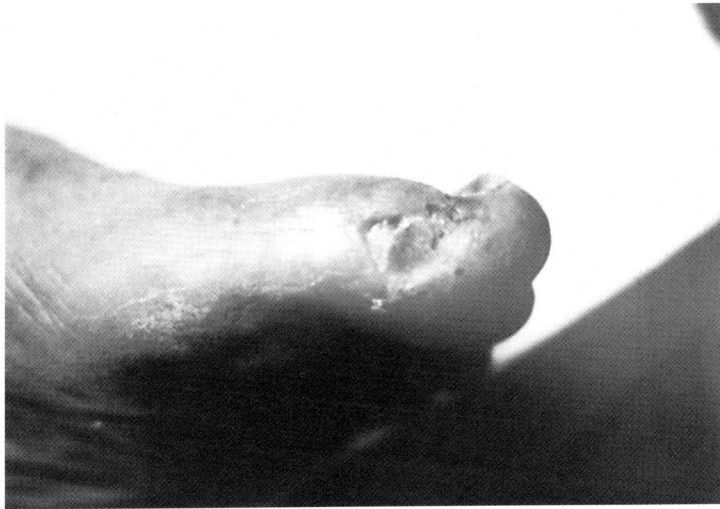

Figure 15-1. Atherosclerotic ulcer. Note distal presentation, pale base, and little periwound erythema.

in all three vessel layers. As postinflammatory fibrosis binds all elements of the neurovascular bundle, venous and neurologic symptoms develop. The ensuing phlebitis is usually of the superficial migratory type. TAO patients are generally free of diabetes mellitus, connective tissue disease, hypercholesterolemia, or hyperlipidemia. Hands become involved in addition to the feet, which does not occur in atherosclerosis. Painful ulcers begin on the toes but, if the patient continues to smoke cigarettes, can develop more proximally. Progressive tissue loss is the rule unless smoking is discontinued.

Because small vessels are involved, the diagnosis is usually made on clinical grounds; arteriography is inconclusive and therefore not recommended.

Atherosclerosis, Takayasu's disease, vasculitis, and arterial emboli form the list of differential diagnoses. Takayasu's disease should be considered in patients who have involvement of the upper extremity, eye, brain, or leg (in young women), are febrile, and present an elevated erythrocyte sedimentation rate.

Vasculitis is often differentiated by the presence of multisystem disease (see below).

Arterial emboli usually occur in older patients, spare the upper extremities, and are sometimes accompanied by fever.

Livedo reticularis. Foot ulcers result from spastic or structural narrowing of cutaneous arterioles with resultant dilatation of capillaries and venules. Livedo reticularis is often idiopathic but can occur in association with numerous diseases.

Livedo ulcerations begin as painful violaceous infarcts in areas of skin demonstrating the classic livedo pattern. Once the skin has broken down, a persistent, cyanotic mottling of the periulcer skin made more intense by cold exposure is often noted. Women between the ages of twenty and forty years of age are most often affected. Although these ulcerations heal slowly, their prognosis is generally good. Of course, the healing rate can be affected by the presence of underlying disease. Severe livedo reticularis with early ulceration is a fairly reliable clue that underlying disease exists.

Hypertension. These ulcerations usually affect females between the ages of fifty and sixty years who relate a chronic history of hypertension. It is believed that this hypertension causes arteriolar changes that result in diminished blood flow to an area. Trauma or severe vessel changes then result in infarction with ulceration.

Ulcerations begin as violaceous papules or plaques that transform into hemorrhagic vesicles or bullae and finally ulcers. These ulcers are painful, exhibit little granulation tissue, have a cyanotic or purpuric rim, and heal slowly. The lateral malleolus is the most commonly affected site and therefore included in this chapter, but hypertensive ulcers can also involve the posterior or posterolateral calf.

In contrast, venous stasis ulcerations exhibit much more granulation tissue, occur on the medial leg, are not very painful, and demonstrate venous stasis changes in the skin surrounding the ulcer. Atherosclerotic and TAO ulcers occur on the toes or distal foot and are accompanied by ischemic changes in the limb. Chronic pernio ulcers occur during colder months, in crops, and begin in the late teenage years and early twenties.

Chronic pernio. As mentioned, younger patients are affected by this malady, which consists of painful recurring lower *leg* ulcers during the colder months. The extensor and flexor surfaces can be involved, especially those just proximal to the malleoli. Technically, these are not foot ulcers but are being included for the sake of completeness and the potential fortuitous involvement of the foot in severe, extensive cases. Ulcerations begin as red papules that blister and then ulcerate. The lesions occur in crops, present with a hemorrhagic base, and heal spontaneously with depressed, hyperpigmented scars. Histologic findings are consistent with vasospasm.

The differential diagnosis includes erythema induratum, erythema nodosum, vasculitis, and livedo reticularis. Erythema induratum does not occur seasonally, affects the calves instead of the lower legs, and exhibits a tuberculid picture histologically. Erythema nodosum does not ulcerate and is not related to cold exposure. Livedo ulcers are rare, do not appear in crops, are difficult to heal, and do not progress through the erythema-blister-ulceration stages. Vasculitis can also occur independently of cold exposure, affects mostly older women (thirty to forty years of age), is more nodular and painful, usually does not ulcerate, and histologically presents a true vasculitis.

Decubiti (pressure sores). These ulcerations result from prolonged immobilization in skin areas that overlay bony prominences. The immobilization leads to capillary compression with resultant necrosis and ulceration. In a fingernail bed, the average pressure required to occlude blood flow was found to be 32 mmHg, but subsequent studies determined that tissue damage followed a time-pressure curve: i.e., the lower the pressure, the longer the time required for necrosis [5]. Even more recently, patients with pressure sores were found to share a number of epidemiological characteristics, such as incontinence and malnutrition. The role played by these variables in decubital ulcer development is unclear; however, when they were corrected or controlled, healing improved.

In normal volunteers (both young and old), studies of skin compression over bony prominences revealed a compensatory *increase* in dermal blood flow during the period of compression, regardless of age. When the same study was repeated on ill, elderly patients deemed at risk for pressure ulcers, compression produced an inconsistent blood flow response: some increased, others decreased, and still others exhibited no change in dermal blood flow at all. At-risk individuals, therefore, demonstrated much more variability in blood flow response than was previously anticipated [5].

As mentioned earlier, the heel is the most common site for decubital ulcer development, followed by the toes and any other skeletal deformity (e.g., hallux valgus, bunionette). The frequency of heel ulceration is indeed unfortunate, because the soft structures between the skin and underlying calcaneus consist largely of adipose tissue. Once the skin's integrity has been compromised, the relatively avascular fatty layer can do little to ward off the spread of microorganisms and calcaneal osteomyelitis. Prevention of the initial ulceration is therefore of key importance. (See Figure 15-2.)

Venous

These ulcerations typically affect the medial lower third of the leg. Because the foot can occasionally be involved, a brief discussion is warranted. The peripheral venous system can be subdivided into superficial, deep, and communicating components. Valves within these veins maintain flow in a proximal-to-distal, superficial-to-deep direction. Prior thrombophlebitis destroys these valves, resulting in venous hypertension, which in turn causes a series of changes that eventually lead to ulceration.

Venous hypertension initially causes peripheral

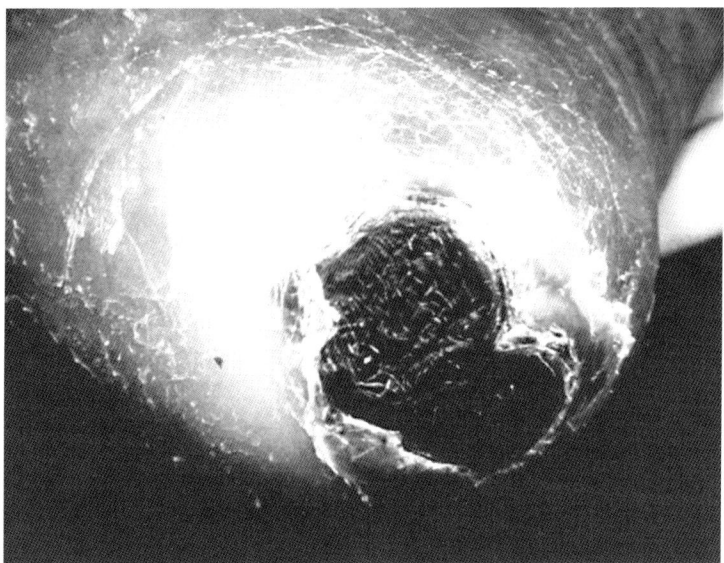

Figure 15-2. Heel decubitus ulcer in a young male with multiple sclerosis. His vascular status was *normal* bilaterally.

edema, which is absent upon arising in the morning and progresses with standing or ambulation. Capillary rupture follows, leading to darkening of skin from hemosiderin deposits left behind by tissue macrophages that have digested extravascular blood. This hemosiderin induces subcutaneous fibrosis, resulting in induration of the already-darkened skin. The fibrosis also worsens the local blood flow, so that the next traumatic event in the affected area forms an ulceration (Figure 15-3).

Venous stasis ulcers are relatively painless, have good granulating bases, and are surrounded by the brown indurated skin described above. Any discomfort associated with them is often relieved by elevation of the leg.

Differential diagnosis includes arteriovenous

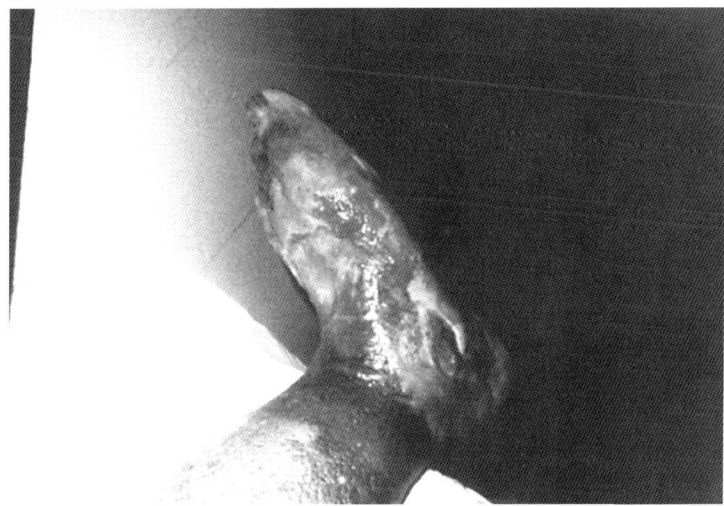

Figure 15-3. Venous stasis ulceration. In contrast to atherosclerotic ulcers, note granulating base and periulcer stasis hyperpigmentation.

fistulae, atherosclerosis, TAO, hypertension, erythema induratum, lymphedema, scleroderma, and pretibial myxedema. Arteriovenous fistulae may present with venous stasis changes, but limb enlargement, thrills, and bruits are also exhibited. Atherosclerotic and TAO ulcers are more painful, occur on the feet and toes, have little granulation tissue, and may be relieved by dependency instead of elevation. Hypertensive ulcers occur in a different location, are painful, and have a cyanotic rim. Erythema induratum occurs on the posterior calf, is bilateral, and does not demonstrate venous stasis changes. Lymphedema exhibits skin thickening, does not subside with elevation, and almost never includes ulceration, venous stasis, or varicose veins. Scleroderma and pretibial myxedema also do not present with stasis changes, do not respond readily to elevation of the leg, and can be differentiated by biopsy.

Lymphatics

Lymphatic vessels ordinarily drain protein-rich tissue fluids that have not reentered capillaries. Congenital absence or malformation of lymphatic channels, as well as secondary obstruction, leads to retention of lymph within tissue spaces. As tissue fluid and its protein content increase, enhanced fibroblastic activity traps the lymph even further, resulting in a markedly edematous (elephantiasis) and firm limb that is vulnerable to ulceration following trauma (Figure 15-4).

Primary forms can either be congenital (Milroy's disease) or develop in young females (lymphedema praecox). Secondary forms are acquired through obstruction via radiation, surgery, trauma, infection, tumor, or filariasis. Chronic cases result in dilated lymphatics (lymphangiectasias) about the toes initially. Ulceration usually does not occur without trauma, unless conversion to lymphangiosarcoma takes place.

Early bilateral cases must be distinguished from cardiac, renal, hepatic, and nutritional causes, and early unilateral cases must be differentiated from venous insufficiency and deep venous thrombosis. This sometimes requires noninvasive vascular testing, venography, or lymphangiography. Ulcerations in lymphedema and venous stasis can appear

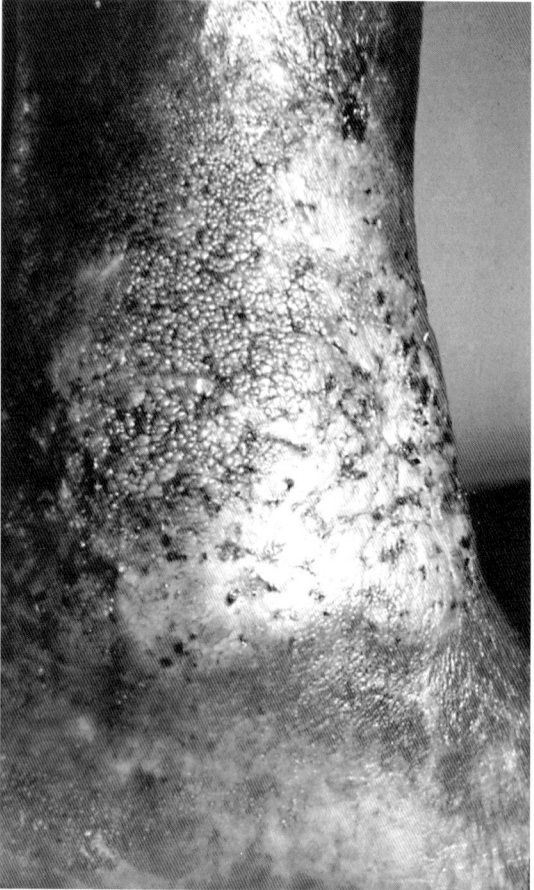

Figure 15-4. Ulceration in a patient with chronic lymphostatic skin changes. The etiology was a pruritic dermatosis of twenty years duration.

similar, but the different appearance of the limb in each disorder facilitates diagnosis.

Arteriovenous fistulae can cause limb enlargement, but are also markedly different in terms of their clinical appearance. A condition known as lipedema also belongs in the differential diagnosis and results from excess adipose tissue. In contrast to lymphedema, lipedema *spares* the foot.

Vasculitis

The **vasculitides** represent a group of disorders characterized by involvement of different-sized vessels in skin and various organs. Histologically, one notes a polymorphonuclear infiltrate involving the vessel wall unassociated with emboli, atherosclerosis, or trauma. The end result of this process is vessel occlusion with tissue infarction. Depending upon the vessel(s) involved, this infarction can lead to nonspecific pedal ulceration.

Clues to the presence of vasculitis include synchronous or consecutive involvement of several organ systems, common diseases that present in unusual settings (i.e., peripheral vascular disease in a young patient), constitutional symptoms out of proportion to the physical findings, and the presence of cutaneous rash with multiorgan disease. A rash usually indicates small-vessel vasculitis, whereas the absence of a rash points to medium or large-vessel involvement.

HEMATOLOGIC ABNORMALITIES

As described above, each of these aberrations leads to increased blood viscosity with resultant ulceration, usually about the lower legs or malleoli. As the foot can become involved, some brief comments follow. Ulcerations may or may not be painful.

Sickle cell disease, hereditary spherocytosis, and thalassemia (Mediterranean anemia) deserve mention. Sickle cell ulcers usually occur only in homozygous S disease. The ulcer base is granulating, but healing is poor without normal blood transfusions. Hereditary spherocytosis ulcers require long-standing anemia to develop. Patients with such disorders also present jaundice and splenomegaly. Splenectomy results in rapid ulcer healing. Thalassemia patients with major and intermediate forms of the disease can develop ulcerations; minor disease patients do not ulcerate.

METABOLIC DISEASES

Pretibial myxedema

Mucopolysaccharide deposition in the dermis results in firm, nonpitting plaques and nodules, usually after irradiation or surgical treatment for thyrotoxicosis. These lesions can ulcerate, but rarely do so.

Lichen amyloidosis

Usually a sign of more serious underlying conditions, patients present with firm, cutaneous, red to reddish-brown plaques that may coalesce. They are the result of subcutaneous amyloid deposition. As in pretibial myxedema, the plaques rarely ulcerate.

Pyoderma gangrenosum

These patients develop erythematous papulonodules that enlarge rapidly and then transform into painful ulcerations with rolled borders and a violaceous rim. They most often occur in association with inflammatory bowel disease, ulcerative colitis, and polycythemia vera. Diagnosis usually requires repeated histologic examinations.

Gout

Ulcerations may occur as a result of erosion by gouty tophi through the skin. Fixation of tophi in absolute alcohol will preserve urate crystals for examination; formalin fixation will dissolve them.

Diabetes mellitus

Atherosclerotic, microangiopathic, and neurotrophic ulcerations account for the vast majority of wounds in diabetic patients. They are only listed here; entire sections of this chapter will be devoted to their discussion as a reflection of their frequency in the general population.

Less commonly, ulcerations can result from the diabetic lesions of necrobiosis lipoidica diabeticorum and diabetic dermopathy.

NEUROTROPHIC ULCERATIONS

Neurotrophic ulcerations (malum perforans) occur in those patients whose sensory neuropathy permits them to ambulate beyond the normal tolerance of skin and soft tissues. As a result, subcutaneous hematomas or seromas develop that eventually devitalize normal skin and subcutaneous tissue. These structures slough, resulting in an ulceration of varying depth and severity.

Clinically, patients present with painless ulcers that have a granulating base and keratotic rim. The ulcers most often occur beneath bony prominences, and in the presence of relatively good macrovascular and microvascular flow. Considerable serous drainage from the ulcer macerates the keratotic rim (Figure 15-5).

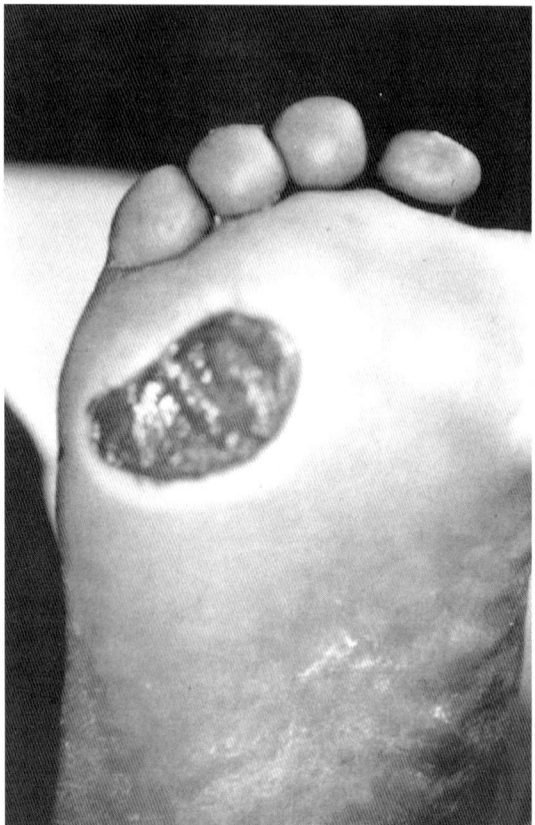

Figure 15-5. Neurotrophic ulceration, diagnosed by its development in an area subject to excessive repetitive trauma.

In today's population, diabetes mellitus is the most common cause of neurotrophic ulcer, but any disease resulting in sensory peripheral neuropathy should be included in the list of differential diagnoses. These include myelomeningocele, myelodysplasia [6], syringomyelia, Hansen's disease (leprosy), spinal bifida, systemic sclerosis [7], and tabes dorsalis (tertiary syphilis). The patient's foot is considered to be "insensate" if the patient can not feel a 5.07-caliber (10-gram) *Semmes-Weinstein* monofilament placed against the sole [8].

ULCERATING TUMORS

All tumors may resemble an ulcer with a granulating base; they are often considered as a diagnostic possibility only when standard therapies fail.

Ulcer borders are more appropriate for biopsy than the necrotic, infected center of the lesion. Ulcerating tumors often lose their characteristic appearance when occurring on the foot. Clues to their existence are keratoses in non-weight-bearing areas, and keratoses accompanied by an erythematous halo.

Tumors that can ulcerate include basal cell epithelioma, keratoacanthoma, squamous cell carcinoma (and verrucous carcinoma, also known as epithelioma cuniculatum [9]), Kaposi's sarcoma, malignant melanoma, fibroma of tendon sheath [10], and the lymphomas. As a complication of multiple myeloma, patients may display foot ulcerations secondary to a rare vasculopathy known as crystalglobulinemia syndrome [11]. Lastly, *any* ulceration of long-standing nature may undergo malignant transformation (broadly referred to as the Marjolin ulcer) (See Figure 15-6).

ULCERATIONS OF INFECTIOUS ETIOLOGY

When faced with a therapeutic stagmire, the clinician should consider an infectious etiology, especially in patients who are immunosuppressed (i.e., those taking corticosteroids or chemotherapeutic drugs) or immunocompromised (i.e., lymphoma patients, and patients who are HIV-positive). Culture and/or biopsy with staining for fungi, viruses, acid-fast bacteria, and parasites are therefore recommended as the next step in care. The recent literature has documented the following etiologies for infectious cutaneous ulceration.

Amoeba

Four genera of amoeba are pathogenic in humans (*Entamoeba, Naegleria, Acanthamoeba,* and *Vahlkampfia*), and must be considered as etiologic agents in HIV-positive patients who present with papulonodules and ulcerations [12]. The correct diagnosis is usually made after cultures and stains for fungi and bacteria are negative and a skin biopsy is performed. In such cases, the skin biopsy reveals amoebic double-walled cysts (often mistaken for macrophages) and trophozoites.

Naegleria fowleri is the only amoeba sensitive to antimicrobial therapy in vivo (amphotericin B). All other amoebae demonstrate in vitro susceptibil-

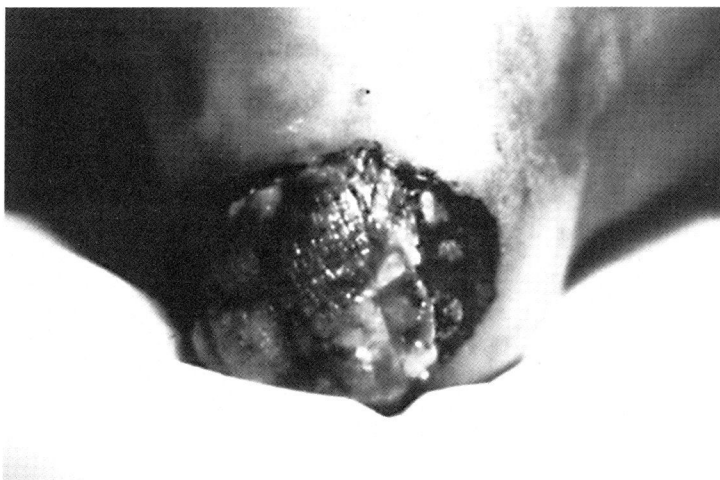

Figure 15-6. Ulceration secondary to advanced acrolentiginous malignant melanoma of the heel.

ity only (*Acanthamoeba* has shown such susceptibility in vitro to ketoconazole, sulfadiazine, flucytosine, pentamidine, and polymyxin B).

These amoebae enter through the nasopharynx, where they form part of the normal oral flora, and then disseminate hematogenously to the central nervous system and the skin. In the central nervous system, encephalitis is the result.

Herpes Simplex Virus

Herpes simplex virus (HSV) [13] infection should be considered in cutaneous ulcerations occurring in HIV-positive, immunosuppressed, corticosteroid-taking patients. Although vesiculation prior to ulceration is a good clinical indicator of HSV infection, violaceous macules may also precede ulceration. Ulcer borders can sometimes worsen when corticosteroid dosage is increased, suggesting an exacerbation of viral activity. Biopsy specimens of the ulcer border for viral culture are often positive for HSV type 2. Patients respond to intravenous acyclovir, followed by 2 grams per day orally for six months.

Nocardia

Three species of this bacterium, all found in soil, account for nearly all human infections: *N. asteroides, N. brasiliensis*, and *N. caviae*. Of the three, *N. asteroides* accounts for most nocardial infections. Over eighty percent of patients present with lung involvement initially, followed by cutaneous dissemination. Only ten percent of patients exhibit lung involvement without skin changes. *Primary* cutaneous nocardiosis usually requires a history of local trauma to the extremity, followed by cellulitis, pustule formation, ulceration, or a lymphocutaneous syndrome resembling sporotrichosis,. Disseminated nocardiosis to the skin usually occurs in an immunocompromised host, whereas primary cutaneous nocardiosis more often occurs in patients that are not immunocompromised. Nocardiosis responds to two grams of sulfadiazine administered every 6 hours. Some cases require as long as two months for resolution.

Fusobacterium

Sports-induced abrasions can sometimes break down to form shallow, painless ulcers with indurated borders. These lesions occur secondary to a spirochete-fusobacterial anaerobic (*Fusobacterium ulcerans*) infection [15], although anaerobes are less frequently isolated from ulcers that last longer than six weeks.

This etiology should also be considered in patients with indolent ulcers returning from the tropics, hence the term *tropic ulcer*.

In either case, penicillin or co-trimoxazole may be effective; flucloxacillin is ineffective.

Secondary Syphilis

Secondary syphilis [16] should be considered in all sexually active patients with persistent ulcerations of the extremities. The clinician should keep in mind that secondary syphilis may also present with guttate keratoses of the palms and soles, as well as a ham-colored maculopapular, generalized rash.

Mycobacteria

In addition to *Mycobacterium leprae*, which causes the ulcerations witnessed in Hansen's disease patients, a number of other mycobacterial species may cause cutaneous ulceration. *Mycobacterium haemophilum* has reportedly caused skin ulceration in immunocompromised patients [17]. Sources of immunocompromise have included renal transplant, AIDS, lymphocytic lymphoma, and Hodgkin's disease. There have also been a few idiopathic (these patients were *immunocompetent*) cases in children. Clinically, *M. haemophilum* ulceration begins as an erythematous or violaceous nodule that may progress to form first an abscess, and secondarily an ulcer. The ulceration seems to have a predilection for the extremities, limiting itself to the skin and underlying tissues. The fact that the organism restricts it own spread to these borders indicates the organism's preference for growth in cooler climates.

Mycobacterium ulcerans infection causes its own variety of skin ulceration [18]. First described in Uganda in 1887, a cluster of cases was discovered in a Ugandan area known as Buruli in the 1960s; hence, the lesion is often referred to as the Buruli ulcer. The lesion begins as a subcutaneous nodule that becomes attached to skin, or as an intradermal pustule. Over the course of weeks to months, the lesion progresses to a necrotizing panniculitis with ulceration, the latter having a wood-hard necrotic base with extensive undermining of the wound edges. The surrounding skin is shiny and hyperpigmented. The lesion is relatively painfree and not warm as would be expected in bacterial infection. When the ulceration heals, it does so with a deeply sunken scar due to the loss of subcutaneous tissue, and overhanging borders of normal skin.

Four clinical stages of the Buruli ulcer exist: I (subcutaneous nodule), II (panniculitis), III (ulceration), and IV (Buruli scar). *M. ulcerans* grows at 32–33°C, explaining its preference for the subcutaneous tissue layer at body temperature like other mycobacteria. *M. ulcerans* is different, however, in that it produces an immunosuppressive/cytotoxic substance that is heat labile. It is this toxin that causes tissue destruction, rather than host defenses.

The natural habitat of *M. ulcerans* is unknown, but it seems to occur where large bodies of water exist. Infection can occur at all ages, but children (usually between the ages of five and fifteen years) are more commonly affected [19]. Ulceration occurs most frequently on the limbs (sparing the palms and soles), but it has also been described as appearing on the head, neck, or trunk. Despite extensive ulceration, little constitutional change occurs. Clinicians must remember that the Buruli ulcer is *not* a disease limited to the poor and malnourished—it can pose a significant new threat to HIV-positive patients. Case-to-case transmission is unusual, even amongst family members sharing the same environment. It has been reported in Africa, South America, Southeast Asia, and the Central Pacific (Australia) [20].

To date, there is no effective treatment for the Buruli ulcer other than supportive measures, preventing superinfection, and allowing the disease to run its natural course. Antibiotics, ulcer excision and grafting, heat treatments, and hyperbaric oxygenation have all been used with mixed results.

Retained Bee Stinger

Although not technically infectious, the retained bee stinger is included in the differential diagnosis because it has been reported to present with cutaneous ulceration. On biopsy, pseudoepitheliomatous hyperplasia can be found, suggesting squamous cell carcinoma. Dermal eosinophilia, also found on histologic examination, will suggest foreign body reaction. Only with persistence was the retained bee stinger found within the dermis on histologic section. [21].

Pseudomonas putrefaciens ulceration

This organism can apparently present as one of two syndromes: benign disease in chronic ulceration, and fulminant disease resembling Gram-negative septicemia. It is because of this latter presentation that *P. putrefaciens* ulceration is included in the infectious category, because its septic shock-like syndrome (mental obtundation, hypotension) in the absence of demonstrable bacteremia suggests exotoxin production. Exotoxin could possibly account for spread of the ulceration and cellulitis. In the reported case, cellulitis began after an ulceration of the lateral malleolus [22].

Epithelioid Angiomatosis (Cat-Scratch Disease)

In immunocompetent individuals, this disease presents with usually no more than a papule at the site of inoculation, regional lymphadenopathy, fever, myalgias, and arthralgias. Recovery is usually spontaneous and occurs within two to four months, although morbidity may last as long as two years. Antibiosis is not of much benefit. In immunocompromised patients, however, the disease is more widespread and fulminating, with cutaneous ulceration necrosis as well as a poorer prognosis. Also, immunocompromised hosts may improve with antibiotic usage. Criteria for clinical diagnosis include a history of cat scratch, regional lymphadenopathy in the absence of other causes for lymphadenopathy, characteristic histopathologic changes in a biopsied lymph node, and a positive cat-scratch disease (CSD) skin test (or histologic diagnosis demonstrating the cat-scratch *bacillus* using Warthin-Starry silver impregnation staining). The organism has been recorded as sensitive to cefotetan, cefotaxime, gentamicin, amikacin, tobramycin, netilmicin, mezlocillin, and ciprofloxacin.

Cat-scratch disease should be added to the list of possible infectious ulcerations occurring in immunocompromised (e.g., AIDS) patients.

MISCELLANEOUS CAUSES

Drugs

Halogens (bromides, iodides) can cause fungating ulcerations on the skin that resemble erythema nodosum or a syphilitic gumma. Ergot administration may result in bullae and pustules that progress to gangrenous ulceration. Ulceration of preexisting psoriatic lesions can occur in patients taking methotrexate.

Burns

Chemical, thermal, and radiation injury can lead to ulceration. Radiation injury can be thought of as acute radiodermatitis (ulceration occurs within weeks of exposure), chronic radiodermatitis (resulting cutaneous atrophy leads to ulceration following minor trauma), and radiation cancer (occurring many years after exposure). Radiation was once a popular therapy for many cutaneous lesions, including plantar warts!

Primary dermatoses

Acrodermatitis chronica atrophicans and the ulcerobullous form of lichen planus comprise this category. The latter condition is confined to the feet and toes and results in chronic, painful ulcerations that are often surrounded by atrophic, depigmented skin.

Factitial ulcerations

These ulcerations are the result of self-inflicted wounds in malingerers or mentally disturbed patients. They are to be suspected in ulcerations that present with striking regularity in shape and/or size (when a single instrument was used to create the wounds), or when the pattern is so bizarre as to not resemble any other known disease.

INFECTED ULCERATIONS

Although the clinical recognition of cutaneous ulcerations is fairly straightforward, determining when an ulcer has become secondarily infected is less easy. Unfortunately, cultures of ulcers often produce only benign, saprophytic microorganisms. The purpose of this section, therefore, is to provide an algorithmic approach to this vexing problem.

HISTORY

In addition to the format espoused in standard physical diagnosis texts, patients with suspected infected cutaneous ulcers should be questioned with regard to recent travel, immigration status, immunologic status, vascular status, and change in the ulceration over time. Personal and business travel is so commonplace that infectious diseases endemic to the visited locale may appear stateside. Adventurous patients take their vacations in obscure regions of the world and may not be familiar with universal precautions regarding health and sanitation. Unless considered, these details may escape the clinician's probe and lead to a delayed or faulty diagnosis.

The same warning applies to a patient who has immigrated, especially when the patient comes from an underdeveloped nation.

In an era of acquired immunodeficiency syndrome (AIDS), resurgent tuberculosis, and widespread chemotherapy use for neoplastic disease, knowledge of the patient's immunologic status is vital to understanding the pathogenesis and treatment of infected ulcerations. Immunocompromise invites tissue destruction by saprophytes and rarely encountered organisms even in those who have never traveled outside the country. Immunocompromise also places more responsibility on extrinsic methods for cure, as the patient's intrinsic systems are either malfunctional or nonfunctional.

Of all the body systems, a patent vascular tree is key to preventing and treating infected skin ulcerations. Tissue nutrition, oxygenation, foreign body phagocytosis, and repair all rely on adequate blood within the macro- and microcirculations. Like immunocompromise, vascular compromise (both arterial *and* venous) interferes with homeostasis sufficiently to warrant its correction before all other measures. The history should therefore exclude or detect symptoms such as intermittent claudication, rest pain, and coldness of feet.

Duration is the final factor to be considered, but always in relationship to progression. *Together, these variables represent the sum total of the body's ability to heal the infected lesion.* An ulcer that has existed for some time without worsening is a sign that, collectively, the host's protective systems are properly functioning. On the other hand, relentless progression in a short interval carries a grave prognosis, often to the point of replacing continued care of the infected part with removing it entirely (i.e., amputating).

PHYSICAL EXAMINATION

Physical examination of the infected ulcer should begin with visual inspection. Location is

an important etiologic clue (e.g., tips of toes in atherosclerotic ulcers), leading the clinician away from considering an infectious cause. On the other hand, atypical locations may signal the presence of primary infection leading to ulceration. Regardless of the cause, the number of ulcerations is directly proportional to the severity of the pathologic process.

Each ulcer's base should be inspected next. Noninfected ulcers should have clean, moist, granulating bases. Alternately, atherosclerotic ulcers may have clean but desiccated bases covered by a tenacious eschar. Deeper structures, such as tendon or bone, may be visible. Their ability to resist bacterial colonization is generally considered to be less than that of adjacent soft tissues; hence, the exposure of these structures to the external environment may contribute to the development of infection, necessitating their surgical removal. This will be discussed at greater length in other chapters of this text. Exposure of these structures, especially in the absence of other features to be discussed, does not automatically imply that the ulcer is infected.

In infected ulcers, the base takes on a different appearance, with tissue necrosis predominating. Such necrosis can be recognized by the grey color of normally-white tissues, the watery consistency of usually-firm tissues, and a foul odor [24]. Necrotic tissues provide nutrition for invading microorganisms, thereby facilitating the necrotic process. The ulcer base should be probed for deep sinuses, with natural tissue planes and gravity providing clues as to which path the infectious process would most likely take. This discussion of sinus tracts will be continued in greater detail in a later section of this chapter dealing with sinography.

Once the skin's continuity has been broken, it is normal for tissue fluids to escape. These fluids are usually odorless, and of a serous or serosanguinous quality. If the ulcer's cross-sectional area is large, the amount of drainage can be appreciable. These findings are normal and do not represent infection. True infection presents with purulence of varying color and/or odor. Even anaerobic infections, which are famous for their thin, watery discharge (often confused with serous drainage) are usually malodorous.

The ulcer border deserves special examination

as well. Undermined borders suggest an infectious organism capable of growing at cooler temperatures (e.g., *Mycobacteria*). As a result, the process extends laterally rather than vertically. Infected ulcers may also demonstrate undermining in the form of a sinus tract; however, if the host defenses permit such undermining, there is a strong chance that deep, vertical sinuses will be present as well.

Finally, the clinician should make special note of the inflammatory changes in the surrounding skin and soft tissues. All clinicians are aware of the parameters that comprise inflammation (warmth, redness, etc.), but probably few practitioners actually grid the border of each change. This is a little-used, yet invaluable, clinical tool, as it provides some objective assessment as to whether the therapeutic plan is having its desired effect: Are borders receding or enlarging? Infected ulcers will present with marked periulcer changes, including cellulitis, lymphangitis, tissue crepitation, and lymphadenopathy. Noninfected ulcers generally present with little more than a mild erythematous border that remains fairly stabilized. If severe enough, infected ulcerations will be accompanied by constitutional symptoms (i.e., malaise, fever), whereas noninfected ulcers will not.

The examination for periulcer changes carries a special warning. The changes just discussed will be seen in patients with uncompromised vascularity. In the case of poor arterial supply, however, infection may cause tissue necrosis *without* the anticipated host defense responses. There will be little purulence, erythema, or edema. At times, the only change may be an increase in the diameter of the pain border or the severity of pain. In cases of sensory neuropathy *and* vascular compromise, *progressive* tissue necrosis should be recognized as a signal that an infected ulcer exists. When noninvasive vascular studies have been performed or are available, an absolute toe pressure of less than 30 mm Hg is considered insufficient for healing. Periwound transcutaneous oxygen tension (TcPO$_2$) of less than 20 mm Hg is also considered a poor prognostic sign [25]. (See Figure 15-7.)

MICROSCOPY

The taking of a thorough history and the performance of a complete examination as described above should provide the clinician with enough data to diagnose an infected cutaneous ulcer. Determination of the pathogenic organism(s) is next in order, and may be rapidly assessed using a Gram stain. Although not as specific as a culture and

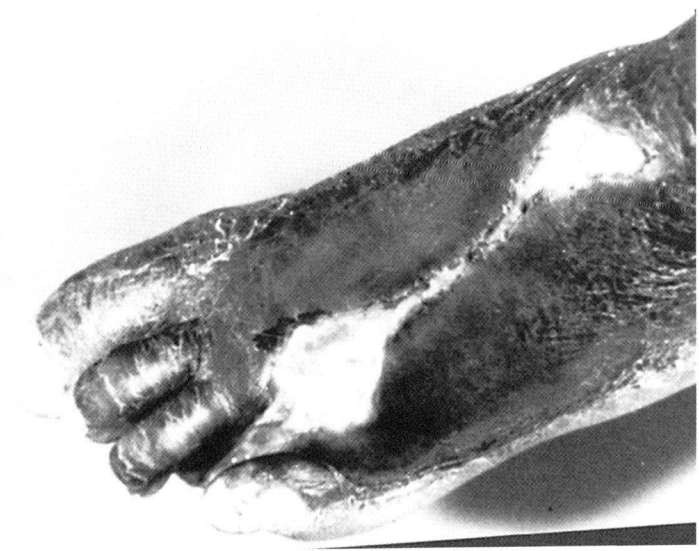

Figure 15-7. Ulceration following an extensor tenectomy to avert proximal cellulitic spread. The ulcer's pale base indicates vascular compromise. The cellulitis spread, and the limb was lost.

sensitivity or **bacteria count and sensitivity**, combining a knowledge of the most frequently encountered flora with a Gram stain permits the initiation of reasonably accurate empiric therapy. Keep in mind that anaerobic infections may present with multiple organisms on a Gram stain, but only one cultured isolate. Gram stains that exhibit bacteria only usually represent contamination; Gram stains that show bacteria *and* polymorphonuclear leukocytes indicate true infection [24].

The bacterial organisms most frequently encountered in foot infections in various patient populations have been published and *replicated* in a number of series. Infected *diabetic* ulcerations have received the greatest literary attention; however, it is probably safe to extrapolate these data to the general population. These organisms are therefore listed in Table 15-1. The reader should use this table as a reference to pinpoint the predominant organism(s). The method of sample collection is vital to ensuring that the organisms seen on Gram stain (or grown in culture) are the ones responsible for the infected or infectious ulcer.

Cutaneous ulcerations in patients with Raynaud's disease or phenomenon are usually associated with yeasts and a variety of bacteria.

Immobile and/or incontinent patients with decubital ulcers often develop contamination of the ulcers with fecal and urinary debris; however, *Staphylococcus aureus* is still the most common

Table 15-1. Most Commonly Encountered Bacteria in Diabetic Foot Ulcerations and Infections

Aerobes
  Gram-positive cocci
    Staphylococcus aureus
    Staphylococcus epidermidis
    Enterococci
    Group B streptococci
  Gram-negative bacilli
    Enterobacteriaceae
    Pseudomonas aeruginosa
    Proteus species

Anaerobes
    Bacteroides species
    Peptococcus species
    Peptostreptococcus species

Sources: Lipsky et al. [67] and Joseph [68].

isolate. In hospitalized patients, *Pseudomonas* species and *Escherichia coli* can occur.

In virtually all cases, ulcer healing is closely related to a decrease in bacteria count.

SINOGRAPHY

The extent, depth, and route of a sinus may be visualized through sinography. Simply stated, this procedure involves the instillation of a radiopaque material into the entire course of the sinus, after which some form of imaging (e.g., a standard radiograph) is employed. The radiopaque dye obscures detail of other tissues in the area, so sinography is best employed after images not using the dye are taken. A silver nitrate stick, moistened and inserted into the sinus, may be used in lieu of the radiopaque dye (personal communication, Randy Cohen, D.P.M.). Although critics of sinography may argue that probing at the bedside or chairside is adequate to map the sinus, sinography may be superior for the initial visualization of tortuous channels and communications with deeper foot compartments. Care must be taken against instilling the radiopaque dye with too much force, as the possibility of opening potential spaces and introducing bacteria exists.

CULTURE AND BIOPSY

Microorganisms can be recovered from any ulcer surface. The organisms collected, however, may not be the true pathogens. Swab cultures are notorious for gathering the "wrong" microbes, and therefore should be used only when deeper methods of culture are contraindicated (i.e., when they would cause harmful extension of the ulcer). Specimens should be collected before antibiotics have been administered, or if possible, after an antibiotic-free period of 48 hours has elapsed [24].

Pus, when available, signifies an intact host response to the presence of infection and provides reliable material for culture. A thin layer of collagen substance usually covers all skin ulcers; this is not to be confused with true purulence. A useful clinical axiom to remember in all culture samplings is that deeper cultures are more reliable cultures. Superficial cultures gather contaminants, and often miss anaerobes (as in the center of an abscess, where anaerobes can thrive). When material from abscesses is to be sampled, anaerobes, aerobes, and a Gram stain should be obtained, in that order [24]. If only fluid is to be obtained, it should be retrieved from the deeper portions of the collection. If tissue from an ulcer base or margins is to be cultured, the tissue should be obtained via curette scrapings of the ulcer base, margin, or the deepest portions of a sinus. All things considered, curette scrapings probably form the most reliable cultures. Curettage should be gentle, however, and not gouge the wound or result in extensive hemorrhage. Do not rely on sinus cultures if osteomyelitis is suspected (bone cultures are required in these instances) except in the case of *Staphylococcus aureus*, which is recovered in the sinus tract and bone approximately 70% of the time [26].

Aspiration has been touted as an alternate culture method, especially when little purulence is present (such as in the advancing edge of cellulitis). Aspiration cultures are performed by using a large-bore needle (15 or 18 gauge) to inject or irrigate the tissue to be cultured with a small amount of sterile water or saline. This fluid is allowed to mix with the adjacent tissues momentarily and is then aspirated through the same needle, hopefully carrying with it the true pathogens. Time has not supported the extensive use of aspiration cultures, as reliable results have been obtained only 10% of the time.

Up to this point, our discussion has focused on aerobic bacteria. Infected and infectious ulcers may also present with and be caused by anaerobes, fungi, acid-fast bacteria, spirochetes, and viruses. If any of these are suspected, special collection containers (although often cumbersome and unreliable) or procedures may become necessary. The microbiology laboratory should be consulted in these instances. When that is not possible, the safest transport system (except for anaerobes) may consist of sterile saline or water. In cases of suspected syphilitic ulceration, serum antibody tests (i.e., VDRL, FTA) take the place of darkfield examinations for the spirochete; in these cases darkfield examinations are nearly impossible to obtain.

Biopsy of infected or infectious ulcers may become necessary when traditional therapy is ineffective, or malignant degeneration is suspected. Except for these two instances, biopsy should probably be considered a technique of last resort because it will always increase the ulcer's size. When necessary, ulcer biopsy should always include a full thickness of the base and/or margin. When the ulcer is problematic and very small, complete excisional biopsy with flap or free graft coverage may be preferred from a diagnostic and therapeutic standpoint.

WOUND CARE

Discussions of osteomyelitis, diagnostic imaging, and antibiotics are beyond the scope of this chapter and will not be included here. Instead, the next several sections will concentrate on wound care, ulcer dressings and ancillary techniques such as hyperbaric oxygenation and the use of growth factors. One comment will be made, however, regarding the use of imaging. The literature espouses one nuclide or another for early detection of infection or differentiation of osteomyelitis from neuropathic joint disease. None is 100% sensitive and specific; thus, clinicians are often left in a quandary. Rather than exposing patients to sometimes frustrating and equivocal examinations, bone biopsy may be the most expeditious choice. T_2-weighted images (the "water image") can be extremely useful in identifying fluid collections like deep abscesses.

The measure of clinical effectiveness is outcome. Using the inflammatory parameters described earlier and the wound changes to be presented below, one should be able to quantify steady, progressive improvement. Each redressing should begin with repeating the physical examination discussed at the beginning of this section. Once the findings have been noted and recorded, attention is next directed to the ulcer surface.

DEBRIDEMENT

The goal in caring for an infected or infectious ulcer surface is to convert it to one consisting only of clean granulation tissue. Such a surface facilitates epithelialization or provides a ready receptacle for grafting. The ulcer surface should therefore be debrided of necrotic debris at each and every dressing change. The method of debridement will vary, depending on the amount and type of necrotic tissue as well as the wound's ability to withstand aggressive therapy. At first presentation, extensive debridement may be necessary, and may require use of a hospital operating room. Nonviable tissue should be removed if (a) it is painful, (b) it provides a nutritional bed for microorganisms, fostering further infection, and (c) it is occluding drainage (Figure 15-8). Necrotic tissue that is especially tenacious, extremely painful to remove, and fails to meet the other aforementioned tests can often be left in place until a natural liquefactive process occurs beneath it. Some clinicians would disagree with this approach, preferring instead to surgically debride the eschar. It is the opinion of the authors' that this methodology is inadvisable, because it further injures the wound. As long as the above tests are unmet, it is gentler to allow the wound to discharge the necrotic material naturally. This can sometimes be a tedious procedure requiring much more patience, but it does not add insult to injury.

As alternates to sharp, surgical debridement, or after such initial debridement has been performed, one might employ simple curettage, the "gauze curette," wet-to-dry dressings, or topical enzymatic debriding agents. Simple curettage should be performed with a large bone curette to remove the loose debris that collects between dressing changes. This curettage should extend down to granulation tissue or other normal tissues in the area. Curettage should not gouge the wound or create hemorrhage.

The weight of the instrument itself should suffice in terms of gauging how much force to use during debridement. Normal tissues have a tough, fibrous feel to them, and dragging the curette across the wound will gather very little material.

"Gauze curettage" may be employed in those wounds that cannot tolerate surgical debridement or traditional curettage. This procedure involves the use of a dry gauze pad or one that has been moistened with an antiseptic solution. Antiseptic scrubs are not used because they make the gauze pad too slippery, interfering with the mechanical action desired. Once prepared, the gauze pad is rubbed back and forth across the wound; when the gauze has become saturated with debris, the pad is replaced with a new one.

As another alternative, the wound may be debrided using standard wet-to-dry dressings. Removal of the dried dressing debrides the wound by lifting debris that has adhered to the dressing during the drying process. This can sometimes be a painful procedure and should be therefore be used only in those patients who can tolerate it.

A variety of topical enzymatic debriding agents exist that may be selected when more aggressive methods of debridement are not feasible. Ointment-based enzymes should probably not be used in purulent wounds, as the ointment is occlusive and therefore inhibits needed drainage.

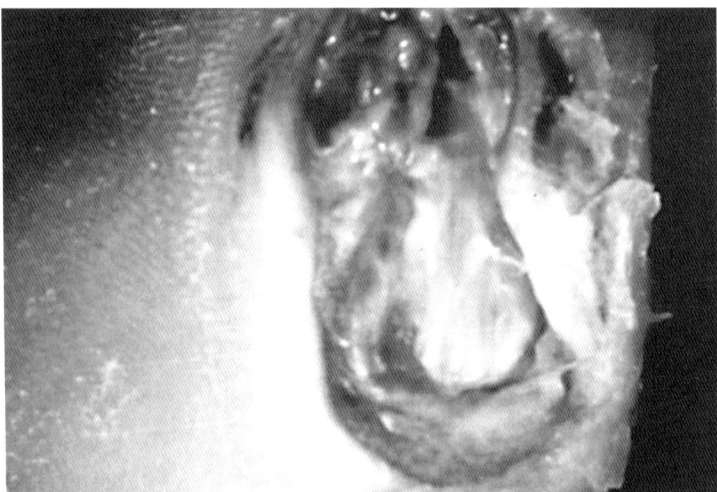

Figure 15-8. Exposure of the flexor tendon in a Wagner II neurotrophic ulceration beneath the first metatarsal head. The tendon's continued vitality helps to determine whether it is debrided or left in place.

While there is general consensus within the medical community as to the indications for sharp surgical debridement, less agreement is encountered concerning the additional debridement methods just described. One school of thought favors regular wound debridement, while another advocates that this manipulation may be disrupting an immature epithelial layer that is attempting to form. The authors contend that, in a patient whose wound and vascular status can tolerate it, regular, scheduled debridement promotes a clean granulating wound that will rapidly epithelialize or can be covered with an appropriate graft. Extensive collections of debris between redressings indicate that the last debridement was not thorough enough, the wound is deteriorating, or that more frequent debridement and dressing changes are required.

IRRIGATION

Following debridement, the ulcer should be irrigated, both to flush away remaining debris and to restore some of the natural moisture that has been lost during debridement. One must keep in mind that ulcers will always drain because the skin's integrity has been lost. This compromise allows normal tissue fluids to escape. Maintenance of a moist wound base is therefore considered necessary for healing of the ulcer. Allowing a wound to desiccate will only promote tissue necrosis.

The choice of irrigant is of less importance than the mechanical benefit to be gained, so simple saline is used in many centers. Nevertheless, clinicians prefer using a microbistatic or microbicidal agent in the irrigant solution. In large ulcerations with extensive sinuses and undermining, a 1:10,000 potassium permanganate solution (0.01%) provides an inexpensive alternative to dilute povidone-iodine mixtures, and in infinitesimal in cost compared to commonly used aminoglycoside irrigants. Potassium permanganate irrigant can be pharmacy prepared by the gallon, increasing its cost effectiveness. Whatever the irrigant, it should be applied with a bulb or other syringe to permit thorough flushing with a modest amount of pressure.

One word of caution should be offered when using hydrogen peroxide irrigants. Their effervescent quality can create compartment syndrome-like changes if employed in small, deep ulcerations with sinuses. This occurs because the gas liberated by the peroxide has nowhere to escape. Such irrigations are therefore more safely used in broad, shallow ulcerations and in those with short, relatively straight sinuses and little undermining.

KERATOTIC RIM

Approximately every 48 hours, the ulcer border becomes covered by a keratotic rim. This keratosis interferes with advancing epithelialization and it should be removed by lifting it with a surgical forceps and picking it off much as one opens the tops of certain packages (Figure 15-9). This maneuver may cause some slight bleeding at the wound edge, which should be of little concern as long as the hemorrhage is of minimal degree. Extensive hemorrhage is a sign that more than the keratotic rim was removed. This is contraindicated, for it causes further injury and the extensive hemorrhage provides a medium for bacterial growth.

DRAINS

After the ulcer has been debrided, cleansed, and irrigated, drains should be inserted into the depth of *every* sinus and underneath each undermined border. Sterile packing gauze is adequate, but iodinated gauze packing may be used as well. The drains may be numerous at times, depending upon the number of sinuses. The drains not only facilitate drainage and oxygenation, but also prevent the maceration that can occur between two granulating surfaces. Drains should be placed, and not packed, into position—packing will inhibit rather than promote drainage. Each day, sinus depth and ulcer border undermining should decrease if the wound is healing normally.

A principle often employed by thoracic surgeons, but of equal benefit in those caring for draining wounds, is postural drainage. Simply stated, this principle requires that the patient or part be positioned so that gravity will aid in draining the wound as well as prevent spread into deeper regions of the area (Figure 15-10). The best pictorial analogy to illustrate this concept is a glass of water that

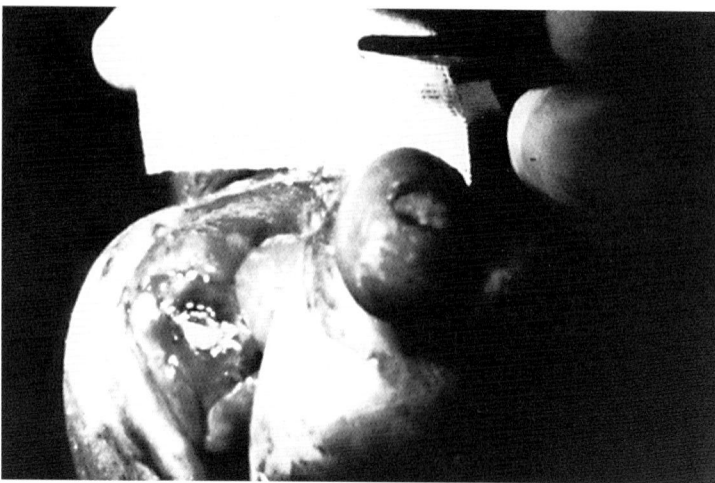

Figure 15-9. Removal of keratotic rim from wound margin every 48–72 hours facilitates epithelialization.

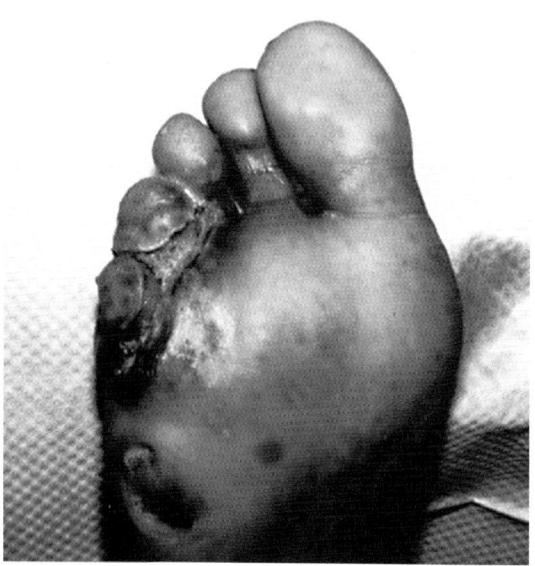

Figure 15-10. This patient must be placed prone and not supine if postural drainage is to prevent proximal spread.

has been left standing upright. In this position, its contents will never drain other than by evaporation. This is the scenario in patients with distal ulcerations who are instructed to remain supine. In this position, fluid will usually dissect proximally and laterally. The lateral migration of fluid occurs be-

cause the lower limbs naturally assume an externally rotated position when the body is supine. The glass of water described above will empty only if it is turned on its side or upside down. In like manner, patients with distal, draining wounds should be placed on the appropriate side or in a prone position.

Another aspect of postural drainage dictates whether the limb should be held elevated, horizontal, or in a dependent position. Lower extremities held in a dependent position for long periods will soon become edematous, a condition that interferes with normal tissue perfusion. This state becomes exacerbated in patients with venous incompetence.

On the other hand, lower extremity elevation may be detrimental in cases of arterial compromise, where an already limited blood supply must now combat the forces of gravity.

Given these circumstances, horizontal positioning of the limb may be best advised, for it neither produces edema nor resists arterial inflow.

MOBILIZATION OF WOUND MARGINS

As the infected or infectious ulcer becomes more healthy and granulating, the clinician must begin to consider the prospect of accelerating wound closure. Although the topic of grafts and flaps is beyond the scope of this chapter, mobilization of wound margins can greatly decrease the size of the wound to be repaired. On occasion, large defects can be closed primarily without the need for further surgery.

Mobilization of wound margins is made possible by the normal elasticity of soft tissues. Injectable or implantable tissue expanders function on this same principle, which results in the production of additional skin and subcutaneous tissues when those structures are placed on prolonged stretch. Clinically, this effect can be achieved by massaging the wound margins just prior to applying the ulcer dressing. The massage should encompass nearly the entire wound margin, and move toward the center of the wound. In approximately five minutes, the available degree of mobilization should have been achieved. Tincture of benzoin or another suitable adhesive is painted on each side of the wound, and the mobilized wound edges are held in place using adhesive tape strips. The placement site of each adhesive strip should be changed to avoid skin maceration. Excessive tension can lead to vascular compromise, and therefore should not be placed on the mobilized wound margin. Excessive tension can be recognized by blanching, cyanosis, and coolness of the skin in the wound margin itself. At each redressing, the wound margins should be more easily mobilized and retain more of their new position without the aid of adhesive strips.

If wound margins are not mobilized at the appropriate time, they will more than likely undergo fibrosis in their existing position. Surgical undermining, larger grafting, or more extensive flaps may therefore become necessary.

WOUND DRESSINGS

The past decade has witnessed an explosion of wound dressing products. In infected and/or infectious cutaneous ulcerations, the wound dressing should serve several vital functions: (1) it should protect the wound from contamination by microorganisms, yet allow cytokines (growth factors) to concentrate beneath it, (2) it should maintain a warm, moist ulcer base to avoid desiccating the wound, (3) it should be absorbent enough to remove excessive drainage that would otherwise cause maceration and foster bacterial growth, but not so absorbent as to cause drying of the wound, (4) removal of the dressing should not cause pain or trauma to

the wound, and (5) the dressing should allow gaseous exchange: i.e., wound oxygenation. Obviously, no single ulcer dressing can perform each of these functions interchangeably (some newer products do, however, profess to have "intelligence"—see Table 15-2). The clinician must be familiar with each of the available dressings and must be prepared to alternate one dressing type with another depending upon the ulcer's condition (Figure 15-11). Ulcer dressings do not cause healing; they merely facilitate natural reparative processes.

Table 15-2. Occlusive Wound Dressings

Semipermeable adhesive transparent polyurethane films
- Change every one to seven days
- Wound can be inspected without removal of the dressing
- Use on shallow wounds with minimal drainage
- Excessive wound drainage may need to be aspirated
- Use skin adherent to protect adjacent skin from maceration

Hydrogel sheets and wafers
- Conform well to wound surface and surrounding skin
- Require a secondary dressing or tape to hold them on
- Absorb a limited amount of wound drainage
- Use on lightly draining wounds
- Usually consist of a polyethylene lattice containing a hydrated cross-linked polymer: e.g., polyethylene oxide
- Retention of any polyethylene film backing makes the dressing occlusive; removal of the backing makes the dressing permeable
- Should be changed every one to three days
- Will dry out when used with hyperbaric oxygenation, unless the hydrogel is covered with a transparent film dressing
- Must be secured with a secondary dressing
- Suitable for rehydration of dry eschar

Calcium alginates
- Derived from brown seaweed
- High absorbency makes them ideal for wounds with extensive drainage
- Interaction with wound fluid produces a viscous hydrogel
- Available as sheets for shallow wounds, or ropes that can be inserted in cavities (the latter will gel to take on the shape of the wound)
- Are biodegradable, so complete removal is unnecessary
- Change every one to three days
- Discontinue use once epithelialization has begun (is more cost effective to use a dressing that can be left on for several days)

Continued

Table 15-2. *Continued*

- Are contraindicated in dry wounds

Nonadherent hydrophilic polyurethane foams
- Must be secured with a secondary dressing
- Highly conformable to irregular surfaces
- Variable ability to absorb wound fluid
- Saturated dressings can leak fluid at their lateral margins ("lateral strike-through")

Hydrocolloids (occlusive wafer dressings)
- Change every one to seven days
- Contain hydrophilic colloidal particles
- Absorb light to medium drainage by particle swelling
- Fairly conformable
- Usually adherent, but may require a secondary dressing
- As wound fluid is absorbed and interacts with dressing, results in the formation of an offensive, yellow-brown liquid that can be confused with pus
- Available as powders and pastes for deep wounds
- Most are opaque; the wound can not be inspected
- Dressing should extend at least 2 cm beyond the wound edge

Moist, saline-soaked gauze
- Change two to three times daily
- Must be secured with a secondary dressing
- Gauze is not impermeable to microorganisms
- Easily removed
- Maintenance of moisture is difficult
- Should not be packed or stuffed into wound

Absorptive powders, beads, pastes, and gels
- All contain absorptive materials (e.g., starch, pectin)
- Change every one to three days
- Do not use in patients with dry eschar
- Highly absorbent, so use in wounds with extensive drainage
- Powders and beads are more absorbent but are difficult to handle and remove
- Unless premixed, preparation may be too wet or dry
- Mixture may be difficult to confine to wound cavity
- Must be used with a secondary dressing

Paraffin gauze dressings
- Use in noninfected, granulating wounds
- Also useful in pink, epithelializing wounds
- Can be left in place for seven days

Sources: Mulder et al. [69], Jeter and Tintle [70], and Carver and Leigh [71], [72].

Table 15-2 compares most of the wound dressings marketed today. In spite of the wide variety of products available, hydrocolloids and simple saline dressings appear to predominate. Saline dressings supply moisture and are easy for patients to self-

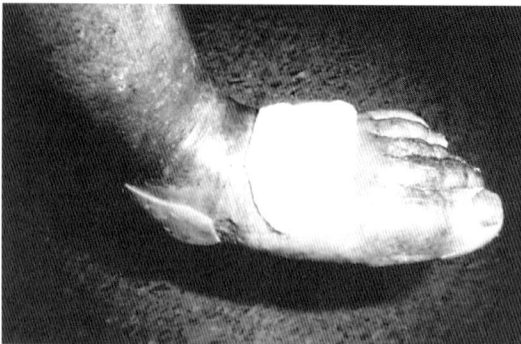

Figure 15-11. Biologic dressings must be changed as the nature of the wound changes. Here, an alginate and hydrocolloid are used in combination for heavily draining, but noninfected, wounds.

administer, but the woven gauze that comprises them does not prevent contamination by microorganisms. Hydrocolloids are also easy to administer, retain wound moisture, are effective barriers against contamination, and may be left in place for long periods, obviating the need for frequent, costly dressing changes. Decades of research have shown that occlusive dressings are superior to permeable ones in noninfected wounds. During infection, however, frequent wound evaluation and redressings are recommended over a reliance on biologic dressings (and total contact casts) left in place for several days.

HYPERBARIC OXYGENATION

First popularized in burn patients, hyperbaric oxygenation of wound was widely utilized in a variety of nonburn wounds. The successes reported in the early years of its use in these circumstances have now waned, regardless of whether whole-body or more-readily-available extremity chambers are employed. Presently, an adequate vascular supply is considered more beneficial than hyperbaric oxygenation. Removal of necrotic debris, drainage of abscesses, copious use of hydrogen peroxide (see warning above), and exposure of deep wound recesses to room air are more reliable in eliminating anaerobic growth.

Patients with infected ulcers in documented sickle cell disease or other conditions made worse by hypoxia may benefit from hyperbaric oxygenation.

TRANSCUTANEOUS ELECTRICAL STIMULATION

Not long after transcutaneous electrical nerve stimulation (TENS) was introduced for pain relief, interest in the effects of electricity on wound healing flourished. No published reports have indicated any beneficial effect on infected or infectious ulcerations. A recent study, however [27], demonstrated a significant increase in transcutaneous partial oxygen tension (PO$_2$) in ischemic and pressure ulcers exposed to chronic (up to nine weeks) alternating current (AC). No significant PO$_2$ changes were noted when direct current (DC) was used, or when the exposure to either current was acute (not more than one hour). The clinician must therefore determine whether this ancillary modality would aid healing of a noninfected ulcer on a case-by-case basis.

SUPPORT SURFACES

Pressure is a well-documented cause of skin breakdown, so it is wise to assume that some part of ulcer healing will rely upon removal of pressure from the wound, especially in the case of neurotrophic ulcerations. The most effective way to do this is to have the area suspended in air. In bedridden, compliant patients this is often easily accomplished. Ambulating patients should be non weight bearing on the affected foot or site. In neuropathic patients, this requires protection of the nonulcerated foot as well, because breakdown of that foot is accelerated by the fact that total body weight is now borne on only one limb. Total contact casts [28], total contact splints, half-shoes [29], felted foam [30], silicone injections [31], extra-depth shoes with accommodative innersoles (for feet that are not deformed), and custom-molded shoes with accommodative innersoles (for deformed feet) allow weight bearing but with pressure distributed over a broader area (Figure 15-12). The durometer measure of accommodative innersole materials must approach that of skin, which requires them to be more soft than firm. Because these inlays fatigue earlier, they must be replaced two or three times per

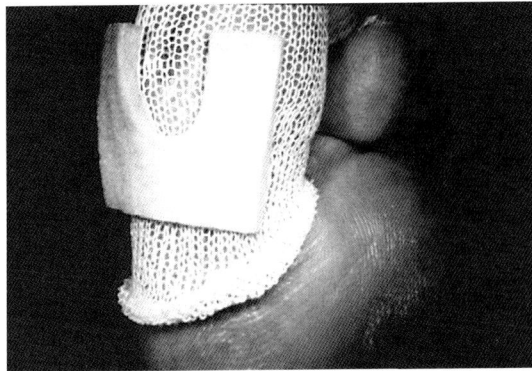

Figure 15-12. Dispersive adhesive felt padding about a neurotrophic ulcer. This is an inexpensive measure that pays great dividends.

year. Orthotist/pedorthist consultation is extremely valuable in this regard, and highly recommended.

In patients who cannot or will not comply with these requirements (those who are comatose, mentally incompetent, stubborn, etc.), the clinician must resort to the wide variety of commercial devices designed for this purpose. Even socks with a thin silicone layer sewn into the sock's plantar surface have been used, and with encouraging results [32]. The therapeutic goal should always be a pressure-free environment, not just one that is rhythmically alternating but never pressure free. This need was underscored by a recent study comparing rhythmically alternating support surfaces with static pressure support surfaces [33]. The study failed to detect a significant difference in mean skin blood perfusion when normal patients were exposed to either surface for 60 minutes.

On occasion, surgical intervention is required to create an even weight-bearing surface. Tendo Achilles lengthening procedures are often used to heal recurrent ulcerations in transmetatarsal amputees who also have equinus deformity [34]. Partial calcanectomy has been advocated for large ulcerations of the heel [35].

GROWTH FACTORS

During wound repair, the wound is nourished by an exudate of mitogens, chemoattractants, and protein-inducing agents. Collectively, these are known as growth factors. As these growth factors initiate more than cell proliferation, they are more appropriately referred to as *cytokines*. In most cases, these cytokines were named after the cells or target that led to their discovery. As a result, their names are misleading, because they do not describe the full activity of the factor. These cytokines can also induce the transcription of oncogenes, and therefore may be tumorigenic [36, 37]. A single growth factor apparently can be either stimulatory or inhibitory based upon which other growth factors are present.

Growth Factor (Cytokine) Production/Mechanism of Action

The cytokines synthesized and released during wound repair [38, 39] may be subdivided into three types: mitogens, chemoattractants, and transforming factors. Cytokines are synthesized and secreted in endocrine, paracrine, and autocrine fashions. As polypeptides (proteins), the cytokines do not easily cross cell membranes. Instead, they seem to work by attaching to receptors that sit across the cell membrane. The binding of two or more adjacent receptors to the same growth factor appears to be necessary for activation. Once activated, a message is sent to the nucleus DNA to create the target proteins that cause cell division, tumorigenicity, etc. In experimental animals, cytokines have helped to heal wounds caused by diabetes mellitus, glucocorticoids, irradiation, or chemotherapy [40].

Mitogens signal cellular proliferation and can be subdivided into *competence* types (which stimulates cells to progress from the resting state to a readiness state and finally to cell division) and *progression* types (which allow continuation of the cell cycle after cell division).

Chemoattractants stimulate cellular migration. They can be subdivided into *chemotactic* (inducing the target cell to move in a given direction) or *chemokinetic* (increasing the rate of cellular migration) types.

Transforming factors alter a cell's phenotypic expression.

Growth factors that exist but do not appear in trials for skin wounds (ulcers) include human growth hormone (hGH), insulin-like growth factor-1 (IGF-1), erythropoietin (normally produced in the kidney in response to hypoxia; it stimulates bone marrow to increase RBC production), tumor necrosis factor (TNF; cachectin), interleukins, and colony-stimulating factors (CSFs).

Individual Growth Factors

Fibroblast Growth Factor (FGF). Two separate subtypes of this peptide exist: basic FGF (bFGF) and acidic FGF (aFGF) [38]. Of the two, bFGF is the more useful because of the high number of target cells it can affect. In clinical trials, the effective dose was determined to be 0.5 µg/day in single or multiple doses. It (bFGF) appears to "turn itself off" once reepithelialization has occurred. Basic FGF is angiogenic, whereas aFGF is nonangiogenic. Both forms have been isolated from endothelial cells.

Transforming and Epidermal Growth Factors (TGF, EGF). Transforming growth factor exists in an alpha and beta form, both of which are angiogenic [38, 42]. The alpha form is more angiogenic than epidermal growth factor (EGF), and shares the same cell receptor as EGF.

Platelets are the most abundant source of the beta form, which seems to regulate the effect of other growth factors so as to control "overproduction." The most important feature of EGF is its angiogenic properties.

Platelet-Derived Growth Factor (PDGF). PDGF is the major human serum growth factor [41]. It was originally discovered in platelets, but it has also been found in other cells. Its mitogenic action is dependent on other growth factors, but its chemotactic activity functions independently.

Normal Wound Healing

Wound repair [36] is a complex, multicellular event that begins when a break in the skin occurs, ends when tissue continuity is restored, and consists of cell recruitment, cell proliferation, and protein synthesis. Coagulation for the purpose of hemostasis is the first event and is made possible by endothelial cells and platelets. The next phase is that of debris removal by leukocytes, and the final component results in tissue replacement (i.e., matrix and epidermal regeneration) involving macrophages, endothelial cells, fibroblasts, and epithelial cells (keratinocytes). Unfortunately, wound repair results in disorganized fibrosis with regenerated epidermis only; adnexal glands/structures are lost.

Granulation tissue replaces the injured area, but is not as good as the original matrix, as it consists of small-diameter collagen fibers only. As the wound matures, collagen of different types and diameters is placed, with various and increased linkages designed to restore normal integrity. Granulation tissue facilitates cellular remodeling.

In the initial response to injury (inflammation phase), normal hemostasis and microvascular occlusion during repair cause gradients that worsen as one gets closer to the wound's center. Repair must therefore occur in a milieu of hypoxia, hyperlacticacidemia, and hypoglycemia.

The cooperative ability of hemoglobin to bind oxygen lowers the cardiac output required to bring oxygen to the tissues. Rapidly metabolizing tissues have lower tissue oxygen pressures, so extraction of oxygen from hemoglobin is facilitated by the gradient created. Therefore, in *uninjured* tissues, the tissues in higher demand have greater access to supply. In wounded tissues, however, this gradient is enhanced by the distance away from the capillary source of oxygen and the presence of fibrin (a barrier to oxygen movement).

Arteriolar dilatation and increased capillary permeability are also observed during the initial phase; at the same time venules constrict. These processes facilitate a pooling of fluids and cells within the area.

Injury allows plasma to interact with tissue protein, causing a number of cascades to come into play: the intrinsic/extrinsic clotting cascade, the fibrinolytic cascade, the complement pathway, the kinin system, and prostaglandins.

The clotting cascade leads to thrombin formation, which converts fibrinogen to fibrin. Fibrin is the major coagulation-promoting component and also plays a role in necrotic tissue removal, chemotaxis, and angiogenesis. Thrombin interacts with platelets to cause the release of platelet-derived growth factor (PDGF). Platelets not only plug the vessel tear, but also release substances that stimulate cell proliferation, migration, and protein synthesis (alpha granules of platelets release TGF-β, PDGF, and EGF).

The kinin system forms bradykinin, which causes much-needed microvascular dilatation at the wound edge.

The complement cascade creates C5a, which attracts neutrophils and monocytes (the first cells to occupy the wound healing space for the first two days after injury). Neutrophils (polymorphonuclear leukocytes, or PMNs) primarily neutralize bacteria and begin debridement of the ischemic matrix. Circulating monocytes differentiate into tissue macrophages and lymphocytes, and appear in the wound at two days postinjury. They join neutrophils in bacterial neutralization and debridement, and these monocytes also orchestrate granulation tissue formation, especially in an "ischemic" environment (hypoxia and lactate stimulate macrophages to secrete angiogenic factors, which promote capillary growth into the repair zone).

The fibrinolytic cascade converts circulating plasminogen (inactive) to plasmin (active), which breaks fibrin clots into fibrin degradation products. The beginning of clot resolution signals the end of the inflammatory phase and the beginning of the repair/regeneration phase of wound healing. Fibrin degradation products are biologically active, functioning as chemoattractants for monocytes (the predominant cell throughout repair) and endothelial cells, as well as collagen synthesis.

As mentioned earlier, fibrinolysis (blood clot resolution) marks the end of the inflammatory phase and the beginning of the tissue repair phase. Fibroblasts appear in the wound site from three days postinjury onward. They proliferate and migrate into the wound site, synthesizing and secreting collagen. The high-lactate, low-oxygen character of healing wounds seems to enhance this process.

In addition to collagen formation, angiogenesis and epithelialization are significant and necessary processes of the repair phase of wound healing. Angiogenesis includes capillary endothelial cell migration and proliferation, protease production, and differentiation into tubes. In addition to wound healing, angiogenesis occurs during (a) fetal development, and (b) tumor growth [41]. Angiogenic growth factors seem to work directly on endothelial cells, or indirectly (via macrophages, which can secrete a direct-acting growth factor) [42]. In theory, angiogenesis is discontinued as the wound heals, probably in response to the restoration of normal tissue oxygen pressure by a now-normal circulation (tissue macrophages are stimulated by hypoxia and lactate to produce an angiogenesis factor; the absence of hypoxia and lactate will therefore "turn off" the macrophage).

As vascular permeability decreases, growth factors (cytokines) probably decrease because of decreased plasma and cell leakage. Epithelialization and the production of angiogenesis-inhibiting factors may also inhibit angiogenesis factor activity.

Platelet-Derived Wound Healing Formula (PDWHF)

This solution [38] was developed out of the landmark research conducted by Knighton et al., who use a naturally occurring mix of growth factors obtained from the patient's own platelets: PDGF, platelet-derived angiogenic factor (PDAF), platelet-derived EGF, TGF-B, and platelet factor 4 (PF-4). This technology is currently marketed as PROCUREN by CuraTech, Inc., Stony Brook, New York.

In the first trial by Knighton et al., 49 patients with 95 wounds were studied. The age range of the patients was from eleven to eighty years, and the duration of conventional treatment extended from one week to thirty-five years (mean 3.8 years). Almost half of the wounds were attributed to diabetes, the remaining wounds being secondary to venous stasis, nondiabetic peripheral vascular disease, trauma, and miscellaneous causes. Wounds were categorized according to severity and subjected to a protocol of debridement, revascularization (where necessary), PDWHF for 12 hours followed by Silvadene or another topical antibiotic for 12 hours, custom-molded shoes, patellar-tendon-bearing prostheses, and instruction in nutrition/blood sugar control/meticulous wound care. In an average of 7.5 weeks (range 1–22 weeks), complete healing was recorded in 90% of the patients and 97% of the wounds. No harmful side effects, no excessive scarring or connective tissue growth, and no malignant transformation were observed.

Knighton et al. next conducted a double-blind, crossover, placebo-controlled trial. The positive group consisted of 13 patients, with 17 of 21 wounds healing in an average of 8.6 weeks. In the placebo group, on the other hand, only 2 of 13

wounds healed in 8 weeks. When crossed over, the remaining 11 wounds healed in an average of 7.1 additional weeks.

Doucette et al. confirmed these results in a retrospective study, concluding that limb salvage could be positively affected using this protocol.

Knighton and his team believe that PDWHF works by promoting rapid growth of granulation tissue to cover the wound, after which rapid epithelialization will occur.

PDWHF is currently in use in at least 20 wound care centers nationwide. Autologous preparations are expensive; preparations through recombinant DNA technique, impregnation in sutures and bandages, and oral/parenteral administration may all occur in the future. Recombinant DNA techniques make the mass production of growth factors more feasible. In this process, the amino acid sequence of the growth factor in question is identified, from which reverse messenger RNA (mRNA) probes are constructed. These probes screen human DNA for the correct gene, which is then separated out and spliced into bacterial DNA. The bacteria secrete the factor into culture media, which is then harvested. A human DNA gene is not always required; some growth factors are not species specific and therefore may be isolated from other mammals [43].

Some barriers to these advances exist, however, and include (a) the chemically unstable nature of these compounds, (b) potential degradation of cytokines by the proteolytic factors found in normal wounds, and (c) uncertainty regarding optimal dosage levels, as different amounts can be either suppressive or stimulatory.

In summary then, the first response to injury is coagulation to limit the loss of blood. Platelets participate in this effort, and release EGF, PDGF, TGF-α, TGF-β, and IGF-1 from their alpha granules. These growth factors have chemotactic and mitogenic qualities.

Inflammation follows this stage, with neutrophils (PMNs) and macrophages infiltrating the wound. Macrophages secrete TGF-α, TGF-β, PDGF, bFGF, and interleukin 1. These chemotactic factors and other chemotactic factors (C5a, bacterial products) cause fibroblast migration into the wound.

Fibroblasts secrete growth factors that (a) produce extracellular matrix components (i.e., proteo-glycans, fibronectin, collagen), and (b) are the most likely source of endothelial cell migration and pro-liferation.

Endothelial cells establish blood supply and se-crete PDGF and bFGF.

Finally, remodeling processes such as collagen synthesis, collagenase synthesis, and collagen cross-linking reestablish the architecture of the wound.

Alterations in the above system can lead to im-paired healing or excessive deposition of connec-tive tissue with fibrosis. Once the infected or infec-tious ulceration has been brought under control, these substances may play a future role in promot-ing wound healing and closure.

Cultured Epithelial Autografts (CEAUs) and Allografts (CEALs)

These grafts [44] are prepared in vitro after a sample has been harvested from the donor. In the case of autografts, the donor and graft recipient (host) are the same person; allografts come from a different person. While in culture, the grafts have a mucoid consistency, are transparent, and consist only of an undifferentiated epidermal layer. Within a week of applying the graft to a granulating bed, however, it assumes the macroscopic and histologic characteristics of normal epidermis. Even more re-markably, the dermal layer underlying the CEAU transforms from a scar-like appearance to one with a normal bilaminar arrangement (i.e., papillary and reticular dermis) of collagen fibrils. CEAUs also seem to possess the unprecedented feature of site specificity: that is, the ability to generate the same type of skin (epidermis and dermis) found at the donor site regardless of where the graft is placed. CEAUs obtained from the sole of the foot will therefore recreate plantar skin *wherever the CEAU is placed*.

Although cutaneous adnexa (hair, glands) are not recreated by the CEAU, dermal development is clearly directed by the epidermis. This finding disproved the prior belief that the dermis directed events within the epidermis. The epidermis' ability to perform these incredible functions has been at-tributed to epidermal cytokines, including acidic and basic-FGF, which has already led researchers to consider CEAUs as favored wound dressings and natural vehicles for the administration of growth factors. Allografts (CEALs) are more easily ob-tained but are rejected soon after their application. As a result, they do not survive long enough to demonstrate the dermal remodeling and site-spe-cific changes witnessed with autografts. Neverthe-less, they do stimulate re-epithelialization until the time of rejection.

SURGICAL INTERVENTIONS

Although beyond the scope of this chapter, these techniques involve foot reconstruction and wound coverage utilizing flaps, microvascular free grafts, and muscle transposition [45–56]. Each method has its proponents, and each should be attempted only by those with proficiency in the required tech-niques. Interestingly, most failures have been the result of persistent osseous deformities that could not be accommodated (please see the earlier sec-tion, Support Surfaces).

MEDICAL INTERVENTIONS DESIGNED TO IMPROVE MICROCIRCULATORY FLOW

These include intravenous administration of prosta-glandin E_1, topical phenytoin, low molecular weight heparin via subcutaneous injection, lyophilized col-lagen used topically, and transvenous retrograde perfusion of a heparin-local anesthetic-gentamicin-dexamethasone mixture [57–61]. As adjuvant treat-ments, they have demonstrated some degree of suc-cess in attaining wound closure.

CLOSING REMARKS

Decubital ulcers and those complicating diabetes mellitus are the most commonly encountered foot ulcerations. A number of papers have demonstrated that the best therapeusis is prevention [62, 63]. This depends heavily on *lifelong* education and surveil-lance of the feet at risk. In a study of medical risk factors and their influence on the healing of diabetic foot ulcers, the most important risk factors for amputation were the presence of rest pain, peripheral edema, proteinuria, and a systolic toe pressure of less than 30 mmHg [64]. Patients with high foot pressures are definitely at higher risk for developing plantar ulceration [65], irrespective of total body mass [66].

Remarkably, a large majority of foot ulcerations will heal with compression devices and therapy, suggesting that venous stasis may play a greater role than previously recognized.

REFERENCES

1. Meehan, M., National pressure ulcer prevalence survey, *Adv. Wound Care* 1994; 7(3):27–38.

2. Duff, N., The evolving role of primary interdisciplinary care in the podiatric management of diabetes, *The Low Extr* 1994; 1(2):77–80.

3. Wagner, F. W., A classification and treatment program for diabetic, neuropathic, and dysvascular foot problems, in F. W. Wagner, ed., *AAOS Instructional Course Lectures*, St. Louis, MO: C. V. Mosby, 1979.

4. DeLauro, T. M., and Positano, R. G., Lower extremity ulcerations, in D. E. Marcinko, ed., *Medical and Surgical Therapeutics of the Foot and Leg*, Baltimore, MD: Williams and Wilkins, 1992.

5. Frantz, R.; Xakellis, G. C.; and Arteaga, M., The effects of prolonged pressure on skin blood flow in elderly patients at risk for pressure ulcers, *Decubitus* 1993; 6(6):16–20.

6. Maynard, M. J.; Weiner, L. S.; and Burke, S. W., Neuropathic foot ulceration in patients with myelodysplasia, *J Pediatr Orthop* 1992; 12(6):786–8.

7. Sant, S. M., and Murphy, G. M., Neurotropic ulceration in systemic sclerosis, *Clin Exp Derm* 1994; 19(1):65–6.

8. Kumar, S.; Fernando, D. J.; Veves, A.; et al., Semmes-Weinstein monofilaments: A simple, effective and inexpensive screening device for identifying diabetic patients at risk of foot ulceration, *Diabet Res Clin Prac* 1991; 13(1–2):63–7.

9. Soong, C. V.; Hughes, D.; and Stirling, I., Verrucous carcinoma (epithelioma cuniculatum) plantare, *Eur J Vasc Surg* 1992; 6(6):662–4.

10. Chi, H., and Oda, J., Fibroma of tendon sheath with ulceration, *J Dermatol* 1993; 20(11):703–6.

11. Ball, N. J.; Wickert, W.; Marx, L. H.; et al., Crystal-globulinemia syndrome. A manifestation of multiple myeloma, *Cancer*, 1993; 71(4):1231–4.

12. May, L. P.; Sidhu, G. S.; and Buchness, M. R., Diagnosis of *Acanthamoeba* infection by cutaneous manifestations in a man seropositive to HIV, *J Am Acad Derm* 1992; 26 (2 Pt 2): 352–5.

13. Wilson, D. C.; Werth, S. G.; and King, L. E.; Ulcerative lesions and herpes simplex virus type 2 in a patient with Evan syndrome, *Southern Med J* 1990; 83(12):1484–6.

14. Boixeda, P.; Espana, A.; and Suarez, J., Cutaneous nocardiosis and human immunodeficiency virus infection, *Inter J Dermatol* 1991; 30(11):804–5.

15. Webb, J., and Murdoch, D. A., Tropical ulcers after sports injuries (letter), *Lancet* 1992; 339(8785): 129–30.

16. Sharma, V. K.; Sharma, R.; and Kumar, B., Ulcerative secondary syphilis, *Inter J Dermatol* 1990; 29 (8): 585–6.

17. Kristjansson, M.; Bieluch, V. M.; and Byeff, P. D., Mycobacterium haemophilum infection in immunocompromised patients: Case report and review of the literature, *Rev Infect Dis* 1991; 13(5):906–10.

18. Muelder, K., Wounds that will not heal: The Buruli ulcer, *Inter J Dermatol* 1992; 31(1):25–6.

19. Endeley, E. M. L.; Enwerem, E. O.; Holcome, C.; and Patel, R. V., Buruli ulcer, *J Indian Med Assoc* 1990; 88(9):260–1.

20. Muelder, K., and Nourou, A., Buruli ulcer in Benin, *Lancet* 1991; 336(8723):1109–1111.

21. Hur, W.; Ahn, S. K.; Lee, S. H.; and Kang, W. H., Cutaneous reaction induced by retained bee stinger, *J Dermatol* 1991; 18(12):736–9.

22. Chen, S. C. A.; Lawrence, R. H.; and Packham, D. R., Cellulitis due to Pseudomonas putrefaciens: Possible production of exotoxins, *Rev Infect Dis* 1991; 13(4):642–3.

23. DeMarco, M. J.; Soroko, T. A.; Kirsh, S.; and Smith, L., Epithelioid angiomatosis, *J Foot Ankle Surg* 1993; 32(1):20–26.

24. Joseph, W. S., *Handbook of Lower Extremity Infections* New York: Churchill-Livingstone, 1990.

25. Pecoraro, R. E.; Ahroni, J. H.; Boyko, E. J.; et al., Chronology and determinants of tissue repair in diabetic lower-extremity ulcers, *Diabetes* 1991; 40 (10):1305–13.

26. Bartolomei, F. J., Subcutaneous infections, in C. Abramson, D. J. McCarthy, and M. J. Rupp, eds., *Infectious Diseases of the Lower Extremity*, Philadelphia: Williams and Wilkins, 1991.

27. Likar, B.; Poredos, P.; Preseren, M.; Vodovnik, L.; and Klesnik, M., Effects of electric current on partial oxygen tension in skin surrounding wounds, *Wounds* 1993; 5(1):32–36.

28. Myerson, M.; Papa, J.; Eaton, K.; et al., The total contact cast for management of neuropathic plantar ulcerations of the foot, *J Bone Joint Surg* 1992; Am vol. 74(2):261–9.

29. Chantelau, E.; Breuer, U.; Leisch, A. C.; et al., Outpatient treatment of unilateral diabetic foot ulcers with "half-shoes," *Diabet Med* 1993; 10(3):267–70.

30. Ritz, G.; Kushner, D.; and Friedman, S., A successful technique for the treatment of diabetic neurotrophic ulcers, *J Am Podiatr Med Assoc* 1992; 82(9):479–81.

31. Balkin, S. W., and Kaplan, L., Silicone injection management of diabetic foot ulcers: a possible model for prevention of pressure ulcers, *Decubitus* 1991; 4(4):38–40.

32. Murray, H. J.; Veves, A.; Young, M. J.; et al., Role of experimental socks in the care of the high-risk diabetic foot. A multicenter evaluation study. American Group for the Study of Experimental Hosiery in the Diabetic Foot, *Diabet Care* 1993; 16(8):1190–2.

33. Mayrovitz, H. N.; Regan, M. B.; and Larsen, P. B., Effects of rhythmically alternating and static pressure support surfaces on skin microvascular perfusion, *Wounds* 1993; 5(1):47–55.

34. Barry, D. C.; Sabacinski, K. A.; Habershaw, G. M.; et al., Tendo Achilles procedures for chronic ulcerations in diabetic patients with transmetatarsal amputations, *J Am Podiatr Med Assoc* 1993; 83(2):96–100.

35. Smith, D. G.; Stuck, R. M.; Ketner, L.; et al., Partial calcanectomy for the treatment of large ulcerations of the heel and calcaneal osteomyelitis, An amputation of the back of the foot, *J Bone Joint Surg—* 1992; Am vol. 74(4):571–6.

36. Skover, G. R., Cellular and biochemical dynamics of wound repair. Wound environment in collagen regeneration, *Clin Podiatr Med Surg* 1991; 8(4):723–756.

37. Ehrlichman, R. J.; Seckel, B. R.; Bryan, D. J.; et al., Common complications of wound healing. Pre-

vention and management, *Surgical Clin N Am* 1991; 71(6):1323–1351.

38. Servold, S. A., Growth factor impact on wound healing, *Clin Podiatr Med Surg* 1991; 8(4):937–953.

39. Herndon, D. N.; Hayward, P. G.; Rutan, R. L.; et al., Growth hormones and factors in surgical patients, *Adv Surg* 1992; 25:65–97.

40. Kingsworth, A. N., and Slavin, J., Peptide growth factors and wound healing, *Brit J Surg* 1991; 78:1286–1290.

41. Heldin, C. H.; Usuki, K.; and Miyazono, K., Platelet-derived endothelial cell growth factor, *J Cell Biochem* 1991; 47(3):208–210.

42. Hom, D. B., and Maisel, R. H., Angiogenic growth factors: Their effects and potential in soft tissue wound healing, *Ann Otol Rhinol Laryngol* 1992; 101(4):349–354.

43. Blitstein-Willinger, E., The role of growth factors in wound healing, *Skin Parmacol* 1992; 4(3):175–182.

44. Compton, C. C., Wound healing potential of cultured epithelium, *Wounds* 1993; 5(2):97–111.

45. Milanov, N. O., and Adamyan, R. T., Functional results of microsurgical reconstruction of plantar defects, *Ann Plast Surg* 1994; 32(1):52–6.

46. Ferreira, M. C.; Besteiro, J. M.; Monteiro, Jr., A. A.; et al., Reconstruction of the foot with microvascular free flaps, *Microsurgery* 1994; 15(1):33–6.

47. Sakai, S., A distally based island first dorsal metatarsal artery flap for the coverage of a distal plantar defect, *Brit J Plast Surg* 1993; 46(6):480–2.

48. Goldberg, J. A.; Adkins, P.; and Tasi, T. M., Microvascular reconstruction of the foot: Weightbearing patterns, gait analysis, and long-term follow-up, *Plast Reconstr Surg* 1993; 92(5):904–11.

49. Lai, C. S.; Lin, S. D.; Chou, C. K.; et al., *Aspergillosis* complicating the grafted skin and free muscle flap in a diabetic, *Plast Reconstr Surg* 1993; 92(3):532–6.

50. Graziano, T. A.; Baratta, J. B.; Menditto, L.; et al., A surgical alternative in the management of chronic neurotrophic ulcerations of the foot, *J Foot Ankle Surg* 1993; 32(3):295–8.

51. Majoroh, T. O., Chronic plantar ulcer of a leprosy patient treated by fasciocutaneous instep flap transfer. Preliminary result, *Trop Geograph Med* 1993; 45(1):39–40.

52. Koshima, I.; Moriguchi, T.; Soeda, S.; et al., Free

thin parumbilical perforator-based flaps, *Ann Plast Surg* 1992; 29(1):12–7.

53. Kurata, S.; Hashimoto, H.; Terashi, H.; et al., Reconstruction of the distal foot dorsum with a distally based extensor digitorum brevis muscle flap, *Ann Plast Surg* 1992; 29(1):76–9.

54. Stern, H. S., and Nahai, F., The versatile superficial inferior epigastric artery free flap, *Brit J Plast Surg* 1992; 45(4):270–4.

55. Eren, S.; Matejic, B.; and Hettich, R., Indication, technique, and results of plantaris medialis neurovascular island flaps, *Ann Plast Surg* 1992; 28 (2):152–9.

56. Gavern, P. E., Heel ulcer in leprosy treated with fasciocutaneous island flap from the instep of the sole, *Scand J Plast Reconstr Surg Hand Surg* 1991; 25(2):155–60.

57. Menezes, J., Rajendran, A., Jacob, A. J., et al., The use of topical phenytoin as an adjunct to immobilization in the treatment of trophic leprosy ulcers, *Southeast Asia J Trop Med Publ Health* 1993; 24 (2):340–2.

58. Jorneskog, G.; Brismar, K.; and Fagren, B., Low molecular weight heparin seems to improve local capillary circulation and healing of chronic foot ulcers in diabetic patients, *Vasa J Vasc Dis* 1993; 22(2):137–42.

59. Di Mauro, C.; Ossino, A. M.; Trefiletti, M.; et al., Lyophilized collagen in the treatment of diabetic ulcers, *Drugs Exp Clin Res* 1991; 17(7):371–3.

60. Seidel, C.; Richter, U. G.; Buhler, S.; et al., Drug therapy of diabetic neuropathic foot ulcers: Transvenous retrograde perfusion versus systemic regimen, *Vasa J Vasc Dis* 1991; 20(4):388–93.

61. Muthukumarasamy, M. G.; Sivakumar, G.; and Manoharan, G., Topical phenytoin in diabetic foot ulcers, *Diabet Care* 1991; 14(10):909–11.

62. Apelqvist, J.; Larsson, J.; and Agardh, C. D., Long-term prognosis for diabetic patients with foot ulcers, *J Intern Med* 1993; 233(6):485–91.

63. Litzelman, D. K.; Slemenda, C. W.; Langefeld, C. D.; et al., Reduction of lower extremity clinical abnormalities in patients with non-insulin-dependent diabetes mellitus. A randomized, controlled trial, *Ann Intern Med* 1993; 119(1):36–41.

64. Apelqvist, J.; Larsson, J.; and Agardh, C. D., Medical risk factors in diabetic patients with foot ulcers and severe peripheral vascular disease and their influence on outcome, *J Diabet Compl* 1992; 6 (3):167–74.

65. Veves, A.; Murray, H. J.; Young, M. J.; et al., The risk of foot ulceration in diabetic patients with high foot pressure: A prospective study, *Diabetologia* 1992; 35(7):660–3.

66. Cavanagh, P. R.; Sims, Jr., D. S.; and Sanders, L. J., Body mass is a poor predictor of peak plantar pressure in diabetic men, *Diabet Care* 1991; 14 (8):750–5.

67. Lipsky, B. A.; Pecoraro, R. E.; and Ahroni, J. H., Foot ulceration and infections in elderly diabetics, *Clin Geriatr Med* 1990; 6(4):747–769.

68. Joseph, W. S., Treatment of lower extremity infections in diabetics, *J Am Podiatr Med Assoc* 1992; 82(7):361–369.

69. Mulder, G. D.; Mason, R.; and Tepelidis, N., Ulceration and osteomyelitis, *Clin Podiatr Med Surg* 1990; 7(4):733–742.

70. Jeter, K. F., and Tintle, T. E., Wound dressings of the nineties: Indications and contraindications, *Clin Podiatr Med Surg* 1991; 8(4):799–816.

71. Carver, N., and Leigh, I. M., Synthetic dressings, *Inter J Dermatol* 1992; 31(1):10–18.

72. ———, Local applications to wounds—II. Dressings for wounds and ulcers, *Drug Therap Bull* 1991; 29(25):97–100.

16

MODIFIED PLANTAR MEDIAL APPROACH FASCIOTOMY TO TREAT DIABETIC FOOT WITH COMPARTMENT SYNDROME

Bok Y. Lee, M.D., V. J. Guerra, M.D., and Irfan M. Jameel, M.D.

INTRODUCTION

It was not until recently that the idea of acute compartment syndromes of the leg became recognized as a unified concept [1, 2]. Compartment syndrome is now a well-described clinical entity that results from increased pressures within a myofascial compartment. Mubarak and Hargens [2] were the pioneers of this concept in the foot. They first suggested the presence of compartment syndrome in the foot by focusing on the interosseous compartment and presenting a possible treatment by decompression performed by longitudinal incisions of the dorsum of the foot. Whitesides [3] anecdotally described isolated compartment syndrome of the foot secondary to burns and direct trauma and recommended decompression of the compartments by the plantar medial approach as described by Henry [9].

The signs and symptoms of compartment syndrome of the foot appear to be similar to those of compartment syndromes in general. A degree of pain that is out of proportion to the injury appears to be the first symptom. An early clinical sign reported by Bonutti and Bell [13] was paresthesia in the distribution of the digital nerves of the toes, especially to pinprick, two-point discrimination, and light touch. Pain and passive dorsiflexion of the toes are also important signs, although direct trauma may cause similar symptoms. Pallor, paresthesia, and a palpable tense compartment have also been reported.

In the presence of infection, bacteria spread from one compartment to another via the proximal calcaneal convergence or by direct perforation through the intercompartment septa. However, because each compartment is bound by rigid fascial separations in the medial-to-lateral and dorsal-to-plantar directions, lateral or dorsal spread of infection is a late sign of infection. Based on the anatomy of the foot, deep space foot infections frequently show deceptively little plantar or dorsal foot abnormality. Therefore, a patient presenting with mild swelling of the foot, but toxic systemic symptoms, must be evaluated for an occult deep space infection. As in the hand, the deep potential spaces or compartments of the foot can allow spread of bacteria from the plantar surface or web spaces of the foot to the ankle and the lower leg regions [14].

Compartment syndrome of the foot is a sequela of an overwhelming infection of the foot, such as a diabetic foot infection. This condition is caused by increased compartment pressure, producing a reduction in tissue arterial blood flow and venous return that produces a diminished local arteriovenous gradient. The sequential elevation in tissue pressure causes increased tissue anoxia and reduction in nerve and muscle function. Although the incidence of this entity is high, compartment syndrome of the foot is often overlooked or unrecognized and, if not promptly treated by reducing intracompartment pressures by fasciotomy, prognosis is poor and can lead to amputation.

Early surgical decompression of the foot by fasciotomy is the only effective means of preventing the late consequences of a compartment syndrome, such as myoneural ischemia [1, 4]. If not properly treated by effective fascial decompression technique of the foot, the end result of the ischemic process is a clawfoot deformity with permanent loss of function, contracture, weakness, sensory disturbance, and gangrene formation [5–8].

Even though surgical decompression is the only reliable method for preventing these long-term ischemic complications, the techniques of fasciotomy of the foot have not been well described. Mubarak suggested two longitudinal dorsal incisions over the metatarsals [2]. The plantar medial approach for surgical decompression of the foot was originally described by Henry, who used it for decompression of the medial and central compartments of the foot [9]. Decompression of the lateral and interosseus compartments can be achieved by a similar separate lateral approach [10]. Grodinsky [11] and Loeffler and Ballard [12] described a long medial plantar utilitarian incision for decompression of established infections of the foot. The latter approach was used more recently by Bonutti and Bell [13] for management of an isolated compartment syndrome of the foot.

We present a stepwise description of fasciotomy of the foot using a single incision plantar medial approach. Such an approach provides for the simultaneous decompression of all four fascial compartments of the foot (Figure 16-1). This approach involves surgical dissection mostly in non-weight-bearing regions of the foot.

ANATOMY OF THE PLANTAR STRUCTURES

There are four fascial compartments of the foot: the medial, central, lateral, and interosseous compartments. The floor of three of these compartments (medial, central, and lateral) consists of the rigid plantar fascia. The roof of these compartments is formed by the metatarsal bones and the interosseous fascia, which is the fourth fascial compartment.

The muscles are the key to surgical exposure. There are four muscle layers in the foot starting from the skin to the bone. Layers 1 and 3 are both triads; each consists of three muscles—a central belly flanked by two companions. Layer 1 consists of the abductor hallucis, flexor digitorum brevis, and abductor digiti minimi. Similarly, layer 3 consists of the flexor hallucis, adductor hallucis, and flexor digiti minimi. Layers 2 and 4 consist of two long tendons plus short muscles. Layer 2 consists of the flexor hallucis longus, flexor digitorum longus, lumbricals, and quadratus plantae. Layer 4 consists of the peroneus longus, tibialis posterior, and interossei.

When standing on a level surface, the foot with its skeleton forms a vaulted cage that opens widely at the inner side. The door that keeps it closed is the abductor hallucis. If the upper fastenings of the abductor and that hinge the belly of the abductor hallucis solewards are freed, then the contents of the cage (although for the moment, these may be screened by fascia) can be reached. Even when opened, the muscles are so packed and linked that until parted cleanly, the view is worthless [8].

There are bands that hold the plantar layers close against the tarsal vault and (behind the layers) to each other. The master knot controlling this assembly is found approximately 2 cm lateral to the navicular tubercle. At this point, the flexor tendons are tied against the summit of the vault.

THE OPERATION

Position. The foot is positioned on its outer edge and the knee is partly flexed. The surgical technique of plantar medial decompression of fascial compartments of the foot involves a series of well-defined steps of dissection, as outlined in Table 16-1.

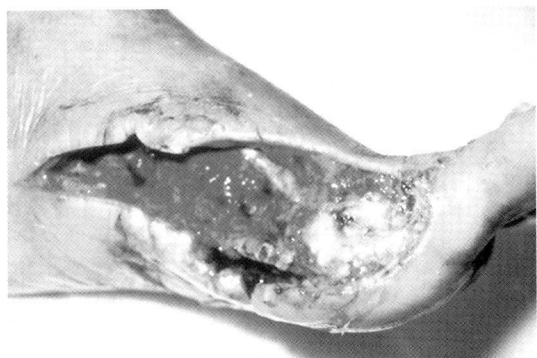

Figure 16-1. Plantar medical incision dividing the skin and subcutaneous tissue between tuber calcanei and first metatarsal.

Step 1 Incision of skin and subcutaneous tissue. A plantar medial incision is made that divides the skin and superficial fascia at the inner side of the foot, from the ball of the great toe to the heel. This follows the length of the plantar surface of the first metatarsal and curves up to cross the tuberosity of navicular bone (Figure 16-2 Color Plate 1). The limits of the incision are the tuber calcanei and the head of the first metatarsal. Care should be taken to avoid pressure points. Subcutaneous tissue is incised along the skin incision to visualize the medial extension of the plantar aponeurosis. Veins are identified and hemostasis is obtained using ligatures. Electrocautery use should be limited.

Step 2 Decompression of medial compartment. The medial extension of the plantar aponeurosis is incised longitudinally to decompress the medial compartment (Figure 16-3 Color Plate 1).

Step 3 Dissection through the medial compartment. After opening the plantar aponeurosis, the abductor hallucis tendon is identified at the inner side of the first metatarsal (Figure 16-4 Color Plate 2). This tendon is mobilized, taking care to leave intact the adjoining fleshy fibers of flexor hallucis brevis. The tendon is used as a guide for separation of the less distinctive margins of the abductor belly. This belly is detached, first from its fascial band with the navicular tuberosity, and then from the indefinite anterior part of the vague annular ligament. The detachment is continued down to the inner tuberosity of calcaneous. The muscle is then hinged solewards through a full right angle, taking

Table 16-1 Plantar Medial Fasciotomy of the Foot Using a Single Incision

Step 1	Plantar medial incision dividing the skin and subcutaneous tissue between tuber calcanei and first metatarsal
Step 2	Decompression of the medial compartment
Step 3	Dissection through the medial compartment muscles (guide to the cage door)
Step 4	Identification of the plantar master knot
Step 5	Cutting off the plantar master knot and releasing the muscles held by it
Step 6	Decompression of the central compartment
Step 7	Decompression of the interosseous compartment by several incisions in the plantar interosseous fascia
Step 8	Decompression of the lateral compartment
Step 9	Wound care after fasciotomy

care to spare the pair of small branches coming from the medial plantar nerve. Both branches lie close to the hinge, 2 and 3 cm, respectively, behind the tuberosity of the navicular.

Step 4 Identification of the master knot. The abductor hallucis muscle is retracted inferiorly (Figure 16-5 Color Plate 2). When this is done, a partial screen of fascia is observed. Located within this defective fascia are the plantar nerves and vessels. These form two bundles, the medial and lateral. These bundles first diverge approximately 3 cm behind the tuberosity of navicular.

Step 5 Releasing the structures bound by the master knot. Next the master knot is cut loose

(Figure 16-6 Color Plate 2). The master knot is an aponeurotic band attached a 1=cm lateral to the tuberosity of the navicular, which attaches the two long second-layer tendons to the vault (flexor hallucis longus and flexor digitorum longus). This step allows for the exposure of the medial intermuscular septum.

Step 6   Decompression of the central compartment. The medial intermuscular septum is exposed and opened longitudinally, decompressing the central compartment (Figure 16-7 Color Plate 2). Digital and blunt dissection are carried out, staying close to the roof formed by the metatarsals.

Step 7   Decompression of the interosseous compartment. The interosseous compartment is decompressed by longitudinally incising the plantar interosseous fascia superior to the quadratus plantae muscle (Figure 16-8 Color Plate 2). The dissection between the quadratus plantae muscle and the lumbrical muscles is deepened, and a second incision in the interosseous fascia allows further decompression of the interosseous compartment. Technical considerations are the preservation of the neurovascular bundle in the postero-medial aspect and the bifurcation of the posterior tibial artery into the medial and lateral plantar arteries, which give rise distally to the superficial arch. This travels medially and connects through the first interosseous space with the dorsalis pedis artery.

Step 8   Decompression of the lateral compartment. Dissection between the lumbrical muscles and the flexor digitorum brevis muscle allows incision of the lateral intermuscular septum and decompression of the lateral compartment (Figure 16-9 Color Plate 2).

Step 9   Wound care after fasciotomy. After decompression of the four compartments, debridement should be minimal and hemostasis established because the decompressed vessels can rebleed. The skin and all the fascial layers are left open. Steps should be taken to ensure that the wound is absolutely dry. The foot should be kept elevated. The wound is bandaged with fixed, firm, and sterile dressings. It has been observed in patients treated with fasciotomy, that when the drainage incision is longitudinal and opens the fascia of the infected compartment, wound healing is considerably accelerated.

REFERENCES

1. Matsen, F. A., III, Compartmental syndrome. A unified concept, *Clin Orthop* 1975; 113:8–14.

2. Mubarak S. J., and Hargens, A. R., *Compartment Syndromes and Volkmann's Contracture,* Philadephia: W. B. Saunders, 1981.

3. Whitesides, T. E., *Disorders of the Foot,* Philadelphia: W. B. Saunders, 1982.

4. Whitesides, T. E. Jr.; Harada, H.; and Morimoto, K., Compartment syndromes and the role of fasciotomy: Its parameters and techniques, *AAOS Instructional Course Lectures,* vol. 25. St. Louis: C. V. Mosby, 1977:179–196.

5. Chuinard, E. G., and Baskin, M., Claw-foot deformity, *J Bone Joint Surg* 1973; 55A:151–162.

6. Cole, W. H., The treatment of claw foot, *J Bone Joint Surg* 1940; 22A:895–908.

7. Jones, R., An address on Volkmann's ischemic contracture with special reference to treatment, *Brit Med J* 1928; 2:639–642.

8. Tsuge, K., Treatment of established Volkman's contracture, *J Bone Joint Surg* 1975; 57A:925–929.

9. Henry, A. K., *Extensive Exposure,* 2nd ed., New York and Edinburgh: Churchill-Livingstone, 1982.

10. Myerson, M. S., Acute compartment syndrome of the foot, *Bull Hosp Dis Orthop Inst* 1987; 47:251–261.

11. Grodinsky, M., A study of fascial spaces of the foot, *Surg Gynecol Obstet* 1929; 49:739–751.

11. Grodinsky, M., A study of fascial spaces of the foot, *Surg Gynecol Obstet* 1929; 49:739–751.

12. Loeffler, R. D., and Ballard, A., Plantar fascial spaces of the foot and a proposed surgical approach, *Foot Ankle* 1980; 1:11–14.

13. Bonutti, P. M., and Bell, G. R., Compartment syndrome of the foot. A case report, *J Bone Joint Surg* 1986; 68A:1449–1451.

14. Bridges, R. M., and Deitch, E. A., Diabetic foot infections. Pathophysiology and treatment, *Surgical Clin N Am* 1994; 74:537–555.

15. Bryce T. H. Quain's Elements of Anatomy. 11th ed. p. 248 1923.

17

TECHNIQUE IN THE SURGERY OF PRESSURE SORES

Alex J. Keller, M.D., and Randall S. Feingold, M.D.

Skin, subcutaneous tissue, fascia, and muscle overlying a bony prominence all sustain injury to a varying degree when subject to the forces of pressure, friction, or shear [1]. Tissue loss is often the result in a patient with altered sensibility or motor function. Although pressure remains the single most important factor leading to this tissue loss, nutritional deficiency and generalized sepsis play contributory roles [2]. Even though the surgeon can provide soft tissue coverage to replace this loss, recurrence is likely unless there is a change in the underlying conditions that are causative to the development of the ulcer.

ANATOMIC DISTRIBUTION

Almost all pressure sores develop in the lower part of the body [3–5]. Dansereau and Conway, in 1964, reported on 2000 pressure sores in paraplegics [6]. The anatomic distribution in this series was: ischial tuberosity (28%), greater trochanter (19%), sacrum (17%), heel (9%), and other sites to smaller degrees.

The site of development is directly related to patient positioning, and thus positioning, mobilization, and periods of pressure relief are critical in the postoperative period and for long-term success of surgical wound closure. The patient lying supine

and on the side is predisposed to pressure ulceration of the sacrum, trochanter, calcaneus, interscapular region, and occiput. Prone positioning, although less common, results in pressure sores of the iliac crest, knees, tibias, and elbows. Patients sitting in bed or for prolonged periods in a wheelchair transfer their weight to the buttocks and ischial tuberosities, resulting in ischial pressure sores.

PATHOLOGY

The visible skin wound of the pressure sore is merely the tip of the iceberg: 70% of the ulcer is below the skin [7]. Pressure is transmitted from the skin through each layer of tissue to the bony prominence so that an inverted cone of tissue destruction is created.

Although the tendency is to think of pressure sores only in terms of their chronicity, they have an acute phase [8]. The first stage is that of transient circulatory disturbance characterized by erythema and edema, but without tissue destruction [9]. This stage is reversible if the pressure is relieved. If pressure continues, the second stage, permanent damage to cutaneous tissue, ensues. Erythema and congestion of the skin continue, leading to induration and gradual excoriation. This may resemble an abrasion or may be deeper, with destruction of full-thickness skin, leaving a dry, black necrotic eschar. A sloughing ulcer follows. The third stage consists of deep penetrating necrosis. Necrotic fat and muscle lead to wet gangrene and periostitis, and osteomyelitis follows. The suppurative process may track along fascial planes, establish sinus tracts, or penetrate joint cavities. In the most advanced cases, dislocations and pathologic fractures are present.

The long-standing chronic ulcer has now passed through cycles of healing and breakdown and may show marginal scar epithelium of a shiny nature with surrounding zones of dense scar tissue. Because of the progressive vascular constriction at the base and margin of the ulcer secondary to dense scarring, the granulation tissue may show little sign of activity.

Bacterial invasion and tissue breakdown form a foul-smelling purulent discharge. Common infecting organisms are *Proteus, Escherichia coli,* or *Pseudomonas* [10, 11]. In a series by Hentz [12], 80% of the patients with positive blood cultures showed anaerobic organisms, with *Bacteroides fragilis* predominating.

PRINCIPLES OF SURGICAL THERAPY

The strategy in the surgical treatment of pressure sores consists of excision of the wound and provision of soft tissue coverage. Successful outcome is dependent upon following sound principles of pre-, intra-, and postoperative care. This includes systemic preparation of the patient, local preparation of the pressure sore, and adherence to specific operative conduct.

A variety of systemic considerations should be addressed prior to surgery. Relief of pressure is mandatory through the use of specialized mattresses or the air-fluidized bed [13]. This is used in combination with preoperative positioning. Counseling prepares the patient for the same postoperative requirement. Spasms should be treated with appropriate pharmacologic agents. Flexion contractions may require release. Nutritional status must be checked and supplementation given to restore positive nitrogen balance and obtain satisfactory serum protein levels [14]. Anemia must be corrected with

diet, medication, or transfusion to increase the red cell mass [15]. Radiographs including sinograms help identify heterotopic calcification, and underlying osteomyelitis, extensive tracking of suppuration, and communication of the ulcer into the femoral neck or hip joint space.

Preparation of the pressure sore consists of surgical debridement, dressing changes, and control of infection. Serial surgical debridement can be done at the bedside, but extensive debridement should be done in the operating room. The need for blood replacement is often underestimated. Wet-to-dry dressing changes are well suited for the removal of necrotic material and for maintaining a surgically clean wound. These may employ saline, acetic acid, or Dakin's solution [16]. Antibiotics have limited utility in the treatment of pressure sores. Topical application is usually ineffective, and although systemic administration may be appropriate for generalized sepsis, the scarred environment around the wound limits access of the drug to the ulcer site.

Once the patient and the wound have been prepared, surgical treatment can proceed. The conduct of the operation is a modification of the principles described by Conway and Griffith in 1956 [4]. These are:

1. Excision of the ulcer, surrounding scar, and underlying bursa to achieve a surgically clean margin with vigorous blood supply. This creates a new wound for closure, and this "true" defect is appreciated to be substantially larger than the preoperative "apparent" defect.

2. Resection of underlying bony prominence as needed to spread out the pressure.

3. Removal of heterotopic soft tissue calcification.

4. Hemostasis and insertion of suction drains.

5. Flap closure to fill dead space and provide well-vascularized padding and coverage.

6. Flap design that avoids placing suture lines over bony prominences and preserves options for utilizing other flaps, should they be needed in the future.

RECONSTRUCTIVE OPTIONS FOR WOUND CLOSURE

The method of soft tissue coverage is one of the most important decisions of the surgeon. Some of the following options were historically common and suffer from high failure rates and frequent ulcer recurrence.

1. Split-thickness skin grafts on a granulating bed.
2. Simple excision and approximation under tension.
3. Stellate closure with sliding flaps.
4. Bipedicle flaps.

A greater variety of methods for soft tissue coverage have become available, not only producing better results, but also giving the surgeon a greater choice in planning the reconstruction:

1. Primary closure without tension for small defects.
2. Large local skin and fasciocutaneous rotation flaps.
3. Muscle transposition covered by split-thickness skin graft or a skin flap.
4. Myocutaneous advancement, rotation and island flaps.
5. Neurovascular flaps.

Muscle or myocutaneous flap reconstruction is the most frequent and possibly the most durable method of coverage of a large defect. The earliest application of muscle flaps in pressure sores was reported by Blocksma in 1949 [17] followed by a second report by Conway and Griffith in 1956 [4]. This concept was subsequently reintroduced and popularized by Ger in the 1970s [18, 19]. He stated the following advantages of muscle transposition, compared to a purely cutaneous flap: increased blood supply, leading to accelerated wound healing; bulk that will fill the cavity of the pressure sore; and bulk that provides a compressible cushion over the underlying bony framework. Note that in choosing a muscle flap in the nonparalyzed patient, there must be ample synergistic muscles to compensate for the loss of function.

More recently, a highly detailed understanding of the specific patterns of muscle and myocutaneous vascular supply has been mapped into a classification system by Mathes and Nahai [20, 21]. These collective reviews, as well as that of McCraw and Arnold [22], depict the now commonplace applications of these flaps in reconstruction of all areas of the body.

TREATMENT OF THE MOST COMMON PRESSURE SORES

Treatment of sacral, trochanteric, and ischial pressure sores is presented to highlight the most useful options for flap reconstruction at each site, including step-by-step operative procedure. More exhaustive lists of reconstructive options are available that include historical and esoteric flaps [21–23].

SACRAL ULCERS

After excision of the ulcer and its bursa, partial ostectomy should include the prominent portions of the sacral spines, the posterior iliac spines, the sacral ligaments, and occasionally the coccyx.

The gluteus maximus muscle or myocutaneous flap is the flap of choice for sacral defects [24]. This muscle supplies the local skin of the buttock via musculocutaneous perforators from the superior and inferior gluteal arteries. Unilateral or bilateral rotation or V-Y advancement flaps may be employed. The muscle can be mobilized by dividing its origin from the sacrum and posterior iliac crest, and its insertion into the iliotibial tract. When used as a unilateral myocutaneous flap, large flaps (in case rerotation becomes necessary) that are inferiorly based and do not encroach upon the ischial or trochanteric areas should be planned. This is illustrated in Figure 17-1 (See Color Plates 3 and 4). The superior, nondominant pedicle can be divided to increase flap mobility. For larger defects, bilateral rotation flaps may be necessary, as illustrated in Figure 17-2 (See Color Plate 4). Bilateral V Y advancement flaps are illustrated in Figure 17-3 (see Color Plate 4).

TROCHANTERIC ULCERS

The ulcer, along with part of the underlying greater trochanter of the femur, should be excised as a unit. The typically large bursa should be excised while preserving normal overlying skin.

Muscle or myocutaneous flaps based on the rectus femoris and vastus lateralis can be used, but the flap of choice is the tensor fascia lata myocutaneous flap described by Nahai et al. [25]. The flap is superiorly based on the lateral femoral circumflex artery, a branch of the profunda artery. Sensibility is possible via the lateral cutaneous nerve of the

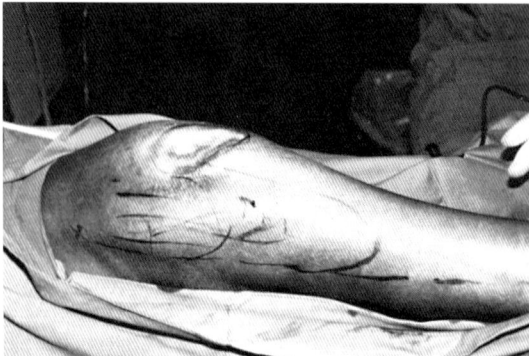

Figure 17-4 (a). A trochanteric pressure sore and the outlines of the tensor fascia lata myocutaneous viewed from the top. (The patient is in the lateral decubitus position.)

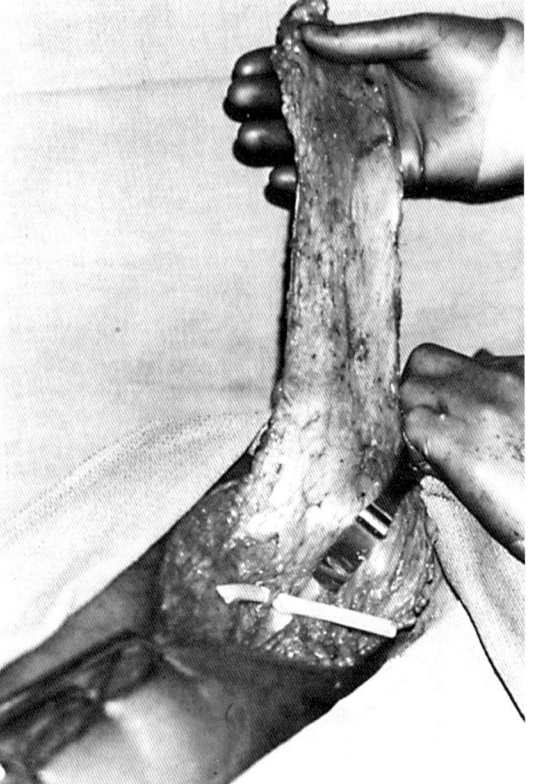

thigh. The flap is durable, and for extra padding, the tip of the flap may be deepithelialized and folded upon itself. The secondary defect in the anterior thigh may be either closed primarily or skin grafted. This flap is illustrated in Figure 17-4. It can also be used as an island flap, a V-Y flap, and a bipedicle flap. Other types of closure are available; however, they are less useful in view of the preceding options. These include an anteriorly based spiral thigh flap elevated below the level of the fascia lata, the groin flap based on the superficial circumflex iliac artery, a bipedicle sliding flap, and the gluteal thigh flap.

Figure 17-4 (b). The tensor fascia lata myocutaneous flap elevated with the lateral circumflex femoral pedicle demonstrated.

ISCHIAL ULCERS

Ulcer excision should be accompanied by some degree of ischiectomy. Early advocates of total ischiectomy argued that partial excision does not remove enough of the bony prominence [6, 26]. However, total ischiectomy is plagued by complications of perineal ulceration, urethral diverticula, and contralateral ischial ulceration [10, 27]. This leads to the suggestion of prophylactic total bilateral ischiectomy [26]. Bors and Comarr [28] reported a 58% incidence of perineal diverticula in bilateral ischiectomy patients. Therefore, it seems prudent to remove the bony prominence by partial rather than total ischiectomy.

The gluteal thigh flap [29] and the inferior glu-

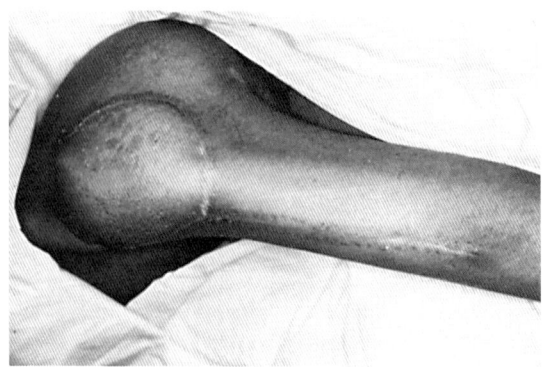

Figure 17-4 (c). Healed result of the transposed flap. Note the primary closure of the donor area.

teus maximus myocutaneous flap [24] are the best choices for reconstructing the ischial pressure sore. The gluteal thigh flap is the flap of choice because it does not preclude using the gluteus for sacral or secondary ischial procedures. This fasciocutaneous flap is based on the descending branch of the inferior gluteal artery, located midway between the ischium and the greater trochanter. Traveling with it is the posterior femoral cutaneous nerve, which allows sensibility to the flap. This flap is illustrated in Figure 17-5 (See Color Plates 4 and 5). Secondary flaps include hamstring [30] and biceps femoris [31] myocutaneous V-Y advancement flaps. These flaps transect the inferior gluteal artery extensions to the posterior thigh skin, precluding future use of the gluteal thigh flap. The extended tensor fascia lata myocutaneous flap will also reach the ischium.

NEUROVASCULAR FLAPS

The possibility of covering a defect with a sensate flap to help decrease the recurrence rate has also been explored. Depending upon the spinal level of disability, an intercostal neurovascular island flap can be designed to provide sensation in the sacral area [32]. The extended tensor fascia lata flap has been used in meningomyelocele patients to provide sensation to the sitting area [33].

AMPUTATIONS

Multiple ulcerations may be treated with multiple flaps. Total thigh flaps have been recommended by Georgiade et al. [26] and Royer et al. [34] for closure of combined ulcerations, especially when the ulcerations are large, multiple, and confluent. When all available local tissue has been exhausted, lower extremity amputation is a method to salvage enough soft tissue to close the defect [35–37]. In general, the patient who is offered amputation is poorly motivated toward rehabilitation and is suffering from end-stage disease. The typical patient is bedridden with fused or ankylosed hips, knees, and ankles. Complicating factors might be osteoarthritis, flexion contractures, and pyarthrosis of the hip. The procedure is formidable in magnitude, requires many units of blood and prolonged operating time, and may not facilitate rehabilitation.

POSTOPERATIVE CARE

The postoperative care consists of maintaining the flap in a pressure-free environment for two to three weeks. This may require prone positioning, although good nursing care allows one to modify this rule. Ideally, the patient is placed on an air-fluidized bed, which allows positioning directly on the flap [38]. Naturally, the nutritional status and hematocrit must be maintained. After three weeks there is a gradual increase in activity with a careful monitoring of all pressure points for signs of early breakdown. The flap should be watched for signs of impaired circulation as activity is increased [39]. A critical part of the postoperative (and preoperative) care is the social rehabilitation of the patient. The patient should not remain in the same setting in which the pressure sore developed.

Complications related to surgery may require treatment as well. Flap necrosis is unusual and related to flap design. Hematomas, seromas, spasms, and wound infections may result in new bursa formation or wound dehiscence.

EARLY AND LATE RESULTS OF SURGICAL THERAPY

The ability of surgical treatment to achieve a healed wound is well documented. The largest, most comprehensive series is that of Conway [6] from the Bronx Veterans Administration Hospital from 1950 to 1962. 2000 cases were analyzed, and all patients were followed for at least one year. The best results obtained were as follows: sacral sores had a recurrence rate of 11% on a total of 60 operations; trochanteric ulcers had a recurrence rate of 7% on 73 such cases; and ischial sores had a recurrence rate of 2% on 44 ulcers. Immediate surgical failures were related to poor flap design or the complications listed above.

However, the long-term recurrence rate is very high despite good surgical treatment. Harding [40] in 1961 reported a recurrence rate of 44% within four years of surgery. Griffith [16] in 1961 reported a recurrence rate of 67%. The most common sites of recurrence are the sacrum, trochanter, and ischium. In paraplegics, the ischial sore is the most common because once rehabilitated they have a tendency to sit for prolonged periods of time. Often the recurrences result from poor planning: i.e., a sharp prominence, a secondarily healed thin scar, a skin graft over bone, residual sinus tracts or osteomyelitis, or failure to alleviate spasticity. Other contributing factors include prolonged immobilization, poor hygiene, anemia, and malnutrition.

The application of muscle and myocutaneous flaps in treating pressure sores has not dramatically impacted long-term recurrences. Surgical treatment of pressures sores is merely a partial solution to an acute problem: i.e., the open wound. Although surgical advances allow closure of larger and more difficult defects, the most formidable component of this problem remains the social rehabilitation and custodial management of patients at risk. Real progress in the treatment of pressure sores will only come with better means of prevention.

REFERENCES

1. Dinsdale, S. M., Decubitus ulcers: Role of pressure and friction in causation, *Arch Phys Med Rehabil* 1974; 55:147.

2. Hubay, C. A.; Kiehn, C. L.; and Drucker, W. R., Surgical management of decubitus ulcers in the post-traumatic patient, *Am J Surg* 1957; 93:705.

3. Yeoman, M. P., and Hardy, A. G., The pathology and treatment of pressure sores in paraplegics, *Brit J Plast Surg* 1954; 7:179.

4. Conway, H., and Griffith, B. H., Plastic surgery for closure of decubitus ulcers in patients with paraplegia; based on experience with 1000 cases, *Am J Surg* 1956; 91:946.

5. Petersen, N. C., and Bittman, S., The epidemiology of pressure sores, *Scand J Plast Surg* 1971; 5:62.

6. Dansereau, J. G., and Conway, H., Closure of decubiti in paraplegics. Report on 2000 cases, *Plast Reconstr Surg* 1964; 33:474.

7. Agris, J., and Spira, M., Pressure ulcers: Prevention and treatment, *Clin Symp* 1979; 31:5.

8. Kosiak, M., Etiology and pathology of ischemic ulcers. *Arch Phys Med Rehabil* 1961; 42:19.

9. Berecek, K., Etiology of decubitus ulcers, *Nurs Clin North Am* 1975; 10:157.

10. Vasconez, L. O.; Schneider, W. J.; and Jurkiewicz, M. J., Pressure sores, *Curr Probl Surg* 1977; 14:4.

11. Galpin, J. E.; Chow, A. W.; Bayer, A. S.; et al., Sepsis associated with decubitus ulcers, *Am J Med* 1976; 61:346.

12. Hentz, V., Management of pressure sores in a specialty center, *Plast Reconstr Surg* 1979; 64:683.

13. Artz, C. P., and Hargest, T. S., Air-fluidized bed, in C. P. Artz, and T. S. Hargest, eds., *Clinical and Research Symposium,* Medical University of South Carolina, Milton Roy Company, 1971.

14. Campell, R., and Delgado, J., The pressure sore, in *Reconstructive Plastic Surgery,* Philadelphia: Saunders, 1979; 3763–3799.

15. Matheson, A. T., and Lipschitz, R., Nature and treatment of trophic pressure sores, *South Afr Med J* 1956; 30:1129.

16. Griffith, B. H., and Schultz, R. C., The prevention and surgical treatment of recurrent decubitus ulcers in patients with paraplegia, *Plast Reconstr Surg* 1961; 27:248.

17. Blocksma, R.; Kostrubala, J. G.; and Greely, P. W., The surgical repair of decubitus ulcer in paraplegics, *Plast Reconstr Surg* 1949; 4:123.

18. Ger, R., The surgical management of decubitus ulcers by muscle transposition, *Surgery* 1971; 69:106.

19. Ger, R., and Levine, S. A., The management of decubitus ulcers by muscle transposition, *Plast Reconstr Surg* 1976; 58:419.

20. Mathes, S. J., and Nahai, F., *Clinical Atlas of Muscle and Myocutaneous Flaps,* St. Louis, Mo: C. V. Mosby, 1979.

21. Mathes, S. J., and Nahai, F., *Clinical Applications for Muscle and Myocutaneous Flaps,* St. Louis, Mo: C. V. Mosby, 1982.

22. McCraw, J. B., and Arnold, P. G., *McCraw and Arnold's Atlas of Muscle and Musculocutaneous Flaps,* Norfolk, VA: Hampton Press Publishing, 1987.

23. Colen, S. R., Pressure sores, in J. G. McCarthy, ed., *Plastic Surgery.* Philadelphia: W. B. Saunders, 1990.

24. Minami, R. T.; Mills, R.; and Pardoe, R., Gluteus maximus myocutaneous flaps for repair of pressure sores, *Plast Reconstr Surg* 1977; 60:242.

25. Nahai, F.; Silverton, J. S.; Hill, H. L.; and Vasconez, L. O., The tensor fascia lata musculocutaneous flap, *Ann Plast Surg* 1978; 1:372.

26. Georgiade, N.; Pickrell, K.; and Maguire, C., Total

thigh flaps for extensive decubitus ulcers, *Plast Reconstr Surg* 1956; 17:220.

27. Karaca, A.; Binns, J.; and Blumenthal, F., Complications of total ischiectomy for the treatment of ischial pressure sores, *Plast Reconstr Surg* 1974; 62:96.

28. Bors, E., and Comarr, A. E., Ischial decubitus ulcer, *Surgery* 1948; 24:680.

29. Hurwitz, D. J.; Swartz, W. M.; and Mathes, S. J., The gluteal thigh flap: A reliable sensate flap for the closure of buttock and perineal wounds, *Plast Reconstr Surg* 1981; 68:521.

30. Hurteau, J. E.; Bostwick, J.; Hahai, F.; Hester, R.; and Jurkiewicz, M. J., V-Y advancement of hamstring musculocutaneous flap for coverage of ischial pressure sores, *Plast Reconstr Surg* 1981; 68:539.

31. Tobin, G. R.; Pompi Sanders, B.; Man, D.; and Weiner, L. J., The biceps femoris myocutaneous advancement flap: A useful modification for ischial pressure ulcer reconstruction, *Ann Plast Surg* 1981; 6:396.

32. Daniel, R. K.; Terzis, J. K.; and Cunningham, D. M., Sensory skin flaps for coverage of pressure sores in paraplegics, *Plast Reconstr Surg* 1976; 58:317.

33. Dibbel, D. G.; McCraw, J. B.; and Edstrom, L. E., Providing useful and protective sensibility to the sitting area in patients with meningomyelocele, *Plast Reconstr Surg* 1979; 64:796.

34. Royer, J.; Pickrell, K.; Georgiade, N.; Mladick, R.; and Thorne, F., Total thigh flaps for extensive decubitus ulcers. A 16-year review of 41 total thigh flaps, *Plast Reconstr Surg* 1969; 44:109.

35. Pearlman, N.; McShane, R.; Jochimsen, P. R.; and Shirazi, S. S., Hemicorporectomy for intractable decubitus ulcers, *Arch Surg* 1976; 3:1139.

36. Spira, M., and Hardy, S. B., Our experience with high thigh amputations in paraplegics, *Plast Reconstr Surg* 1963; 31:344.

37. Weeks, P. M., and Brower, T. D., Island flap coverage of extensive decubitus ulcers, *Plast Reconstr Surg* 1968; 42:433.

38. Harvin, J., and Hargest, T., The air-fluidized bed: A new concept in the treatment of decubitus ulcers, *Nurs Clin North Am* 1970; 5:181.

39. Rogers, J., and Wilson, L., Preventing recurrent tissue breakdown after "pressure sore" closures, *Plast Reconstr Surg* 1975; 56:419.

40. Harding, R., An analysis of one hundred rehabilitated paraplegics, *Plast Reconstr Surg* 1961; 27:235.

18

SURGICAL MANAGEMENT OF DIFFICULT RECURRENT PRESSURE ULCERS

Zahid B. M. Niazi, M.D., and C. Andrew Salzberg, M.D.

INTRODUCTION

Since 1938, when John Staige Davies first reported the need to provide extra "padding" by the use of skin flaps to replace scar epithelium over bony prominences, soft tissue coverage in one form or the other has been used for closure of pressure ulcers by almost all surgeons. Unfortunately for both the patients and the surgeons, surgical correction has a reported recurrence rate ranging from 0% to 91% in different series [1–12]. The recurrent pressure ulcer is a failure in which not all contributing factors may be recognized. Rehabilitation centers struggle with a certain number of recurrences, and these recurrences become an enormous logistic and economic problem as the paralyzed patient population increases annually. It is these difficult recurrent pressure sores that we are going to address in this chapter.

The surgical options for this group of patients are usually limited because of a shortage of available useful tissue and vary with the site of the pressure ulcer, the previous operations performed, and the vascularity and sensibility of the area. As with primary pressure ulcer closure, it is imperative at the time of surgery for all of these chronic wounds that the bursal sac be removed completely, along with partial resection of any bony prominences, to re-duce the likelihood of recurrence. The medical management of the patient lays the groundwork for the success of any surgical procedure carried out. Similarly, the importance of proper postoperative rehabilitation must be emphasized and becomes even more important in the management of the difficult or recurrent pressure ulcer. All patients are given perioperative, culture-specific intravenous antibiotics before surgery and then for one week postoperatively. All patients have a mechanical bowel prep as a part of their preoperative preparation.

Recurrent pressure ulcers are a difficult surgical problem and the patients who develop them because of a failure, albeit uncontrollable in some instances, of the previous surgical procedure, are physically and psychologically impaired to some extent. These patients may present with extensive or multiple ulcers (Figure 18-1 (a)–(c) see Color Plate 5). The surgical repair in these patients who present with paucity of viable tissue, or chronic, extensive, or recurrent postsurgical ulcers necessitates the consideration of additional reconstructive options. Surgeons therefore have to consider the surgical options of tissue expansion, comprising expanded cutaneous or myocutaneous flaps, sensate flaps, filleted leg/thigh flaps, free fasciocutaneous, free muscle, or myocutaneous flaps, any of which may be used as necessary to close these wounds in patients who may be chronically ill. The following algorithm provides some guidelines.

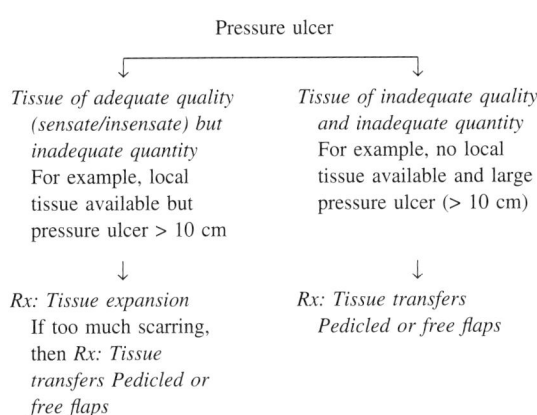

ALGORITHM

Pressure ulcer

Tissue of adequate quality (sensate/insensate) but inadequate quantity
For example, local tissue available but pressure ulcer > 10 cm

Tissue of inadequate quality and inadequate quantity
For example, no local tissue available and large pressure ulcer (> 10 cm)

↓

Rx: Tissue expansion
If too much scarring, then *Rx: Tissue transfers Pedicled or free flaps*

↓

Rx: Tissue transfers Pedicled or free flaps

If tissue transfers are required, then local or distant muscle flaps can be mobilized and transferred as muscle alone or as a myocutaneous transfer [13–18] or one can proceed to free tissue transfer [19–22].

We will now discuss the specifics of the pressure ulcers according to site and the common operative procedures that are usually carried out for their repair, as well as the other surgical options.

PRESSURE ULCERS AND TREATMENT SPECIFIC TO SITE

ISCHIAL ULCERS

These ulcers occur at the posterior inferior aspect of the pelvis and may present with a small area of skin ulceration and with a large undermined cavity as a characteristic feature. The ischium forms the base of the ulcer and will require surgical excision and contour. The patient should have partial ischiectomy if indicated, but never a radical ischiectomy, as this may lead to unnecessary complications [23, 24].

A superiorly based gluteus maximus myocutaneous flap is the primary choice for flap reconstruction of ischial ulcers (Figure 18-2 (a),(b) see Color Plate 6), because of its large size, reliability of its

blood supply, and ability to be rerotated if required for treatment of recurrences. Alternatively, if the skin defect is large, the hamstring may be advanced as a V-Y advancement myocutaneous flap. This provides a large surface that can also be rerotated for future breakdowns. This large muscle-based flap is reliable and will cover larger defects when needed. On rarer occasions, the tensor fascia lata may prove to be useful in covering the ischium and can be utilized to cover both trochanteric and ischial ulcers at the same operative time (see Figure 18-4(b)).

SACRAL ULCERS

These ulcers are centered over the sacral prominence and are usually characterized by a large skin defect with overhanging edges. The ulcers are usually shallow with the sacrum at the base (Figure 18-3(a) see Color Plate 6). An inferiorly based large gluteus maximus myocutaneous flap is the primary choice for these typically broad, yet shallow, ulcers. Random cutaneous flaps have been used in the past; however, they do not provide the reliability, the soft tissue volume, and the increased blood supply inherent in a myocutaneous flap. The gluteus maximus myocutaneous flap may be designed as a V-Y advancement flap (Figure 18-3(b) see Color Plate 6) and for larger defects a bilateral advancement can prove extremely useful. In patients with low-level spinal cord injuries, the potential for reconstruction with a sensate intercostal or tensor fascia lata flap can also be considered.

GREATER TROCHANTERIC ULCERS

These ulcers occur over the most lateral aspect of the femur just distal to the femoral neck. These ulcers may have a modest skin defect overlying a similar deeper defect (Figure 18-4(a) see Color Plate 7). The tensor fascia lata flap is the treatment of choice (Figure 18-4(b) see Color Plate 7). This flap can be used as a transposition or a V-Y rotation advancement flap. The large amount of skin and fascia available for rotation makes this workhorse flap the most utilized and dependable flap. The vastus lateralis muscle flap is a good second choice as it can be turned back into a large femoral cavity or after a girdlestone procedure. It is both reliable and bulky but requires additional skin coverage. The rectus femoris myocutaneous flap can also be used as an island flap (Figure 18-4(c) see Color Plate 7) for treatment of trochanteric ulcers. Keeping future reconstructions in mind, random rotations or transposition flaps (rhomboid flaps) and even bipedicle fasciocutaneous flaps can be designed easily for smaller defects.

Quadriplegics and paraplegics may develop ulcers at other sites: i.e. heel, ankles, knee, iliac crests, elbows, scapula, thoracic spine, and occipital scalp. These patients can be treated on the same principles of pressure ulcer management, and the defects can be covered with local cutaneous, muscle, or fasciocutaneous flaps. However, if no local tissue is available, then a pedicled flap or free tissue transfer reconstruction has to be considered.

MULTIPLE PRESSURE ULCERS

Extensive ulcerations may be associated with complications like osteomyelitis, and perineal and urethral fistulae. Some of these may represent recurrent ulcers or ulcers that have been present for a long time. In the latter situation one needs to be aware of malignant degeneration occurring in these chronic, long-standing ulcers, and a biopsy may be considered to rule out squamous cell carcinoma.

TREATMENT OF THE DIFFICULT OR RECURRENT PRESSURE ULCER

The recurrent pressure ulcer requires new insights into tissue availability and sensibility and remains a challenge for the plastic and reconstructive surgeon. This type of ulcer is a difficult surgical problem because the traditional methods of reconstruction have either already been used or cannot give the appropriate outcome.

The surgical repair of the pressure ulcer in a patient who presents with a paucity of viable tissue, or chronic, extensive, or recurrent postsurgical ulcers, necessitates the consideration of additional reconstructive options. We therefore have to consider tissue expansion, uncommonly used muscle flaps, sensate flaps, free tissue transfers, or flaps

harvested from amputated legs or limbs. The operative procedures are more extensive and time consuming, may require blood transfusions, and are associated with a higher patient morbidity, especially if the patient's condition and the patient selection for that particular procedure have been ill determined previously.

EXPANDED CUTANEOUS OR MYOCUTANEOUS FLAPS

We have utilized the concept of tissue expansion to increase the reconstructive options in order to meet the needs of some of these patients [25–27]. Tissue expansion has been shown to give more tissue of good quality and good vascularity, and even has the ability to bring sensate flaps to the area. This is well documented in the literature, as exemplified by the work of Cherry et al. [26], who demonstrated an increase in blood flow in expanded tissue, caused by an increased vascularity appearing at the interface between the host and capsule tissue. In expanded tissue there is an increase in the number and size of vessels. Studies have shown that expanded flaps have not only an increase in microvascularity [27], but also a demonstrably increased pedicle flow. Furthermore, expanded flaps exhibit an increased survival length of 117% over nonexpanded control flaps [26].

The patients selected for tissue expansion can be both the high spinal cord (quadriplegic) and low spinal cord (paraplegic) injured patients with recurrent pressure sores, patients with a large sore, or those having a limited amount of remaining viable tissue available for reconstructive purposes (Figure 18-5 See Color Plate 7). In some of these patients an expanded sensate flap can be transposed to provide cover.

The tissue expanders need to be defect specific and can be round, rectangular, crescentic, or tubular. Incisions for insertion of the expanders should be made away from the ulcer, usually on the lateral margin of the planned incision of the future flap. Newer techniques now allow for endoscopic placement using remote sites. For removal of the wrinkles, approximately 60–75 cc of sterile saline needs to be injected into the expander at the time of expander insertion. Following one to two weeks of postoperative healing time, they are then injected with amounts varying from 20–50 cc of sterile saline every 4 to 5 days, depending on the degree of skin tension and capillary refill of the overlying skin. The paraplegic patient presents a unique situation to the use of tissue expansion because symptoms of discomfort or pain from overexpansion (ordinarily one of the criteria used as a clinical gauge) cannot be used in these neuropathic individuals. Expansion is continued until enough tissue is created to close the defect. Usually a 550–600-cc expander may require a 6–8-week period for inflation to its maximum, after which the expander is removed, the ulcer is excised, and the expanded tissue incorporated into a standard myocutaneus flap (i.e., gluteus maximus, tensor fascia lata, or any other local myocutaneus flap available) to close the wound. Suction drains are inserted and left in situ for 2 to 3 weeks postoperatively. All patients are given perioperative, culture-specific intravenous antibiotics on call to the operating room and then one week postoperatively. All patients have a preoperative mechanical bowel prep.

The concept of using local myocutaneous tissue of adequate quality but inadequate quantity, expanding it, and creating a larger surface area has been well documented to heal wounds and improve cosmesis in other areas of the body. This principle of tissue expansion was used in recurrent or difficult pressure sores in a prospective series of ten consecutive patients seen over a 24-month period in 1989–1990 at the VA Medical Center in Castle Point, New York [25]. Tissue expansion in this situation resulted in good cover of the defect with a complication rate of 10–15%. In this series, nine patients had the gluteus myocutaneous flap expanded (Figure 18-6(a),(b) see Color Plate 7); in only one patient was the tensor fascia lata flap expanded. Since reporting this consecutive series of patients, we have continued to use this concept of the expanded myocutaneous flap in many different reconstructive situations in the pressure ulcer patient with excellent results and low complication rates.

A similar concept has been utilized by expanding adequate quality sensate skin in an adjacent area to provide soft tissue coverage for pressure ulcers and reduce the recurrence rate. Neves et al. [28] reported using tissue expansion of sensate skin of the back for treatment of pressure ulcers with good results.

MUSCLE FLAPS

In long-standing sacral, ischial, or trochanteric ulcers, patients can develop osteomyelitis of the underlying bone. The treatment of choice in such patients is debridement and reconstruction with a muscle flap, as we well know that muscle flaps improve healing in bone infections and trauma.

Quadriplegic or paraplegic patients with an ischial pressure ulcer commonly develop perineal complications with the development of urethral fistulae and ulcerations. Kauer and Andourach [13] reported a 19-case series using the gracilis musculocutaneous flap to prevent such complications and emphasized that this flap has many advantages. The flap is thick, it protects the urethra from injury, it can be raised as a myocutaneous flap with a large amount of good-quality skin for cutaneous defects, it has an ample arc of rotation, especially as an island flap, the donor can be closed easily, and the posterior musculocutaneous region of the thigh remains uncompromised for use in treating other ulcers. Alternatively, we and others [14, 16] have utilized the inferiorly based rectus abdominis myocutaneous flap (Figure 18-7(a),(b) see Color Plate 8) with good results. Pena et al. [14] utilized an inferiorly based rectus abdominis myocutaneous flap in a series of eight recurrent or chronic perineal and ischial pressure ulcers in neurologically impaired patients, reporting distinct advantages of using this flap in such patients and a low complication rate. Bunkis and Fudem [16] used this inferiorly based pedicled myocutaneous flap to cover perineal and ischial wounds, especially in previously amputated pelvises.

In refractory pressure ulcers with hip joint involvement, Evans et al. [17] reported carrying out a girdlestone arthroplasty in a 15-patient series, with no femoral stabilization, and reconstructed the soft tissue with a vastus lateralis muscle flap with good results.

Paletta et al. [15] in 1993 reported the use of 22

posterior thigh flaps in 21 patients for soft tissue coverage of trochanteric, ischial, and some sacral wounds. They also stated that the posterior thigh flap can be used as a pedicled flap in the management of heel and foot wounds.

SENSATE FLAPS AND REINNERVATION

The concept of reinnervation of the gluteal region in paraplegics by mobilizing intercostal nerves and extending their reach by sural nerve grafts and neurotization of the required area without involving other skin areas is interesting in that it is purported to achieve: (1) reinnervation of skin to gain protective sensibility in the pressure-bearing area, (2) reinnervation of the gluteus maximus muscle to gain voluntary muscle contraction to improve blood flow and diminish ischemia (Hauge [29]).

Mackinnon et al. [30] reported a technique of reinnervating the territory of the lateral femoral cutaneous nerve (the tensor fascia lata musculocutaneous flap) using the medial antebrachial cutaneous nerve of the forearm. This neurotization procedure restored sensibility to the area of the healed pressure sore. We have found that these flaps are technically demanding and usually do not give enough sensation to these patients to warrant their use routinely.

Another sensate flap that has been used for preventing pressure ulcer recurrence is the upper quadrant (intercostal) flap, based on the ninth, tenth, or eleventh intercostal bundles. Spear et al. [31] stated that the flap-covered area with transferred sensibility appears to be protected by referred sensation and recommended its use in certain specific conditions where the benefit of a sensory flap outweighs the price of a more extensive procedure.

Luscher et al. [12] reported a 0% incidence of local recurrence in 19 consecutive neurosensory tensor fascia lata flaps and stated that if the neurological pattern permits a neurosensory flap, then such flaps should be the primary choice of reconstruction to minimize long-term morbidity. This series is commendable for achieving a perfect result in the patients. Neves et al. [28] used tissue expansion of sensate skin of the back for providing adequate tissue coverage of debrided pressure ulcers

without a donor site deficit, but these patients required a two-stage procedure.

SALVAGE FLAPS (FILLETED LEG/THIGH) FROM PARTIAL OR TOTAL LIMB AMPUTATIONS

The concept of using tissue that is to be discarded allows the reconstructive surgeon to treat even the most extensive, difficult, recurrent, or multiple pressure ulcers (Figure 18-8(a),(b) see Color Plate 8). The total thigh flap provides a large bulk of tissue for use when all other options have failed, or the tissue available is inadequate for coverage of a large ulcer. This procedure is sometimes performed to save life, rather than limb, in severely ill patients with uncontrollable infection involving the underlying bone and in whom the ulcer is extensive. The amount of soft tissue required determines the type and length of the flap that is needed. Georgiade et al. [32] suggested making the lower incision at the knee level in carrying out a total thigh flap. For covering large sacral defects, Spira and Hardy [33] suggested a longer length of flap, making the lower incision approximately 9 inches below the knee joint level to allow the flap to reach. Whereas Weeks and Brower [34] used the entire length of soft tissue of the leg down to the level of the malleoli as an island flap for covering extensive ulcers.

MICROVASCULAR FREE TISSUE TRANSFER

Yamamoto et al. [19] in 1992 reported two successful reconstructions of recurrent pressure ulcers with free microvascular fasciocutaneous flaps. In the first case a free lateral thigh pedicled on the first and third direct cutaneous branches of the deep femoral vessels was used to cover a large recurrent sacral pressure ulcer. The vascular pedicle was dissected to the deep femoral trunk proximally and anastomosed to the inferior gluteal vessels. In the second case a free medial plantar flap was transferred to a recurrent ischial pressure ulcer. The vascular pedicle was dissected to the posterior tibial vessels proximally. The long vascular pedicle of the flap was passed through the femoral subcutaneous tunnel, and end-to-side microvascular anastomoses were performed to the superficial femoral trunk without any vein grafts. The authors advocate the use of free tissue transfer for recurrent pressure sore reconstruction.

Daniel et al. [20] reported using a myocutaneous intercostal neurovascular flap that failed on postoperative day 10. Morrison et al. [21] reported using a free medial plantar flap of one side to reconstruct a heel defect of the other foot. Chen et al. [22] reported using a single filleted lower leg myocutaneous free flap to cover multiple extensive pressure ulcers. Free tissue transfers for truncal pressure ulcers are long operative procedures, are technically challenging, and require postoperative monitoring with specialized units to obtain consistent flap survival and healing. Even with these limitations, the use of free flaps should be considered as an option in all reconstructive plans. Our limited experience demonstrates that, although the use of microvascular transfer appears to be a good option, the use of other reconstructive procedures usually provides stable long-term coverage without significant recurrence.

SUMMARY

Initial surgical treatment must be planned so that the flap design does not violate other vascular territories or pedicles that would make future flaps impossible. Recurrent, extensive, or multiple truncal pressure ulcers are a difficult problem to manage; they are a challenge. In centers of excellence, utilizing individual patient-focused treatment and the use of the plastic and reconstructive surgeon's armamentarium, an appropriate long-term stable outcome is possible.

REFERENCES

1. Lamid, S., and El Ghatit, A. Z., Smoking, spasticity, and pressure sores in spinal cord injured patients, *Am J Phys Med* 1983; 62(6):300–6.

2. Evans, G. R. D.; Dufresne, C. R.; and Manson, P. N., Surgical correction of pressure ulcers in an urban center: Is it efficacious? *Advances in Wound Care* 1994; 7(1):40–6.

3. Harding, R. L., An analysis of 100 rehabilitated paraplegics, *PRS* 1961; 27:235.

4. Griffith, B. H., and Schultz, R. C., The prevention and surgical treatment of recurrent decubitus ulcer, *Acta Chir Scand* 1942; 87(76S):207.

5. Dias, J. J.; Curlton, J. M.; and Goldberg, N. H., Efficacy of operative cure in pressure sore patients, *PRS* 1992; 89:272–278.

6. Relander, M., and Palmer, B., Recurrence of surgically treated pressure sores, *Scand J Plast Reconstr Surg* 1988; 22:89–92.

7. Davis, J. S., Operative treatment of scars following bed sores, *Surgery* 1938; 3:1–7.

8. Dansereau, J. G., and Conway, H., Closure of decubitus in paraplegics. Report on 2000 cases, *PRS* 1964; 33:474.

9. Mathes, S. J.; Feng, L. J.; and Hunt, T. K., Coverage of the infected wound, *Ann Surg* 1983; 198(4):420–9.

10. Rubayi, S.; Cousins, S.; and Valentine, W. A., Myocutaneous flaps. Surgical treatment of severe pressure ulcers, *AORN J* 1990; 52(1):40–55.

11. Salzberg, S. A., Recurrence of pressure ulcers in 219 spinal cord injured patients, *Fortieth Annual Conference of the American Paraplegic Society,* Las Vegas, September 1994.

12. Luscher, N. J.; De Roche, R.; Krupp, S.; Kuhn, W.; and Zach, G. A., The sensory tensor fascia latae flap: A 9-year follow-up, *Ann Plast Surg* 1991; 26(4):306–10, discussion 311.

13. Kauer, C., and Andourah, A., Perineal complications and gracilis musculocutaneous flap in patients with paraplegia. Apropos of 19 cases, *Ann Chir Plast Esthet* 1991; 36(4):347–52.

14. Pena, M. M.; Drew, G. S.; Smith, S. J.; and Given, K. S., The inferiorly based rectus abdominis myocutaneous flap for reconstruction of recurrent pressure sores, *Plast Reconstr Surg* 1992; 89(1):90–5.

15. Paletta, C.; Bartell, T.; and Shehadi, S., Applications of the posterior thigh flap, *Ann Plast Surg* 1993; 30(1):41–7.

16. Bunkis, J., and Fudem, G. M., Rectus abdominis flap closure of ischiosacral pressure sore, *Ann Plast Surg* 1989; 23:447.

17. Evans, G. R.; Lewis, V. L., Jr.; Manson, P. N.; Loomis, M.; and Vander-kolk, C. A., Hip joint communication with pressure sore: The refractory wound and the role of Girdlestone arthroplasty, *Plast Reconstr Surg* 1993; 91(2):288–94.

18. Daniel, R. K., and Faibisoff, B., Muscle coverage of pressure points: The role of myocutaneous flaps, *Ann Plast Surg* 1982; 8:446.

19. Yamamoto, Y.; Nohira, K.; Shintomi, Y.; Igawa, H.; and Ohura, T., Reconstruction of recurrent pressure sores using free flaps, *J Reconstr Microsurg* 1992; 8(6):433–6.

20. Daniel, R. K.; Terzis, J. K.; and Cunningham, D. M., Sensory skin flaps for coverage of pressure sores in paraplegic patients, *Plast Reconstr Surg* 1976; 58:317.

21. Morrison, W. A.; Crabb, D. McK.; O'Brien, McC.; and Jenkins, A., The instep of the foot as a fasciocutaneous island and as a free flap for heel defects, *Plast Reconstr Surg* 1983; 72:56–63.

22. Chen, H.; Weng, C.; and Noordhoff, M. S., Coverage of multiple extensive pressure sores with a single filleted lower leg myocutaneous free flap, *Plast Reconstr Surg* 1986; 78:396.

23. Karaca, A.; Binns, J.; and Blumenthal, F., Complications of total ischiectomy for the treatment of ischial pressure sores, *Plast Reconstr Surg* 1974; 62:96.

24. Berlemont, M., and Keromest, R., The dangers of removal of the ischium in the treatment of paraplegic ulcers. A review of 236 case records (translated from French), *Rev Chir Orthop* 1987; 73:656–664.

25. Gray, C. G.; Salzberg, C. A.; Petro, J. A.; and Salisbury, R. E., The expanded flap for reconstruction of the difficult pressure sore, *Decubitus* 1990; 3(2):17–20.

26. Cherry, G. W.; Austed, E. D.; Pasyk, K.; et al., Increased survival and vascularity of random-pattern skin flaps elevated in controlled expanded skin, *Plast Reconstr Surg* 1983; 72:680.

27. Forte, V.; Middleton, W. G.; and Briant, T. D., Expansion of myocutaneous flaps, *Arch Otol* 1983; 11:371.

28. Neves, R. I.; Kahler, S. H.; Banducci, D. R.; and Manders, E. K., Tissue expansion of sensate skin for pressure sores, *Ann Plast Surg* 1992; 29(5):433–7.

29. Hauge, E. N., The anatomical basis of a new method for re-innervation of the gluteal region in paraplegics, *Acta Physiol Scand Suppl* 1991; 603:19–21.

30. Mackinnon, S. E.; Dellon, A. L.; Patterson, G. A.; and Gruss, J. S., Medial antebrachial cutaneous-lateral femoral cutaneous neurotization to provide sensation to pressure-bearing areas in the paraplegic patient, *Ann Plast Surg* 1985; 14(6):541–544.

31. Spear, S. L.; Kroll, S. S.; and Little, J. W., Bilateral upper-quadrant (intercostal) flaps: The value of protective sensation in preventing pressure sore recurrence, *Plast Reconstr Surg* 1987; 80(5):734–736.

32. Georgiade, N.; Pickrell, K.; and Maguire, C., Total thigh flaps for extensive decubitus ulcer, *Plast Reconstr Surg* 1956; 17:220.

33. Spira, M., and Hardy, S. B., Our experience with high thigh amputations in paraplegics, *Plast Reconstr Surg* 1963; 31:344.

34. Weeks, P. M., and Brower, T. D., Island flap coverage of extensive decubitus ulcers, *Plast Reconstr Surg* 1968; 42:433.

INDEX